Dentistry: Oral Assessment, Treatment and Preventive Care

Dentistry: Oral Assessment, Treatment and Preventive Care

Edited by Clifford Moody

hayle medical
New York

Hayle Medical,
750 Third Avenue, 9th Floor,
New York, NY 10017, USA

Visit us on the World Wide Web at:
www.haylemedical.com

ISBN: 978-1-63241-457-1

The publisher's policy is to use permanent paper from mills that operate a sustainable forestry policy. Furthermore, the publisher ensures that the text paper and cover boards used have met acceptable environmental accreditation standards.

Printed in China.

Cataloging-in-Publication Data

Dentistry : oral assessment, treatment and preventive care / edited by Clifford Moody.
p. cm.
Includes bibliographical references and index.
ISBN 978-1-63241-457-1
1. Dentistry. 2. Dental care. 3. Preventive dentistry. 4. Dental therapeutics. I. Moody, Clifford.
RK61 .D45 2017
617.6--dc23

Table of Contents

Preface

This book has been a concerted effort by a group of academicians, researchers and scientists, who have contributed their research works for the realization of the book. This book has materialized in the wake of emerging advancements and innovations in this field. Therefore, the need of the hour was to compile all the required researches and disseminate the knowledge to a broad spectrum of people comprising of students, researchers and specialists of the field.

Oral health care or dentistry is a sub-field of medicinal sciences which is concerned with the proper functioning and wellness of the oral cavity. It includes the diagnosis, treatment and prevention of the disorders and diseases related to dentition and oral mucosa. This book on dentistry traces the progress of this field and highlights some of its key concepts and applications. The topics included in it on oral health care are of utmost significance and bound to provide incredible insights to readers. Coherent flow of topics, student-friendly language and extensive use of examples make this text an invaluable source of knowledge. Students, researchers, experts, dentists and all associated with this field will benefit alike from the book.

At the end of the preface, I would like to thank the authors for their brilliant chapters and the publisher for guiding us all-through the making of the book till its final stage. Also, I would like to thank my family for providing the support and encouragement throughout my academic career and research projects.

Editor

1

Nonsurgical Endodontic Retreatment of Advanced Inflammatory External Root Resorption Using Mineral Trioxide Aggregate Obturation

Shivani Utneja,[1] Gaurav Garg,[1] Shipra Arora,[2] and Sangeeta Talwar[1]

[1] *Department of Conservative Dentistry and Endodontics, Maulana Azad Institute of Dental Sciences, Bahadurshah Zafar Marg, New Delhi 110002, India*
[2] *Department of Periodontics, Maulana Azad Institute of Dental Sciences, Bahadurshah Zafar Marg, New Delhi 110002, India*

Correspondence should be addressed to Shivani Utneja, shivaniutneja81@yahoo.co.in

Academic Editors: J. H. Campbell and D. Ram

Inflammatory external root resorption is one of the major complications after traumatic dental injury. In this case report, we describe treatment of a maxillary central incisor affected by severe, perforating external root resorption. An 18-year-old patient presented with a previously traumatized, root-filled maxillary central incisor associated with pain and sinus tract. Radiographic examination revealed periradicular lesion involving pathologic resorption of the apical region of the root and lateral root surface both mesially and distally. After removal of the root canal filling, the tooth was disinfected with intracanal triple antibiotic paste for 2 weeks. The antibiotic dressing was then removed, and the entire root canal was filled with mineral trioxide aggregate. The endodontic access cavity was restored with composite resin. After 18 months, significant osseous healing of the periradicular region and lateral periodontium had occurred with arrest of external root resorption, and no clinical symptoms were apparent.

1. Introduction

Inflammatory external root resorption (IERR) is a pathologic condition caused by several etiologic factors including traumatic dental injury. Displacement of the teeth, as well as subsequent repositioning or replantation procedures inevitably causes damage to the root, resulting in denuded areas on the root surface which are chemotactic to phagocytes [1]. This inflammatory response can exacerbate in the presence of bacteria and their byproducts inside the root canal system and dentinal tubules after pulp necrosis and in the absence of protection of cementum barrier. If allowed to progress, the resorptive process may lead to rapid tooth loss [2, 3].

Clinically, teeth are usually not symptomatic in the early period of the process. However, as IERR progresses, the teeth may become symptomatic, and periradicular abscess may develop with increasing tooth mobility. Radiographically, radiolucencies can be observed in the external root surface and adjacent to the bone [4]. Endodontic treatment should be initiated promptly to prevent further hard tissue loss and root perforation [5]. In advanced cases, endodontic intervention may require prior repair of the perforation site with a suitable biomaterial [6].

Mineral trioxide aggregate (MTA) has emerged as a reliable bioactive material with extended applications in endodontics that include obturation of the root canal space owing to its superior physiochemical properties [7]. In conjunction with being sterile, radiopaque, and dimensionally stable the material is not sensitive to moisture and blood contamination [8]. MTA also provides an effective seal against dentin and cementum and promotes biologic repair and regeneration of the periodontal ligament [9, 10]. Clinical studies have confirmed the biocompatibility of this material and have shown a hard tissue inductive effect [11, 12]. These favorable properties render MTA a suitable material for the management of tissue damage caused by IERR [13]. Because perforation repair, root end induction, and root end filling are essential forms of partial canal obturation, the orthograde filling of the entire root canal system with MTA is the next logical progression in the evolutionary application of this material [14].

The present case report describes the nonsurgical endodontic retreatment of advanced IERR in a maxillary central incisor, which was treated with complete MTA obturation.

2. Case Report

An 18-year-old male presented with the chief complaint of pain on mastication and recurrent swelling in the labio-gingival aspect of maxillary left central incisor. He gave a history of traumatic injury seven years earlier. For the first three years after trauma the patient did not take any treatment as the tooth remained asymptomatic. Thereafter the patient started experiencing pain in the tooth and underwent root canal treatment in 21 followed by full coverage restoration by a local dentist. Four years after root canal obturation the tooth again became symptomatic, and the patient was referred to our department for endodontic retreatment of 21. There was no relevant medical history. An intraoral examination revealed labial sinus tract with respect to 21. The tooth did not exhibit significant mobility, and there was no gingival sulcular bleeding on probing. 21 was tender to percussion. Radiographic examination of 21 showed extensive lateral and apical root resorption associated with periapical radiolucency and interdental bone loss both mesially and distally in relation to the resorption defect. The root canal space of 21 was inadequately obturated (Figure 1(a)).

Taking into consideration the extent and severity of the resorption, it was planned to do orthograde MTA obturation of the canal space after removing the old root canal filling to arrest the root resorption along the length of the root canal. This internal approach was preferred over surgical management as the latter would have sacrificed the already compromised bone support around 21. Intentional replantation was also not a good option as there was a danger of fracture of the tooth while extraction owing to severity of resorption. The procedure was fully explained to the patient, and informed consent was taken.

The endodontic access opening was made through porcelain fused to metal crown using transmetal bur (Dentspy Maillefer, Ballaigues, Switerland). Previous gutta percha filling was removed using Hedstrom files in conjunction with Endosolv-E (Septodont, Inc., New castle, Delaware, USA). A radiograph taken to ensure complete removal of gutta percha showed uneven radiolucent regions along the external borders of the root, and the outline of original root canal was completely visible (Figure 1(b)). This was highly suggestive of external root resorption. Working length was determined radiographically (Figure 1(c)), and canal preparation was accomplished in a circumferential filing motion using H files while irrigating with copious amount of 1% sodium hypochlorite (Novo Dental Products Pvt. Ltd. Mumbai, India). This was followed by irrigation with normal saline to remove any remnants of hypochlorite. The canal was dried with absorbent paper points and filled with triple antibiotic paste (ciprofloxacin, metronidazole, and minocycline) as described by Sato et al. [15]. The access cavity was sealed with a temporary restorative material (Cavit-G, 3M ESPE, St. Paul, MN, USA). After 2 weeks, when the sinus had healed, intracanal medicament was flushed with distilled water and 1% sodium hypochlorite followed by rinse of saline. 2% chlorhexidine was used as the final irrigant. The canal was dried with absorbent paper points. White MTA (Pro Root Dentsply Tulsa, OK, USA) was mixed according to the manufacturer's instructions and was initially carried to the apical third using MTA carrier and compacted using endodontic plugger, size 5/7 (Dentsply, Maillefer, Ballaigues, Switzerland). After the apical 5 mm of canal was completely filled with MTA which was verified radiographically, a sterile reamer rolled with wet cotton was used to compact the MTA into the resorption cavity. In this way the entire root canal system was filled with MTA. A baseline radiograph was taken which showed that MTA was adequately compacted into the resorption defect with good adaptation to the root contours (Figure 1(d)). Moist cotton pellet was kept in the chamber, and the access cavity was sealed with a temporary restorative material. After one week, the temporary restoration was removed and the access cavity was restored with glass ionomer cement (Ketac Molar Easymix 3M ESPE).

The patient was recalled after 6, 12, and 18 months for clinical and radiographic followup. On clinical examination 21 was functional without sensitivity to percussion or palpation. The tooth showed normal physiologic mobility and no periodontal pockets on probing. The periapical radiograph showed regression in the size of periapical radiolucency with signs of osseous repair and no further progression of external resorption. There was initiation of osseous healing adjacent to mesial and distal resorption sites on the root surface (Figures 1(e), 1(f), and 1(g)).

3. Discussion

IERR is initiated by mechanical trauma, resulting in the destruction of cementoblasts and loss of precementum and sometimes cementum in areas of the root surface. The resorptive process is then maintained by bacterial products from the infected root canal which provides the necessary continuous stimulation for the resorbing cells [1]. Thus, the treatment protocol for IERR should involve elimination of bacteria and their byproducts from the root canal system and dentinal tubules to stop the inflammatory processes involving the root surface to allow the regeneration of periodontium [16].

The conventional and preferred treatment protocol for a progressive IERR consists of chemomechanical preparation of the root canal system including a short-term (1 month) dressing of creamy paste of calcium hydroxide ($Ca(OH)_2$) for bacterial disinfection of the root canal space. The process is followed by a long-term dressing of densely packed $Ca(OH)_2$ to provide an alkaline Ph inside the dentinal tubules to kill the bacteria and neutralize the endotoxins, which are potent inflammatory stimulators [4, 17].

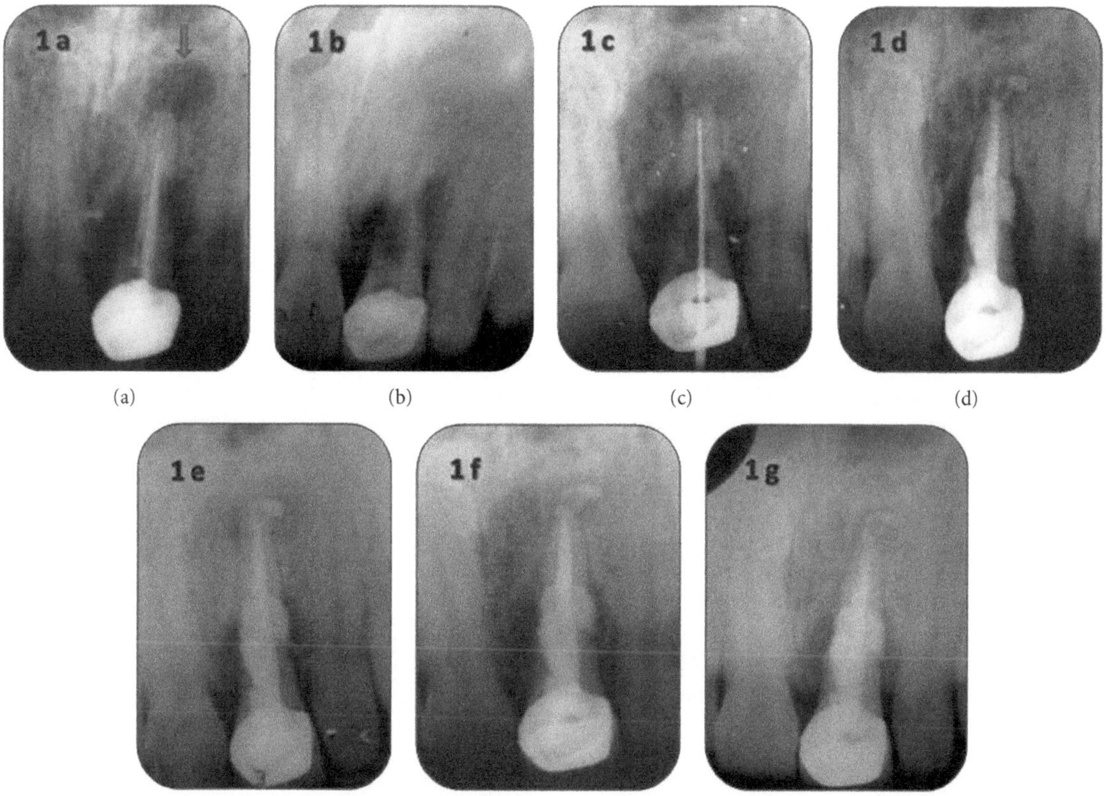

(a) (b) (c) (d) (e) (f) (g)

Figure 1: (a) Preoperative periapical radiograph showing periapical lesion and external apical and lateral root surface resorption in a maxillary left central incisor. The radiograph also reveals previous poor quality obturation. (b) Radiograph after removal of old gutta percha filling showing root canal outline completely visible through resorption defect. Bone resorption adjacent to resorption lacunae on root is also evident. (c) Working length radiograph. (d) Immediate postobturation radiograph showing adequate density of MTA obturation without voids and good adaptation of MTA to root contours. (e) Six-month followup periapical radiograph revealing stability of resorption and periapical healing. (f) Advanced osseous healing of periapical tissues and initiation of repair adjacent to lateral root surface resorption at 12 months. (g) An 18-month radiographic view showing complete regeneration of periradicular tissues and advanced osseous healing evident in the lateral periodontal tissues.

Although this treatment protocol has a high success rate [1], the long-term use of $Ca(OH)_2$ has some disadvantages. Because the treatment includes repeated clinical sessions to replace $Ca(OH)_2$, it demands high cooperation and motivation from the patient. In addition, long-term presence of $Ca(OH)_2$ in root canal space can increase the brittleness of the root dentin and the risk of future cervical root fractures especially in immature teeth [18]. There are studies that discuss the contraindication of $Ca(OH)_2$ use in teeth with damaged cementum because of the necrotizing effects of $Ca(OH)_2$ on periodontal cells that repopulate on the root surface. This necrotizing effect can prevent formation of a normal attachment apparatus and result in replacement resorption and ankylosis [19].

The antibacterial and tissue dissolution action of sodium hypochlorite increases with its concentration, but this is accompanied by an increase in toxicity [20]. As the contact between the irrigant and the surrounding vital tissues cannot be completely avoided in cases of perforating resorption, therefore a dilute concentration of the irrigant that still retains adequate disinfective properties is recommended [21]. In the present case 1% w/v sodium hypochlorite did not cause any caustic effects on periodontal tissues. To further prevent its prolonged contact with surrounding vital tissues, normal saline was used each time after rinsing the canal with sodium hypochlorite [22]. Final rinse before obturation was performed using 2% chlorhexidine solution as the present case was a retreatment case where high proportions of gram-positive bacteria are suspected. Hence use of chlorhexidine as a final irrigant would appear advantageous in such a situation [20]. Placement of an intracanal medicament is crucial in necrotic cases. In our case a mixture of ciprofloxacin, metronidazole, and minocycline was chosen as an intracanal medicament as it has been shown to be very effective in eliminating endodontic pathogens in vitro and in situ [15]. Apart from disinfection, minocycline present in this paste might have also contributed in arresting the inflammatory resorption as it possesses anti-inflammatory property. This has been proved in reimplanted dog teeth after extended dry time that intracanal placement of ledermix paste which contains corticosteroid and tetracycline inhibits inflammatory root resorption [23].

The development of new bioactive materials such as MTA make possible other therapeutic approaches, including the obturation of the root canal space in complex cases of iatrogenic or pathologic root perforation [14]. In the present case, there was severe inflammatory external resorption in the lateral and apical portions of the root associated with periapical pathology. As the tooth was very fragile, treating it by orthograde obturation of the entire canal system with MTA was the only viable option. It has been shown that intracanal application of MTA can also cause release of calcium ions through dentinal tubules into external resorption defect, which may favour the repair potential of the surrounding tissues [24]. Recent research has demonstrated that root canal treated teeth obturated with MTA exhibit higher fracture resistance than their untreated counterparts [14]. This could be attributed to the ability of MTA to prevent the destruction of collagen by inducing the expression of a tissue inhibitor of metalloproteinase 2 in the dentin matrix [25].

In the case described here 6, 12, and 18 month radiographic recall showed osseous repair of periapical pathosis. Although reestablishment of the entire periodontal apparatus did not occur, the resorption site remained stable throughout the 18-month followup period. The patient was asymptomatic, with the tooth exhibiting normal sulcular probing depth, mobility, and function. The patient was also pleased with the treatment outcome as a permanent tooth with otherwise hopeless prognosis was maintained. Orthograde retreatment of the present case with MTA proved to be very conservative as it lead to avoidance of surgical treatment with similar prognostic outcomes. However, longer followup for this case is required to be sure of success.

References

[1] L. Tronstad, *Clinical Endodontics A Textbook*, Theime Medical and Scientific Publishers, 2nd edition, 2002.

[2] A. Sigurdsson, M. Trope, and N. Chivian, "The role of endodontics after dental traumatic injuries," in *Pathways of the Pulp*, S. Cohen and R. C. Burns, Eds., pp. 620–654, Mosby, St. Louis, Mo, USA, 10th edition, 2011.

[3] J. Andreasen and L. Bakland, "Pathologic tooth resorption," in *Ingle's Endodontics*, J. Ingle, L. Bakland, and J. Baumgartner, Eds., pp. 1358–1382, BC Decker, Ontario, Canada, 6th edition, 2008.

[4] Z. Fuss, I. Tsesis, and S. Lin, "Root resorption—diagnosis, classification and treatment choices based on stimulation factors," *Dental Traumatology*, vol. 19, no. 4, pp. 175–182, 2003.

[5] I. Guzeler, S. Uysal, and Z. C. Cehreli, "Treatment of severe inflammatory root resorption in a young permanent incisor with mineral trioxide aggregate," *Journal of the Canadian Dental Association*, vol. 77, article 108, 2011.

[6] G. S. Heithersay, "Clinical endodontic and surgical management of tooth and associated bone resorption," *International Endodontic Journal*, vol. 18, no. 2, pp. 72–92, 1985.

[7] N. K. Sarkar, R. Caicedo, P. Ritwik, R. Moiseyeva, and I. Kawashima, "Physicochemical basis of the biologic properties of mineral trioxide aggregate," *Journal of Endodontics*, vol. 31, no. 2, pp. 97–100, 2005.

[8] R. A. VanderWeele, S. A. Schwartz, and T. J. Beeson, "Effect of blood contamination on retention characteristics of MTA when mixed with different liquids," *Journal of Endodontics*, vol. 32, no. 5, pp. 421–424, 2006.

[9] M. Torabinejad, P. W. Smith, J. D. Kettering, and T. R. Pitt Ford, "Comparative investigation of marginal adaptation of mineral trioxide aggregate and other commonly used root-end filling materials," *Journal of Endodontics*, vol. 21, no. 6, pp. 295–299, 1995.

[10] S. J. Lee, M. Monsef, and M. Torabinejad, "Sealing ability of a mineral trioxide aggregate for repair of lateral root perforations," *Journal of Endodontics*, vol. 19, no. 11, pp. 541–544, 1993.

[11] D. T. Holden, S. A. Schwartz, T. C. Kirkpatrick, and W. G. Schindler, "Clinical outcomes of artificial root-end barriers with mineral trioxide aggregate in teeth with immature apices," *Journal of Endodontics*, vol. 34, no. 7, pp. 812–817, 2008.

[12] J. Mente, N. Hage, T. Pfefferle et al., "Mineral trioxide aggregate apical plugs in teeth with open apical foramina: a retrospective analysis of treatment outcome," *Journal of Endodontics*, vol. 35, no. 10, pp. 1354–1358, 2009.

[13] M. Torabinejad and N. Chivian, "Clinical applications of mineral trioxide aggregate," *Journal of Endodontics*, vol. 25, no. 3, pp. 197–205, 1999.

[14] G. Bogen and S. Kuttler, "Mineral trioxide aggregate obturation: a review and case series," *Journal of Endodontics*, vol. 35, no. 6, pp. 777–790, 2009.

[15] T. Sato, E. Hoshino, H. Uematsu, and T. Noda, "In vitro antimicrobial susceptibility to combinations of drugs on bacteria from carious and endodontic lesions of human deciduous teeth," *Oral Microbiology and Immunology*, vol. 8, no. 3, pp. 172–176, 1993.

[16] L. Levin and M. Trope, "Root resorption," in *Dental Pulp*, K. Hargreaves and H. Goodis, Eds., pp. 425–448, Quintessence, Chicago, Ill, usa, 3rd edition, 2002.

[17] M. Trope, J. Moshonov, R. Nissan, P. Buxt, and C. Yesilsoy, "Short vs. long-term calcium hydroxide treatment of established inflammatory root resorption in replanted dog teeth," *Endodontics & Dental Traumatology*, vol. 11, no. 3, pp. 124–128, 1995.

[18] J. O. Andreasen, B. Farik, and E. C. Munksgaard, "Long-term calcium hydroxide as a root canal dressing may increase risk of root fracture," *Dental Traumatology*, vol. 18, no. 3, pp. 134–137, 2002.

[19] L. E. Massarstrom, L. B. Blomlof, B. Feiglin, and S. F. Lindskog, "Effect of calcium hydroxide treatment on periodontal repair and root resorption," *Endodontics & Dental Traumatology*, vol. 2, no. 5, pp. 184–189, 1986.

[20] M. Zehnder, "Root canal irrigants," *Journal of Endodontics*, vol. 32, no. 5, pp. 389–398, 2006.

[21] M. Hülsmann and W. Hahn, "Complications during root canal irrigation—literature review and case reports," *International Endodontic Journal*, vol. 33, no. 3, pp. 186–193, 2000.

[22] I. C. Mackie, "Management and root canal treatment of non-vital immature permanent incisor teeth," *International Journal of Paediatric Dentistry*, vol. 8, no. 4, pp. 289–293, 1998.

[23] H. Chen, F. B. Teixeira, A. L. Ritter, L. Levin, and M. Trope, "The effect of intracanal anti-inflammatory medicaments on external root resorption of replanted dog teeth after extended

extra-oral dry time," *Dental Traumatology*, vol. 24, no. 1, pp. 74–78, 2008.

[24] H. O. Özdemir, B. Özçelik, B. Karabucak, and Z. C. Cehreli, "Calcium ion diffusion from mineral trioxide aggregate through simulated root resorption defects," *Dental Traumatology*, vol. 24, no. 1, pp. 70–73, 2008.

[25] S. Hatibović-Kofman, L. Raimundo, L. Zheng, L. Chong, M. Friedman, and J. O. Andreasen, "Fracture resistance and histological findings of immature teeth treated with mineral trioxide aggregate," *Dental Traumatology*, vol. 24, no. 3, pp. 272–276, 2008.

2

Combined Treatment with Laser Sintering and Zirconium: A Case Report of Dentinogenesis Imperfecta

Simel Ayyildiz,[1] Cem Sahin,[2] Özlem Marti Akgün,[3] and Feridun Basak[3]

[1] *Department of Prosthodontics, Center of Dental Sciences, Gulhane Military Medical Academy, Etlik, 06018 Ankara, Turkey*
[2] *School of Dental Technology, Hacettepe University, 06100 Ankara, Turkey*
[3] *Department of Pediatric Dentistry, Center of Dental Sciences, Gulhane Military Medical Academy, 06018 Ankara, Turkey*

Correspondence should be addressed to Simel Ayyildiz; simelayyildiz@gmail.com

Academic Editors: P. G. Arduino, W. L. Chai, and M. W. Roberts

Osteogenesis imperfecta (OI) is a heterogeneous disorder of connective tissue that manifests mainly as skeletal deformity and bone fragility. Dentinogenesis imperfecta (DI) is sometimes an accompanying symptom of OI. The treatment protocol of these patients varies according to the clinical appearance. The case report here describes complete mouth rehabilitation of an 18-year-old male patient with OI and DI using direct metal laser sintering (DMLS) technique of metal-ceramic restorations and zirconium all-ceramic crowns. DMLS is an additive metal fabrication technology that is simpler, more precise, and healthier than conventional manufacturing and can be remarkably cost effective. Moreover, the technique affords highly accurate production of fixed partial dentures with ideal marginal fit and excellent mechanical properties. The patient was treated using a multidisciplinary strategy that focused on controlling caries, protecting teeth from further wear, obtaining an appropriate vertical dimension, and providing soft tissue support to return the facial profile to a normal appearance using new technology in the field of prosthetics.

1. Introduction

Osteogenesis imperfecta (OI), also known as "brittle bone", disease is a genetically determined connective tissue disorder that results from mutations of 2 genes (COL1A1 and COL1A2) responsible for the formation of type 1 collagen [1–3].

Clinical features of OI include growth deficiency, blue sclera, bone fragility, joint hypermobility, dentinogenesis imperfect (DI), and the presence of wormian bones on skull radiographs [3, 4]. Additional radiographic findings are osteopenia, scoliosis, and thin cortices. OI is classified on the basis of clinical and radiologic criteria established by Sillence et al. in 1979 (Table 1) [5–7].

DI is an autosomal dominant form of mesodermal dysplasia that affects both primary and permanent dentition. Shields [8] has identified 3 different types of DI as follows: DI-I: DI associated with OI; DI-II: the same clinical radiographic and histological features as DI-I, but without OI; and DI-III: a rare type of DI found only in the triracial population of Brandywine, MD, USA.

DI associated with OI generally affects primary dentition more severely than permanent dentition. Although the enamel appears structurally normal, it is often dislodged, exposing soft, dysplastic dentin to the oral cavity and provoking rapid, extensive attrition [3, 9]. Histologically, exposed dentin is generally characterized by irregular tubules. Radiographically, teeth affected by DI show cervical constriction, bulbous crowns, short roots, short pulp chambers, and obliterated canals [10]. Adult patients with OI frequently exhibit class III malocclusions, anterior or posterior cross-bite, posterior open-bite, and vertical height loss [1, 3, 11].

Conventional casting is the most frequently used technique for manufacturing Co-Cr alloys for the fixed partial dentures. In recent years, modern computer-aided technologies for manufacturing individual prostheses have been gaining popularity in the field of dental technology [12]. Computer-aided design (CAD) and computer-aided manufacturing (CAM) technologies are used frequently in the dental field to fabricate prostheses ranging from crowns to long-span fixed partial dentures and from removable

TABLE 1: Classification of osteogenesis imperfecta.

Type	DI	Clinical severity	Typical features
I	–	Mild, nondeforming OI	Normal height or mild short stature; blue sclera
II	?	Perinatal lethal	Multiple rib and long bone fractures at birth; pronounced deformities; broad long bones; low density of skull bones on radiographs; and dark sclera
III	+	Severely deforming	Very short; triangular face; severe scoliosis; and grayish sclera
IV	+	Moderately deforming	Moderately short; mild-to-moderate scoliosis; and grayish or white sclera
V	–	Moderately deforming	Mild-to-moderate short stature; dislocation of radial head; mineralized interosseous membrane; hyperplastic callus; and white sclera
VI	–	Moderate-to-severe deforming	Moderately short; scoliosis; accumulation of osteoid in bone tissue, fish-scale pattern of bone lamellation; and white sclera
VII	–	Moderately deforming	Mild short stature; short humeri and femora; coxavara; and white sclera

Modified from [5, 7]. DI: Dentinogenesis Imperfecta.

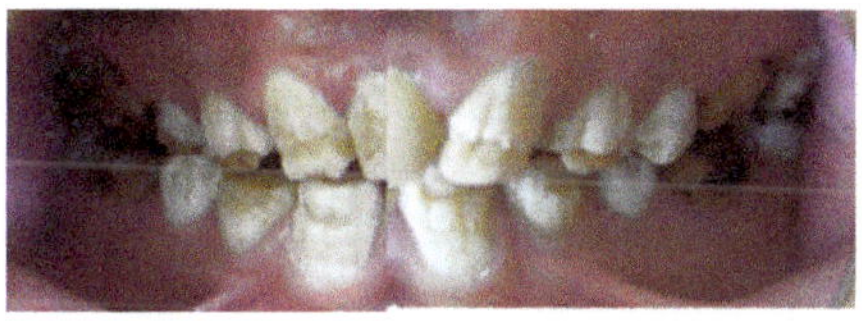

FIGURE 1: Clinical appearance of extensive enamel deformities chipped during mastication.

prostheses to dental implants [13]. The actual fabrication of a Co-Cr product is carried out by computer numerical control (CNC) milling machines or direct metal laser sintering (DMLS) machines [14, 15]. These systems were developed to address a number of disadvantages of the traditional casting method (e.g., increasing cost, manufacturing defaults, and human-aided manufacturing). DMLS is an additive metal fabrication technology that involves the use of a high-power Yb-fiber optic laser [15]. In this technology, metal powder is melted locally with a focused laser beam and fused into a solid part. The parts are built up additively, layer by layer, each of which is 10–30 μm thick [14, 15]. DMLS technology affords highly accurate production of fixed partial dentures with fine marginal adaptation and excellent mechanical properties [13, 16].

This paper presents the multidisciplinary dental treatment of a young patient with DI related to OI. Also, this clinical report explores the use of direct metal laser sintering technique for the fabrication of posterior Co-Cr metal-ceramic fixed partial dentures and zirconium anterior restorations for the treatment of vertical height loss with complete mouth rehabilitation.

2. Case Report

An 18-year-old male patient was referred to the Gulhane Military Medical Academy's Department of Pediatric at the Center of Dental Sciences for examination, evaluation, and treatment of defective and hypersensitive teeth. A detailed dental and medical history was obtained. The medical history indicated that the patient had been diagnosed with OI and was being treated orthopedically.

An extraskeletal clinical examination showed the patient to have moderately short stature, a femoral deformity, and a narrow shoulder breadth. An extraoral examination assessing vertical dimension of occlusion and vertical dimension at rest showed that attrition of the posterior teeth had resulted in an increase in interocclusal rest space (approximately 9 mm). The patient also complained of continuously chipping of teeth in both arches while masticating (Figure 1). Intraoral examination showed that eruption of the permanent teeth was complete and that teeth 16, 26, 36, and 46 had been restored with stainless steel crowns (SSC) (Figure 2). There was extensive destruction of enamel, which was opaque-white in color, whereas dentin was yellowish brown.

A dental history indicated that composite laminate veneers had been applied to the upper anterior teeth by a pediatric dentistry clinic for esthetic reasons 3 years previously (Figure 3). The patient complained about general hypersensitivity; therefore, the SSCs were removed, and an OPG was taken. The radiographic examination revealed secondary caries under the occlusal restorations of teeth 16, 26, 36, and 46. There was no evidence of any periapical pathoses. Extraoral posterior-anterior radiographs showed normal skull morphology. A plain radiograph of the lower extremities showed intramedullary rod fixations in both femurs (Figure 4).

Prior to prosthetic consultations, secondary caries were restored with glass-ionomer cement. In consultations with the Department of Prosthodontics, the decision was made to treat all teeth with fixed porcelain prosthetic restorations in order to restore vertical height and esthetics. An occlusal splint was fabricated to reset the interocclusal distance. A TMJ radiograph was obtained with this splint to examine the condyle-articular eminence, and full-time usage of the splint was proposed in order to adjust the dentoalveolar relation to the new vertical dimension.

After 2 months of usage, the splint was divided into two parts anteroposteriorly, and the left and right sides of the splint were used separately to attain the necessary occlusal reduction. A Bis-GMA-based provisional restorative material

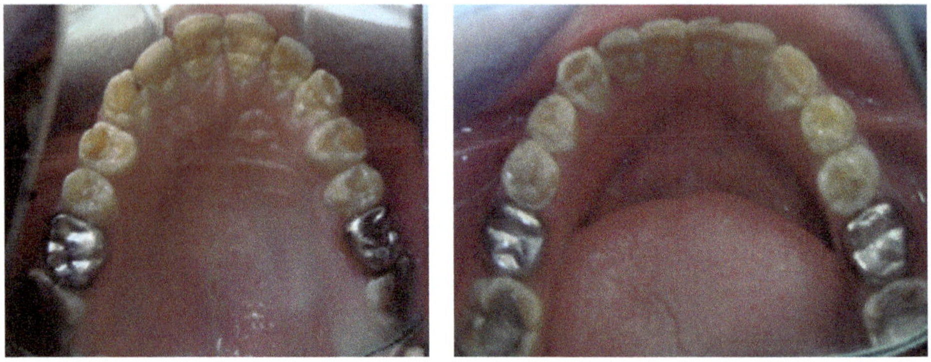

(a) (b)

FIGURE 2: Typical intraoral appearance of dentinogenesis imperfecta. Stainless steel crowns had been applied during mixed dentition to preserve hard tissue.

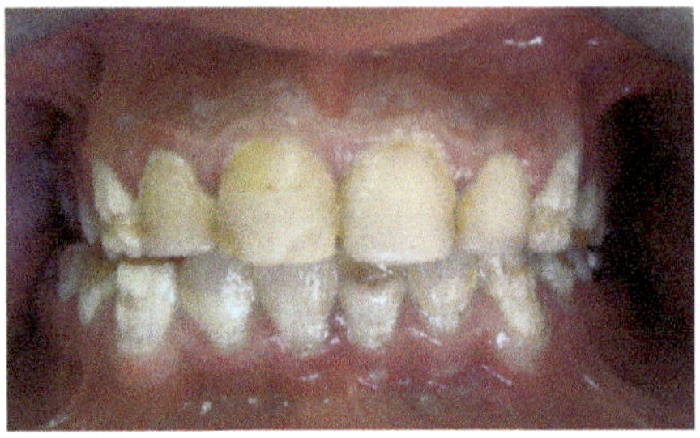

FIGURE 3: Anterior teeth had been restored with composite laminate veneers for esthetic reasons.

(C&B Provilink, Ivoclar Vivadent AG, Schaan, Liechtenstein Germany) was used to obtain an interocclusal record of the right side in order to control the occlusal reduction of molar and premolar teeth on the left side.

Master impressions were made with polyvinyl siloxane impression material (Speedex II, Colténe Whaledent Group, Inc, Mahwah, NJ, USA) to fabricate permanent metal-ceramic crown units. Casts were prepared with type III dental stone. After the recording of maxillomandibular relation, the casts were mounted on a semiadjustable articulator (Artex CT, AmannGirrbach, Germany) using face-bow records, and temporary crowns were fabricated in line with the new occlusal height dimensions. Models were scanned with an optic scanner (Activity 102, Smart Optics, Sensortechnik GmbH, Bochum, Germany) and 3D CAD was performed. Direct Metal Laser Sintering (DMLS) (M2, Concept Laser, Hoffmann, Innovation Group, Lichtenfels, Germany) technology was used to fabricate Co-Cr (Remanium Star CL, Dentaurum, Ispringen, Germany) metal frameworks in the 3D Solid Modelling Center at Gulhane Military Medical Academy (3D SMC-GMMA). After metal try-in of the fixed partial dentures, feldspathic porcelain (Vita VM13, Vita Zahnfabrik, Bad Säckingen, Germany) was fired according to the manufacturer's recommendations.

Occlusal surfaces of posterior restorations were selectively ground during the porcelain try-in stage to attain mutually protected occlusion at the defined vertical dimension. Restorations were cemented with polycarboxylate cement (Adhesor Carbofine, Spofa Dental, Prague, Czech Republic) (Figure 5).

Anterior teeth were prepared one week after the cementation of molars and premolars. Zirconium porcelain was selected as the anterior restoration material for both esthetics and durability. Impressions were obtained using polyvinyl siloxane (Speedex II, Colténe Whaledent Group, Inc., Mahwah, NJ, USA), and the zirconium restorations were fabricated at SMC-GMMA using a five-axis CNC unit (Figure 5). Restorations were cemented with polycarboxylate cement [17] following try-in (Figure 6).

The patient was recalled at 2-month intervals. Clinical and radiographic examinations revealed no pathoses associated with rehabilitation over a 12-month follow-up period. The patient was satisfied with both the functional and esthetic aspects of the restorations.

3. Discussion

OI is a rare disorder that has been reported to be accompanied by DI of varying severity in between 28% and 73% of cases [3, 18, 19]. In such cases, dental, oral and craniofacial variations may be clinically evident [3, 4]. In this case, the patient exhibited signs of OI such as short stature, femoral deformities, and oral manifestations specific to DI.

Skeletal class III malocclusion has been described in many patients with types III and IV OI [3]; however, our patient exhibited an anterior class I occlusal relationship with a unilateral posterior cross-bite. The collapse of occlusal height due to attrition is a typical feature of DI [19] that was present in our case as well.

Patients with DI may have enamel of abnormal thickness, but frequently is dislodged exposing the softer dentin. Dislodging of enamel may be attributed to a smooth dentino-enamel junction that tends to be scalloped in DI patients [9]. Teeth affected by DI do not seem to be more susceptible to caries than normal teeth; in fact, the structure of dentin in teeth affected by DI, namely, the absence of ordinary dentinal tubules, suggests greater caries resistance [20]. Although the

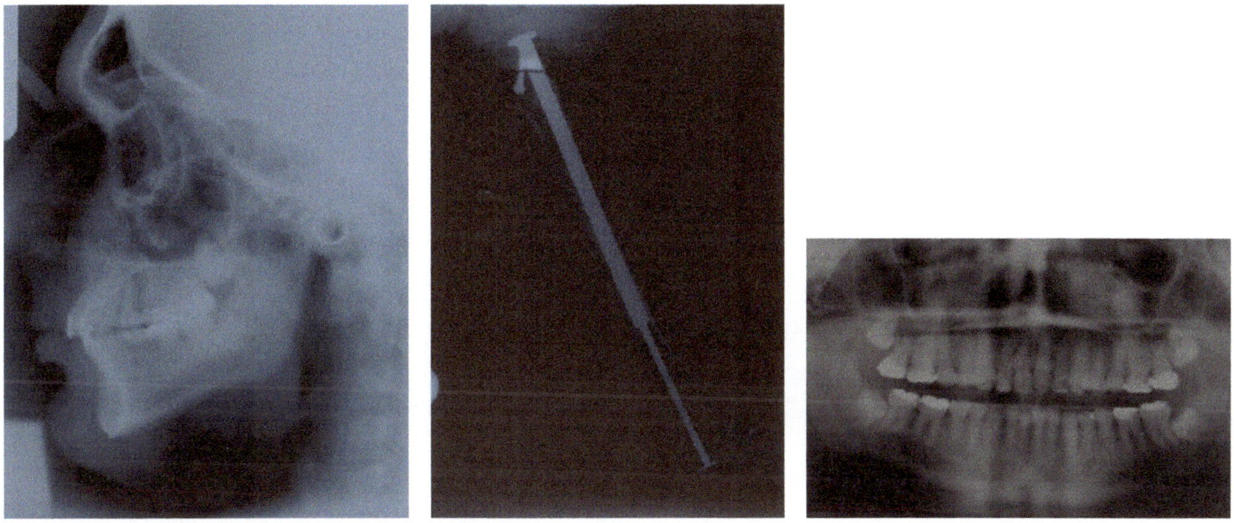

(a) (b) (c)

FIGURE 4: Patient radiographs: Lateral cephalograph (a); plain femoral radiograph (b); and orthopantomograph (OPG) (c).

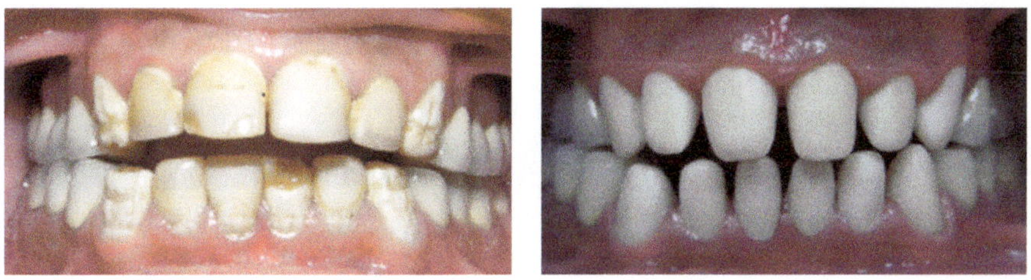

(a) (b)

FIGURE 5: (a) Cemented posterior crowns fabricated from feldspathic porcelain using Laser Sintering technology. Vertical occlusal dimension was established according to the measurements. (b) Zirconium frameworks produced using a 5-axis CNC unit.

permanent teeth of the case presented here confirm this with its absence of dentinal caries, secondary caries was examined under the SSCs. The main reason of this situation may be the coronal microleakage of the prefabricated crowns.

Treatment of patients with DI should focus on protecting teeth from further wear. A multidisciplinary treatment strategy is required to restore appropriate vertical dimension and good esthetics while providing adequate soft tissue support to maintain a normal facial profile. The treatment strategy for this case was to reconstruct all upper and lower teeth with a fixed partial denture in order to protect the remaining hard tissue and achieve sufficient vertical dimensions for function and esthetics. Metal-ceramic crowns were selected for posterior teeth for both stability and economic reasons. A Co-Cr metal framework was fabricated using the rapid manufacturing system of DMLS. Laser sintering forms part of a family of new manufacturing technologies known as rapid prototyping [21]. Laser sintering has applications in a wide range of areas including industrial engineering, the military and aerospace sectors, and medical products. It is gaining popularity in dentistry at last years. Also, DMLS is simpler, more precise, and healthier than conventional manufacturing and can be remarkably cost effective [21]. Moreover, DMLS technology affords highly accurate production of fixed partial dentures with ideal marginal fit and excellent mechanical properties [13, 16]. While both Co-Cr and Ti fine powder alloy mixtures can be used to produce metal frameworks for use in dentistry, because of its ease of fabrication, Co-Cr is most commonly used over porcelain restorations. For this reason, Co-Cr metal-ceramic fixed partial dentures that were manufactured by DMLS technique were chosen for the rehabilitation of posterior region of the presented case.

The anterior teeth of the patient were restored with all-ceramic crowns for esthetic reasons. Zirconium porcelain was selected for its superior resistance when compared to other all-ceramic materials. The main reasons for the selection of zirconium porcelain in this case were to protect the decreased resistance of anterior teeth and to adapt the patient esthetically to the rearranged anterior guidance due to the increased vertical height.

4. Conclusion

Complicated cases such as DI require multidisciplinary treatment to achieve the best results. Early diagnosis and treatment of DI patients may preserve dental tissue and

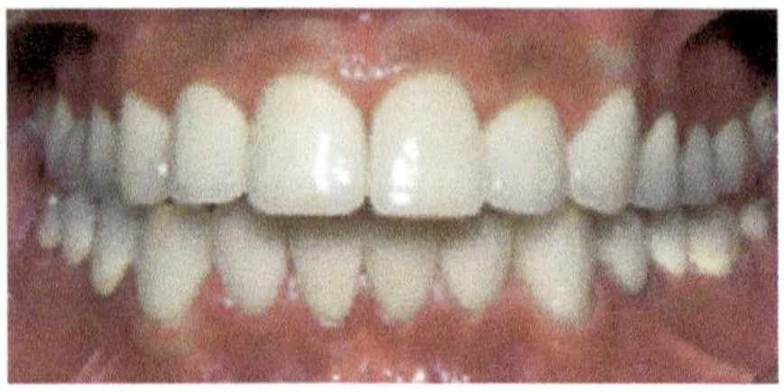

(a)

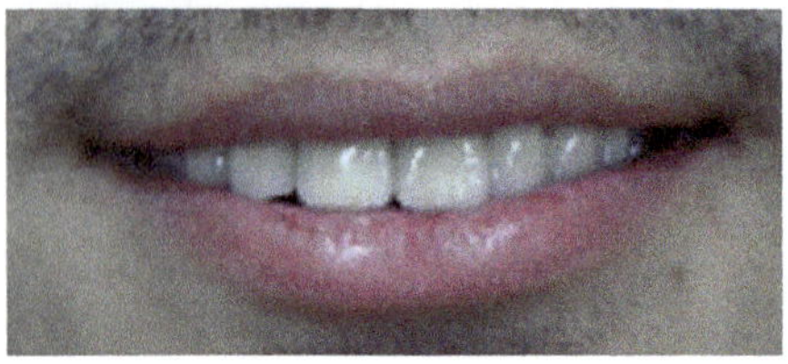

(b)

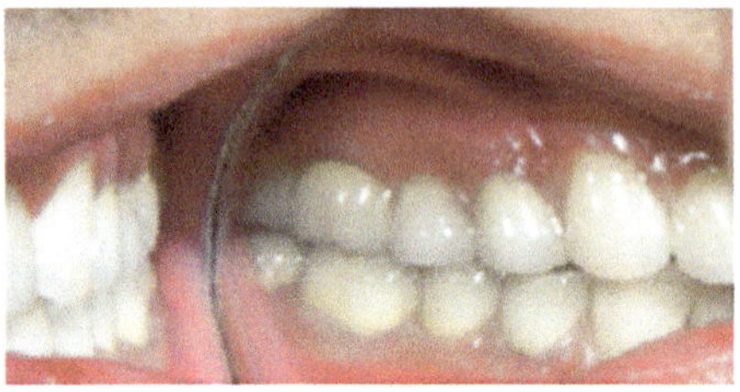

(c)

FIGURE 6: Intraoral appearance of prosthetic restorations.

the stomatognathic system. Appropriate treatment may be required to prevent subsequent restorative problems. In the case presented here, laser sintering technology and a CNC unit were used together to achieve satisfactory function and esthetics, and the patient was recalled for periodical control to extend the longevity of his restorations.

Conflict of Interests

There are no financial or other relationships that might lead to a conflict of interests.

References

[1] J. Kindelan, M. Tobin, D. Roberts-Harry, and R. A. Loukota, "Orthodontic and orthognathic management of a patient with osteogenesis imperfecta and dentinogenesis imperfecta: a case report," *Journal of orthodontics*, vol. 30, no. 4, pp. 291–296, 2003.

[2] F. S. van Dijk, J. M. Cobben, A. Kariminejad et al., "Osteogenesis Imperfecta: a review with clinical examples," *Molecular Syndromology*, vol. 2, no. 1, pp. 1–20, 2011.

[3] A. C. O'Connell and J. C. Marini, "Evaluation of oral problems in an osteogenesis imperfecta population," *Oral Surgery, Oral Medicine, Oral Pathology, Oral Radiology, and Endodontics*, vol. 87, no. 2, pp. 189–196, 1999.

[4] B. Malmgren and S. Norgren, "Dental aberrations in children and adolescents with osteogenesis imperfecta," *Acta Odontologica Scandinavica*, vol. 60, no. 2, pp. 65–71, 2002.

[5] D. O. Sillence, A. Senn, and D. M. Danks, "Genetic heterogeneity in osteogenesis imperfecta," *Journal of Medical Genetics*, vol. 16, no. 2, pp. 101–116, 1979.

[6] F. H. Glorieux, L. M. Ward, F. Rauch, L. Lalic, P. J. Roughley, and R. Travers, "Osteogenesis imperfecta type VI: a form of brittle bone disease with a mineralization defect," *Journal of Bone and Mineral Research*, vol. 17, no. 1, pp. 30–38, 2002.

[7] L. M. Ward, F. Rauch, R. Travers et al., "Osteogenesis imperfecta type VII: an autosomal recessive form of brittle bone disease," *Bone*, vol. 31, no. 1, pp. 12–18, 2002.

[8] E. D. Shields, "A new classification of heritable human enamel defects and a discussion of dentin defects," *Birth Defects*, vol. 19, no. 1, pp. 107–127, 1983.

[9] A. Majorana, E. Bardellini, P. C. Brunelli, M. Lacaita, A. P. Cazzolla, and G. Favia, "Dentinogenesis imperfecta in children with osteogenesis imperfecta: a clinical and ultrastructural study," *International Journal of Paediatric Dentistry*, vol. 20, no. 2, pp. 112–118, 2010.

[10] V. S. Opsahl, C. Gaucher, C. Bardet et al., "Tooth dentin defects reflect genetic disorders affecting bone mineralization," *Bone*, vol. 50, no. 4, pp. 989–997, 2012.

[11] S. R. Shetty, D. Dsouza, S. Babu, and P. Balan, "Osteogenesis imperfecta, (Type IV) with dental findings in siblings," *Case Reports in Dentistry*, vol. 2011, Article ID 970904, 4 pages, 2011.

[12] B. Karpuschewski, H. J. Pieper, M. Krause, and J. Döring, "CoCr is not the same: CoCr-blanks for dental machining," in *Future Trends in Production Engineering: Proceedings of the First Conference of the German Academic Society for Production Engineering, Berlin, Germany, June 2011*, G. Schuh, R. Neugebauer, and E. Uhlmann, Eds., Springer, New York, NY, USA, 1st edition, 2013.

[13] D. Fasbinder, "Using digital technology to enhance restorative dentistry," *Compendium of Continuing Education in Dentistry*, vol. 33, pp. 668–672, 2012.

[14] M. N. Aboushelib, W. A. Elmahy, and M. H. Ghazy, "Internal adaptation, marginal accuracy and microleakage of a pressable versus a machinable ceramic laminate veneers," *Journal of Dentistry*, vol. 40, pp. 670–677, 2012.

[15] M. Figliuzzi, F. Mangano, and C. Mangano, "A novel root analogue dental implant using CT scan and CAD/CAM: selective laser melting technology," *International Journal of Oral and Maxillofacial Surgery*, vol. 41, pp. 858–862, 2012.

[16] R. Castillo-de-Oyagüe, A. Sanchez-Turrion, J. F. Lopez- Lozano et al., "Vertical misfit of laser-sintered and vacuum-cast implant-supported crown copings luted with definitive and temporary luting agents," *Medicina Oral Patologia Oral y Cirugia Bucal*, vol. 17, no. 4, pp. e610–e617, 2012.

[17] M. F. Haddad, E. P. Rocha, and W. G. Assunção, "Cementation of prosthetic restorations: from conventional cementation to dental bonding concept," *Journal of Craniofacial Surgery*, vol. 22, no. 3, pp. 952–958, 2011.

[18] H. Dhaliwal and S. McKaig, "Dentinogenesis imperfecta—clinical presentation and management," *Dental Update*, vol. 37, no. 6, pp. 364–371, 2010.

[19] R. Sæves, L. L. Wekre, E. Ambjørnsen, S. Axelsson, H. Nordgarden, and K. Storhaug, "Oral findings in adults with osteogenesis imperfecta," *Special Care in Dentistry*, vol. 29, no. 2, pp. 102–108, 2009.

[20] N. Shetty, M. Joseph, P. Basnet, and S. Dixit, "An integrated treatment approach: a case report for dentinogenesis imperfecta type II," *Kathmandu University Medical Journal*, vol. 5, no. 18, pp. 230–233, 2007.

[21] U. Iseri, Z. Ozkurt, and E. Kazazoglu, "Shear bond strengths of veneering porcelain to cast, machined and laser-sintered titanium," *Dental Materials*, vol. 30, no. 3, pp. 274–280, 2011.

3

Nonextraction Treatment of Severe Crowding with the Aid of Corticotomy-Assisted Orthodontics

Ali S. Aljhani[1] and Khalid H. Zawawi[2]

[1] *Division of Orthodontics, College of Dentistry, King Saud University for Health Sciences and National Guard Health Affairs, P.O. Box 22490, Riyadh, Saudi Arabia*
[2] *Division of Orthodontics, Faculty of Dentistry, King Abdulaziz University, P.O. Box 80209, Jeddah 21589, Saudi Arabia*

Correspondence should be addressed to Khalid H. Zawawi, kzawawi@kau.edu.sa

Academic Editors: A. Markopoulos and A. Milosevic

This paper illustrates the combined nonextraction orthodontic treatment with the corticotomy technique in an adult patient (age: 25 years and 3 months) with severely crowded arches to accelerate tooth movement and shorten the treatment time. Both her upper lateral incisors were congenitally absent and both upper central incisors' roots were short. Initial fixed orthodontic appliances (bidimensional) were bonded and one week later buccal and lingual corticotomy with alveolar augmentation procedure in the maxilla and mandible was performed. Orthodontic activation to level and align and unravel the crowding was performed every two weeks. The total treatment time was 8 months with no adverse effects observed at the end of active treatment. The addition of the decortication procedure to the conventional orthodontic therapy decreased the duration of treatment significantly. Successful alignment of both arches with ideal overbite and overjet as well as adequate occlusion was achieved.

1. Introduction

An increasing number of adults in recent years are undergoing orthodontic treatment. Correction of malocclusion makes it possible to improve their periodontal health and psychosocial status [1]. It was shown in the Medical Expenditure Panel Survey (MEPS) that orthodontic visits by adults were 23.1% of all orthodontic visits [2]. This was also demonstrated in the fifth study of orthodontic and treatment procedures in 2008 that the percentage of adult active patients was about 20% of the total patients being treated in orthodontic offices in the United States [3]. The duration and management of comprehensive orthodontic treatment for adults is significantly longer compared to adolescent patients [4, 5]. Treatment modifications have been suggested to reduce the treatment time. The technique to accelerate tooth movement was first introduced by Köle, in 1959 [6]. This technique involved a radicular corticotomy and supra-apical osteotomy. The theory was that by creating blocks of bone with vertical buccal and lingual corticotomies and supra-apical horizontal osteotomy connecting cuts, segments of bone with the embedded teeth could be moved rapidly. Later, Anholm and coworkers [7] completed a nonextraction treatment of a case with severe malocclusion in 11 months using corticotomy. Suya [8] suggested modification to the osteotomy cuts with horizontal corticotomy. Gantes et al. [9] presented orthodontic cases treated with corticotomy in which they performed circumscribing corticotomy cuts both facially and lingually around the six upper anterior teeth. The upper first bicuspids were removed and the bone over the extraction sockets was removed both buccally and lingually. Chung et al. [10] removed blocks of medullary bone, block by block, with orthopedic forces. Similarly, Hwang and Lee [11] performed intrusion of unopposed molars by performing a corticotomy procedure and used magnets to deliver the force.

The corticotomy technique was later modified by Wilcko et al. with the addition of alveolar augmentation with resorbable, alloplastic freeze-dried bone to increase the volume of alveolar bone, regenerate bone affected by possible dehiscence and fenestration, and prevent gingival recession. Their justification was that the movement does not result

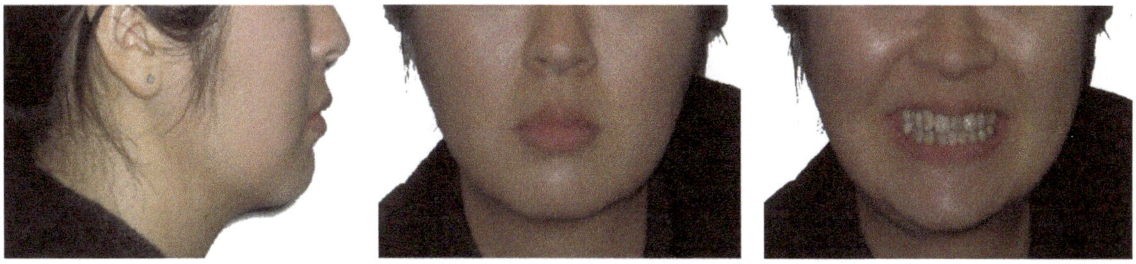

(a) (b) (c)

FIGURE 1: Pretreatment extraoral photographs.

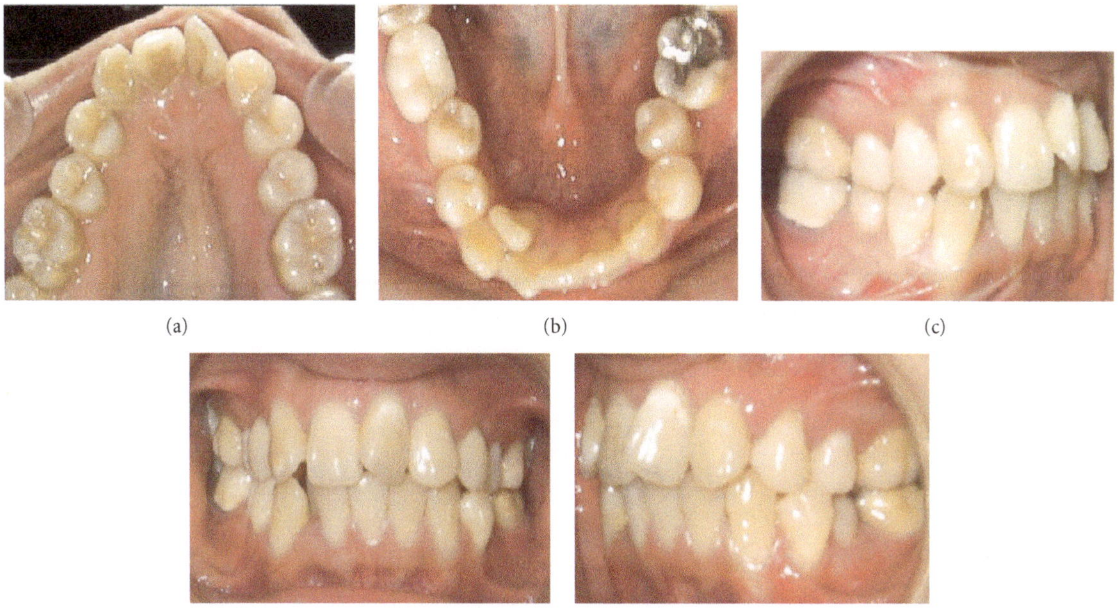

(a) (b) (c)

(d) (e)

FIGURE 2: Pretreatment intraoral photographs.

from repositioning of tooth-bone blocks, but rather from a cascade of transient localized reactions in the bony alveolar housing leading to bone healing [12]. Since then, limited numbers of cases treated with corticotomy were reported in the literature. Germeç et al. [13] reported the treatment of an adult patient with a modified corticotomy technique, in which the lingual vertical and subapical horizontal cuts were eliminated, for the retraction of the lower anterior teeth after the extraction of four premolars. In a preliminary study, Fischer [14] compared the movement of impacted canines after surgical exposure using conventional surgical technique with their contralateral canines exposed using a corticotomy-assisted technique, and he concluded that corticotomy-assisted surgical technique reduced the orthodontic treatment time by 28–33%.

This paper illustrates in detail the effect of rapid orthodontic treatment of a severely crowded case with compromised upper central incisors with the aid of decortication technique and to discuss the surgical and the orthodontic steps involved.

2. Case Report

A female patient (age: 25 years and 3 months) presented with a chief complaint of: *"I want my teeth fixed quickly"*. Her medical was noncontributory and she presented with several restorations, extractions of third molars, and good oral hygiene.

2.1. Pretreatment Evaluation. The patient had a mild convex profile with mild protrusive and competent lips and shows 75% of her upper teeth when smiling. Nasolabial angle was within normal limits (Figure 1).

Dental analysis revealed a full cups class II molars and canines relationships with 4-5 mm overjet and 2 mm overbite; maxillary arch was mildly crowded (4 mm) and mandibular arch was severely crowded (8-9 mm) with the right lateral incisor lingually crowded. Her upper right and left lateral incisors were missing. Upper midline was deviated to the right 2 mm and lower was deviated 4 mm to the right (Figure 2).

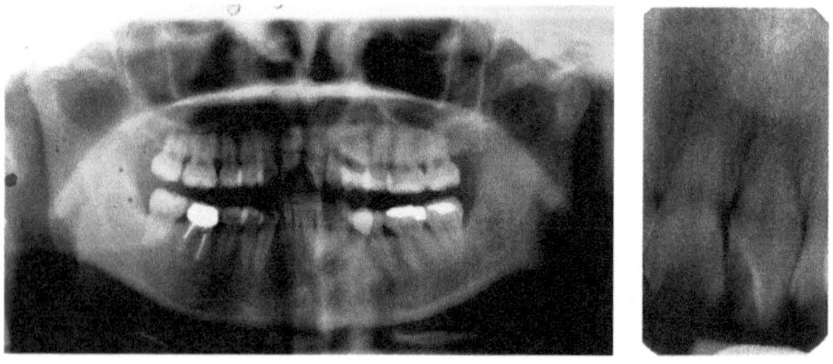
(a) (b)

Figure 3: Pretreatment panoramic and periapical radiographs.

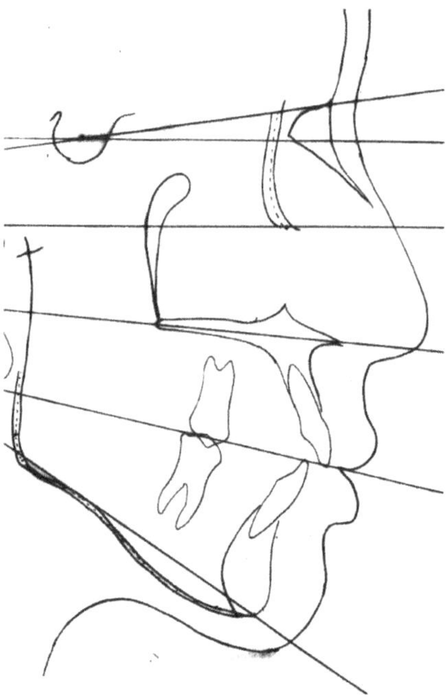

Figure 4: Pretreatment cephalometric tracing.

Table 1: Summary of cephalometric measurements.

Measurement	Norm	Before treatment	After treatment
SNA (degrees)	82	78	78
SNB (degrees)	80	75	74
ANB (degrees)	2	3	4
Wits appraisal (mm)	0	1	1
FMA (degrees)	25	36	35
U1-NA (degrees)	22	22	24
U1-NA (mm)	4	6	7
L1-NB (degrees)	25	30	31
L1-NB (mm)	4	7	7
IMPA (degrees)	90	94	97
Nasolabial angle (degrees)	102	98	94
E-Line-Upper lip (mm)	−4	−2	0
E-Line-Lower lip (mm)	−2	0	2

The panoramic radiograph confirmed the absence of the lateral incisors and showed the existence of short rooted upper right and left central incisors with no pathology. The lower left first molar had a large occlusodistal amalgam restoration. This was confirmed with a periapical radiograph (Figure 3).

Cephalometric measurements showed a skeletal class I with hyperdivergent mandibular plane with moderately proclined and protrusive lower incisors (Table 1 and Figure 4).

2.2. Treatment Plan. The treatment options were discussed with the patient. The initial option of lower premolar extraction to relief the crowding, align the lower arch, and control possible bite opening during treatment due to the hyperdivergent mandibular plane angle. The patient declined this option and showed a genuine interest to have the orthodontic treatment completed as soon as possible and she was not willing to extract any teeth to relieve the crowding. The treatment plan involved the following comprehensive orthodontic treatment with fixed appliances to align the upper and lower teeth and correct the crowding and corticotomy procedure in both arches to accelerate the tooth movement. Due to the congenitally missing upper lateral incisors and lack of space the canines will substitute the missing laterals and first premolars will substitute the canines and finish in class II molar relationship. Also, the patient was informed that the lower left first molar large amalgam restoration could be compromised during treatment.

2.3. Treatment Progress. One week before the surgery, fixed appliances (Clarity, 3 M Unitek, USA, Bi-Dimensional prescription appliances, that is, 0.018×0.025-inch slot brackets for the incisors and 0.022×0.028-inch for the canines and the posterior teeth) and 0.016-inch NiTi arch wires were inserted for initial leveling and alignment. The lower right lateral incisor was not engaged.

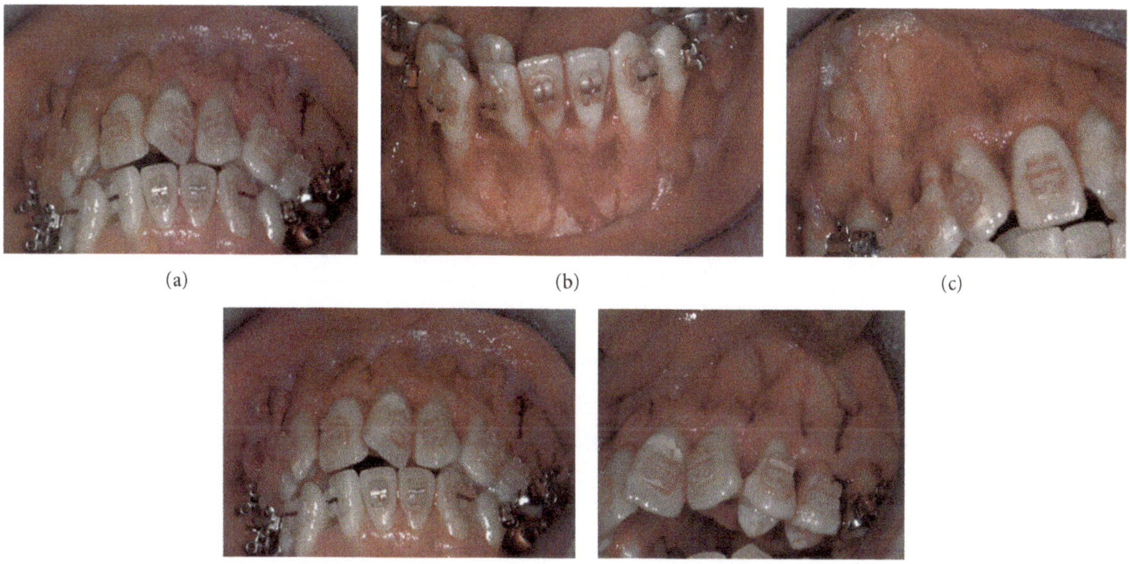

(a) (b) (c)

(d) (e)

FIGURE 5: Maxillary and mandibular corticotomy of the buccal side.

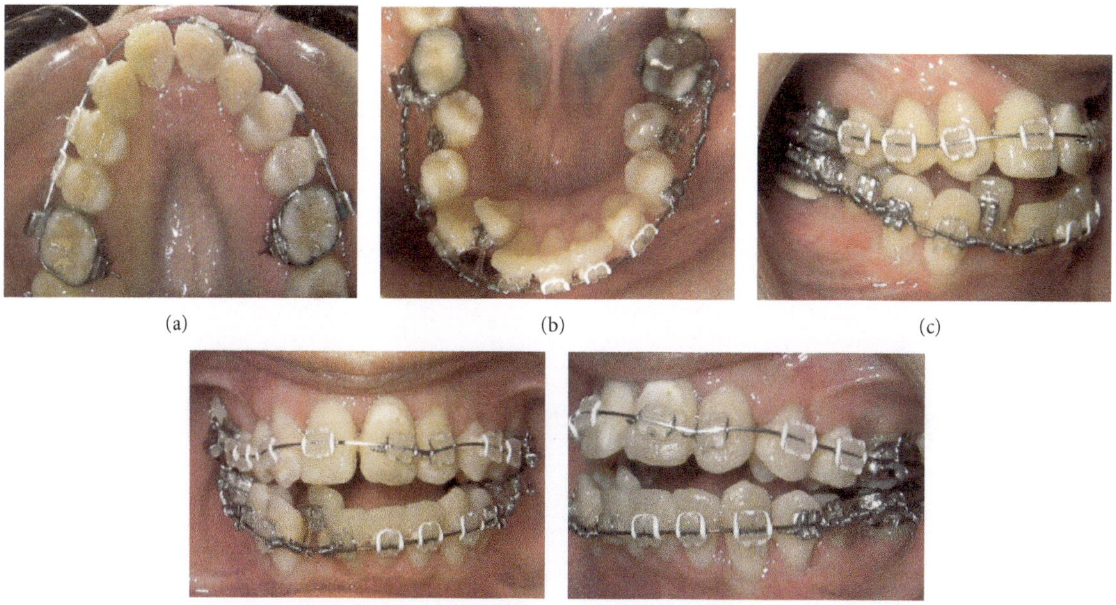

(a) (b) (c)

(d) (e)

FIGURE 6: Intraoral photographs 2 weeks after corticotomy.

2.4. Surgical Procedure. Corticotomy technique as described by Wilcko [12] was performed by a periodontist. Briefly, after administering the proper anesthetic dose, a full thickness flap was reflected sharply both facially and lingually around all erupted teeth, in both arches, from the first molar to the first molar (Figure 5). Each flap was released with a sulcular incision and with papillary preservation technique when possible. The lingual interdental papilla between the maxillary central incisors was not reflected and no vertical releasing incisions were used. Cuts in the alveolus that penetrate the entire thickness of the cortical plate and penetrate just barely into the medullary bone were performed both buccally and lingually around all the teeth in both arches. Vertical decortication cuts were made between the roots of the teeth and they were stopped 2-3 mm shy of the alveolar crest. Horizontal scalloped corticotomy cuts were used to connect the vertical cuts along with perforations in the cortical plate. Bone grafting mixture OraGraft demineralized cortical particulate (LifeNet Health, Inc., Virginia Beach, VA, USA) was then applied to the

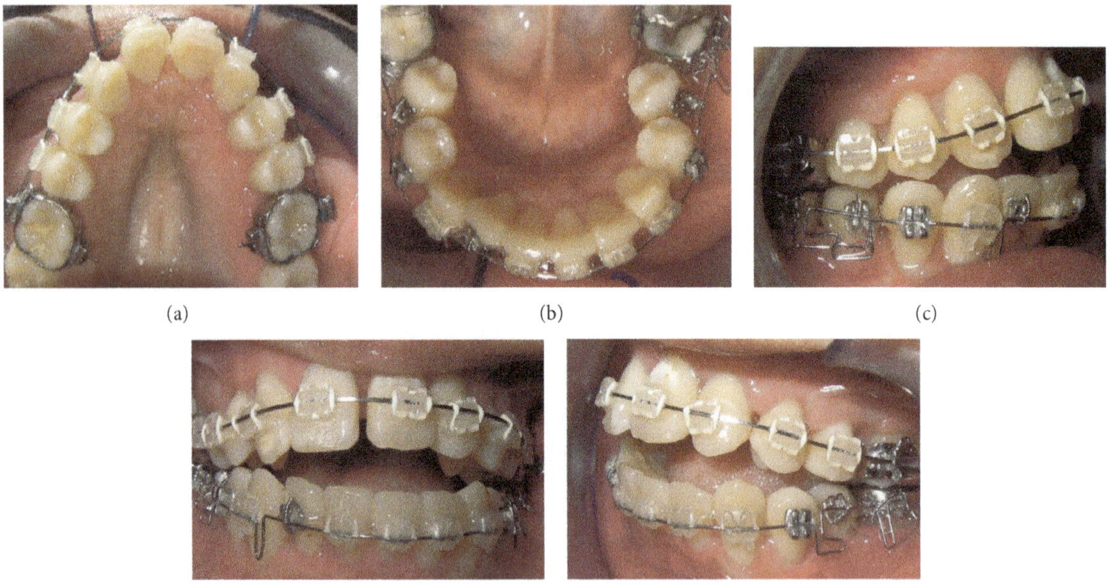

(a) (b) (c)

(d) (e)

Figure 7: Intraoral photographs 10 weeks after corticotomy.

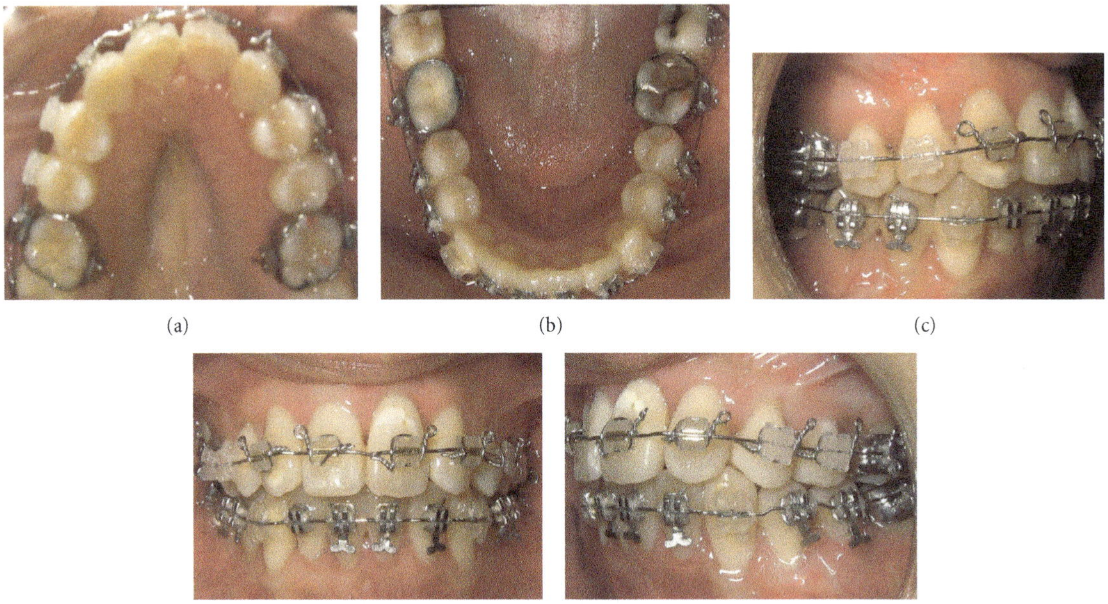

(a) (b) (c)

(d) (e)

Figure 8: Intraoral photographs 28 weeks after corticotomy.

activated cortical plates. Flaps were repositioned to their presurgical positions and sutured with interrupted loop sutures. Nonresorbable sutures (Gore-tex, CV-5, RT-16, from W. L. Gore & Associates, Inc., Medical Products Division, Flagstaff, AZ, USA) were used and the sutures were removed after 14 days from the procedure. The patient was kept under antibiotic for 10 days following the surgery.

At the suture removal appointment, 0.016×0.022-inch NiTi archwire was inserted in the upper arch and 0.016-inch stainless steel was inserted in the lower arch with 150 g NiTi push coil springs to create space for the ectopic lower right lateral incisor (Figure 6).

After 10 weeks, postoperatively, the ectopic lateral incisor was bonded and engaged with a power thread. The patient developed an open bite that was anticipated due to her hyperdivergent mandibular plane and as her lower premolars started to align. Vertical elastics were used to control for the open bite (Figure 7). She was instructed to wear Class II box

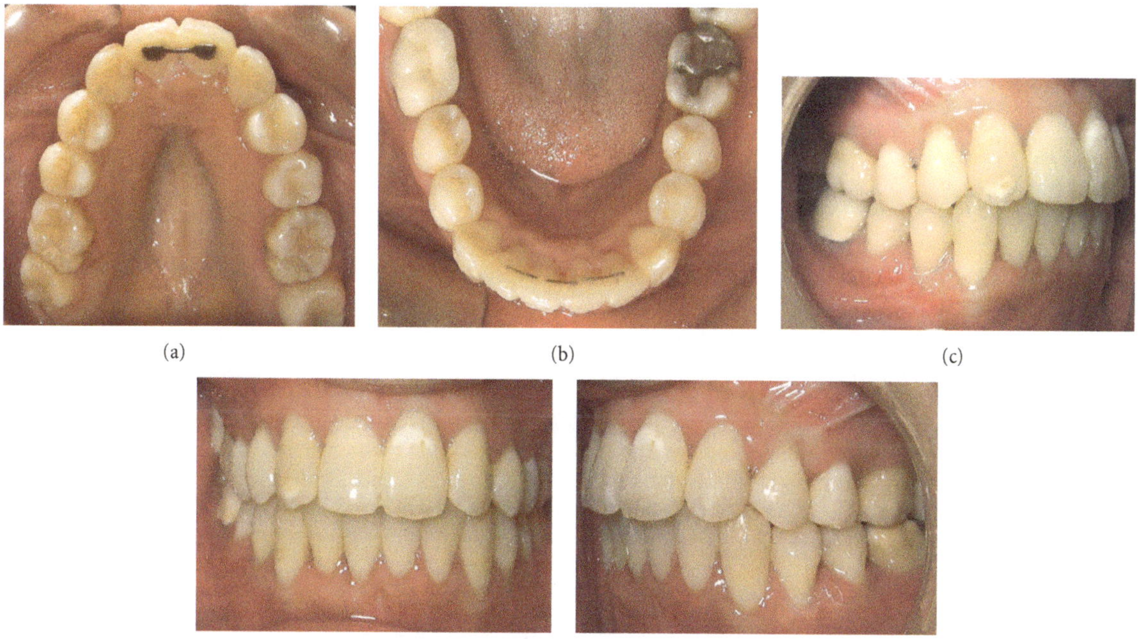

(a) (b) (c) (d) (e)

Figure 9: Intraoral photographs 32 weeks after corticotomy.

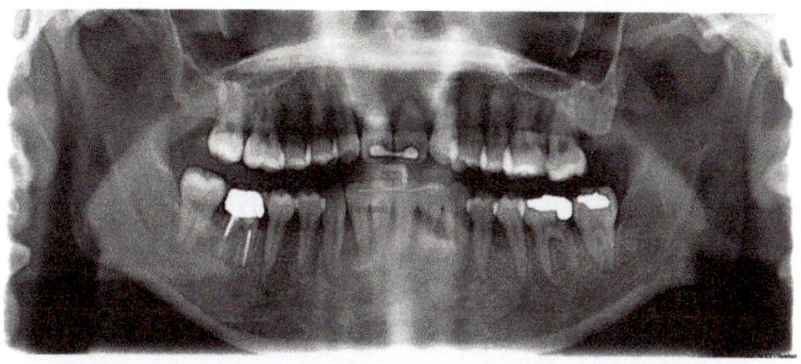

Figure 10: Posttreatment panoramic radiograph.

elastics ("3/16", 4 oz) full-time. The patient was extremely compliant and used the elastic as instructed. During the 28th week postoperatively, the upper and lower arched were leveled and aligned, the ectopic lower right lateral incisor was in proper position (Figure 8).

After 33 weeks of active treatment, the upper and lower crowding and rotations were corrected. The teeth are well aligned with good intercuspal relation. The total treatment period with the fixed appliance therapy was 8 months. After the appliance was removed, lingual bonded retainers were set on both the upper and lower arches and removable upper circumferential and lower Hawley retainers were delivered to be worn full time for the first 6 months (Figure 9).

2.5. Treatment Results. Post-treatment evaluation of the patient revealed a normal overjet and overbite, upper and lower midlines were coincident to one another and to the facial midline. The upper and lower dental arches are well aligned and class II molars and canines relationships

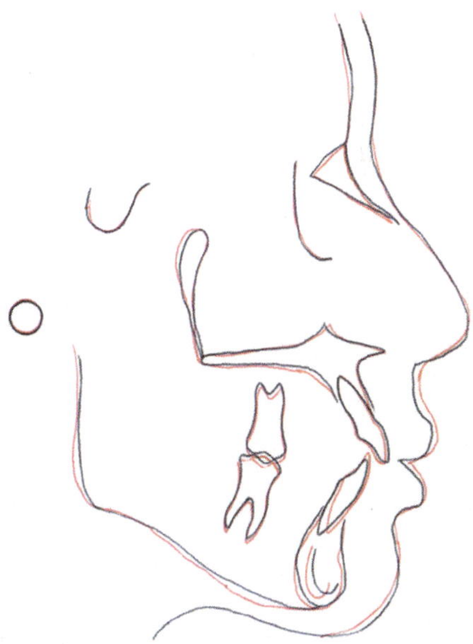

Figure 11: Cephalometric superimposition (pretreatment: black and posttreatment: red).

was achieved as planned. Also, good preservation of the interdental papillae with no gingival recession was evident. Posttreatment panoramic radiograph showed good parallelism of the roots, no significant reduction in the radiographic height of the crestal bone, and no evidence of any significant apical root resorption. Furthermore, the roots of the upper central incisors condition was stable (Figure 10).

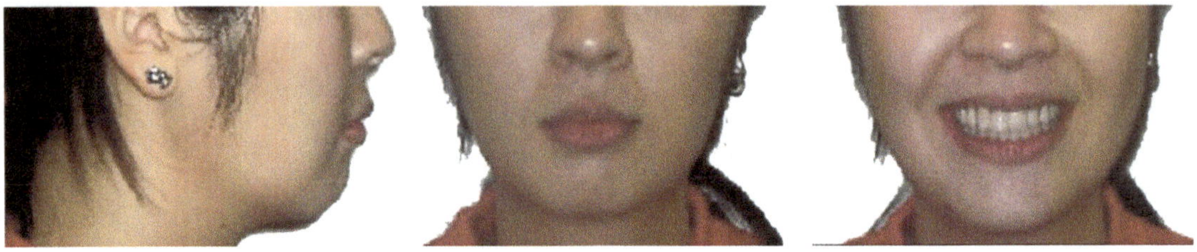

(a) (b) (c)

FIGURE 12: Posttreatment extraoral photographs.

Final lateral cephalometric analysis showed minimal proclination of the upper and lower anterior teeth with mild upper and lower lip protrusion (Table 1 and Figure 11). Eventhough the nasolabial angle decreased, it remained within normal limits (Figure 12).

3. Discussion

The comprehensive orthodontic treatment of this adult patient who presented with severe lower crowding was completed in 8 months which is significantly less than the routine duration that conventional orthodontic treatment of similar cases require. The addition of the corticotomy procedure has been reported to shorten the conventional orthodontic treatment time and it was claimed that teeth can be moved 2 to 3 times further in 25 to 30% less time required for traditional orthodontic treatment [7–11, 15, 16]. The current paper confirms previously published findings and supports this treatment option.

The concept of corticotomy as initially introduced and later adapted by several investigators relied on creating blocks of bone with the embedded teeth that can be moved rapidly with heavy forces [6–10]. On the other hand, conventional orthodontic forces were advocated by Wilcko et al. [12, 15, 16] who explained the rapid tooth movement as an illustration of regional acceleratory phenomenon (RAP). Frost described this process in 1983, and found that the surgical wounding of osseous tissues results in accelerated regional healing process. It can accelerate both hard and soft tissue healing 2 to 10 folds and this leads to decreased regional bone density and accelerated bone turnover [17–19]. This was reported to occur also in intraoral cortical bone by others [20–22]. Wilcko and coworkers showed that transient localized de- and remineralization in the bony alveolar housing occurs and the demineralization of the alveolar bone over the root surfaces leaves the collagenous soft tissue matrix of the bone, which can be carried with the root surface and then remineralizes following the completion of the orthodontic treatment [15]. Initially, the term "Accelerated Osteogenic Orthodontics" was used to describe the combined corticotomy-facilitated orthodontics and periodontal alveolar augmentation [12]. Later, Wilcko et al. [15] modified it to be *"Periodontally Accelerated Osteogenic Orthodontics"* (PAOO) technique. In a recent report comparing the alveolar bone reactions to osteotomy-assisted and corticotomy-assisted tooth movement, Lee et al. [23] found evidence of regional accelerated phenomenon in the alveolar bone of the corticotomy-treated animals and distraction osteogenesis in the osteotomy-assisted tooth movement using micro-Computed Tomography. This confirms the hypothesis of the difference in the healing processes involved in both procedures.

Original corticotomy-facilitated orthodontic treatment involved buccal and lingual osteotomy cuts with orthopedic forces, and the use of alveolar augmentation with demineralized bone graft was advocated to cover any fenestration and dehiscence and to increase in the bony support for both the teeth and the overlying and soft tissues [12, 16]. Surface computed tomographic scans taken before and after the treatment showed a return of the layer of mineralized bone over the roots of the teeth and a general increase of the bone volume [12, 16]. More controlled studies are still warranted to investigate the importance of the alveolar augmentation in the decortication technique and the effects of different grafting materials on the alveolar bone. While osteotomy cuts were recommended on both alveolar surfaces (buccal and lingual) [6, 12, 16], two recently published case reports showed the results of selective corticotomy limited to the buccal and labial surfaces to reduce the operation time and postoperative patient discomfort and avoid the risk of violating vital lingual anatomy [13, 24]. The current case was managed with both buccal and lingual cuts and efficient tooth movement was observed, however, elimination of the lingual cuts should be studied in future trials.

Most of the recently published literature showed no adverse effects of the corticotomy on the periodontium [13, 15, 24–26]. In the present case, no reduction in the crest bone height, gingival recession, and apical root resorption was seen after the orthodontic treatment. The upper central incisors did not exhibit any further resorption and were stable during the treatment. The disadvantages of this procedure are the need for more frequent activation compared to conventional orthodontic treatment, the extra expenses for the periodontal surgery, and the postoperative discomfort were the disadvantages of this technique that the patient need to tolerate for a faster course of treatment.

Since most of what is known about the decortication procedures in orthodontic treatment is based on case reports, more laboratory and clinical studies are necessary to better explain the biological mechanisms involved at both the tissue and molecular level, and most importantly, investigate the long term effects of this procedure.

4. Conclusions

Comprehensive orthodontic treatment with the aid of the decortication technique is an effective treatment option in adults to achieve the desired results in significantly reduced treatment duration.

Conflict of Interests

The authors of the paper do not have any direct financial relation with the commercial identities mentioned in the paper that might lead to a conflict of interests for any of the authors.

References

[1] J. Rusanen, S. Lahti, M. Tolvanen, and P. Pirttiniemi, "Quality of life in patients with severe malocclusion before treatment," *European Journal of Orthodontics*, vol. 32, no. 1, pp. 43–48, 2010.

[2] A. H. Guay, L. J. Brown, and T. Wall, "Orthodontic dental patients and expenditures-2004," *American Journal of Orthodontics and Dentofacial Orthopedics*, vol. 134, no. 3, pp. 337–343, 2008.

[3] R. G. Keim, E. L. Gottlieb, A. H. Nelson, and D. S. Vogels, "2008 JCO study of orthodontic diagnosis and treatment procedures, part 1: results and trends," *Journal of Clinical Orthodontics*, vol. 42, no. 11, pp. 625–640, 2008.

[4] I. Kocadereli, "Changes in soft tissue profile after orthodontic treatment with and without extractions," *American Journal of Orthodontics and Dentofacial Orthopedics*, vol. 122, no. 1, pp. 67–72, 2002.

[5] P. S. Vig, D. Orth, J. A. Weintraub, C. Brown, and C. J. Kowalski, "The duration of orthodontic treatment with and without extractions: a pilot study of five selected practices," *American Journal of Orthodontics and Dentofacial Orthopedics*, vol. 97, no. 1, pp. 45–51, 1990.

[6] H. Köle, "Surgical operations on the alveolar ridge to correct occlusal abnormalities," *Oral Surgery, Oral Medicine, Oral Pathology*, vol. 12, no. 5, pp. 515–529, 1959.

[7] J. M. Anholm, D. A. Crites, R. Hoff, and W. E. Rathbun, "Corticotomy-facilitated orthodontics," *Journal California Dental Association*, vol. 14, no. 12, pp. 7–11, 1986.

[8] H. Suya, "Corticotomy in orthodontics," in *Mechanical and Biological Basics in Orthodontic Therapy*, E. Hosl and and A. Baldauf, Eds., pp. 207–226, Huthig Buch, Heidelberg, Germany, 1991.

[9] B. Gantes, E. Rathbun, and M. Anholm, "Effects on the periodontium following corticotomy-facilitated orthodontics. Case reports," *Journal of Periodontology*, vol. 61, no. 4, pp. 234–238, 1990.

[10] K. R. Chung, M. Y. Oh, and S. J. Ko, "Corticotomy-assisted orthodontics," *Journal of Clinical Orthodontics*, vol. 35, no. 5, pp. 331–339, 2001.

[11] H. S. Hwang and K. H. Lee, "Intrusion of overerupted molars by corticotomy and magnets," *American Journal of Orthodontics and Dentofacial Orthopedics*, vol. 120, no. 2, pp. 209–216, 2001.

[12] W. M. Wilcko, "Rapid orthodontics with alveolar reshaping: two case reports of decrowding," *International Journal of Periodontics and Restorative Dentistry*, vol. 21, no. 1, pp. 9–19, 2001.

[13] D. Germeç, B. Giray, I. Kocadereli, and A. Enacar, "Lower incisor retraction with a modified corticotomy," *Angle Orthodontist*, vol. 76, no. 5, pp. 882–890, 2006.

[14] T. J. Fischer, "Orthodontic treatment acceleration with corticotomy-assisted exposure of palatally impacted canines: a preliminary study," *Angle Orthodontist*, vol. 77, no. 3, pp. 417–420, 2007.

[15] M. T. Wilcko, W. M. Wilcko, and N. F. Bissada, "An evidence-based analysis of periodontally accelerated orthodontic and osteogenic techniques: a synthesis of scientific perspectives," *Seminars in Orthodontics*, vol. 14, no. 4, pp. 305–316, 2008.

[16] W. M. Wilcko, D. J. Ferguson, J. E. Bouquot, and M. T. Wilcko, "Rapid orthodontic decrowding with alveolar augmentation: Case report," *World Journal of Orthodontics*, vol. 4, no. 3, pp. 197–205, 2003.

[17] H. M. Frost, "The regional acceleratory phenomenon: a review," *Henry Ford Hospital Medical Journal*, vol. 31, no. 1, pp. 3–9, 1983.

[18] H. M. Frost, "The biology of fracture healing. An overview for clinicians. Part I," *Clinical Orthopaedics and Related Research*, no. 248, pp. 283–293, 1989.

[19] H. M. Frost, "The biology of fracture healing. An overview for clinicians. Part II," *Clinical Orthopaedics and Related Research*, no. 248, pp. 294–309, 1989.

[20] R. S. Goldie and G. J. King, "Root resorption and tooth movement in orthodontically treated, calcium-deficient, and lactating rats," *American Journal of Orthodontics*, vol. 85, no. 5, pp. 424–430, 1984.

[21] M. S. Shih and R. W. Norrdin, "Regional acceleration of remodeling during healing of bone defects in beagles of various ages," *Bone*, vol. 6, no. 5, pp. 377–379, 1985.

[22] A. Yaffe, N. Fine, and I. Binderman, "Regional accelerated phenomenon in the mandible following mucoperiosteal flap surgery," *Journal of Periodontology*, vol. 65, no. 1, pp. 79–83, 1994.

[23] W. Lee, G. Karapetyan, R. Moats et al., "Corticotomy-/osteotomy-assisted tooth movement microCTs differ," *Journal of Dental Research*, vol. 87, no. 9, pp. 861–865, 2008.

[24] H. Nowzari, F. K. Yorita, and H. C. Chang, "Periodontally accelerated osteogenic orthodontics combined with autogenous bone grafting," *Compendium of Continuing Education in Dentistry*, vol. 29, no. 4, pp. 200–218, 2008.

[25] S. Iino, S. Sakoda, and S. Miyawaki, "An adult bimaxillary protrusion treated with corticotomy-facilitated orthodontics and titanium miniplates," *Angle Orthodontist*, vol. 76, no. 6, pp. 1074–1082, 2006.

[26] D. D. Oliveira, B. F. de Oliveira, H. H. de Araújo Brito, M. M. G. de Souza, and P. J. Medeiros, "Selective alveolar corticotomy to intrude overerupted molars," *American Journal of Orthodontics and Dentofacial Orthopedics*, vol. 133, no. 6, pp. 902–908, 2008.

4

Effect of Preorthodontic Trainer in Mixed Dentition

Pallavi Pujar[1] and Suryakanth M. Pai[2]

[1] *Department of Pedodontics, Maratha Mandal's Dental College, Belgaum 590010, Karnataka, India*
[2] *Department of Pedodontics, College of Dental Sciences, Davangere 577004, India*

Correspondence should be addressed to Pallavi Pujar; pallavi.pujar@yahoo.co.in

Academic Editors: R. S. Brown and M. W. Roberts

Background. This paper reports a case with end-on-molar relation with maxillary anterior teeth proclination, lower anterior teeth crowding, and deep bite. The case was successfully treated in a short span. Clinically significant improvement in the dimensions of the maxillary and mandibular dental arch forms and sufficient space for the eruption of permanent teeth was observed. *Conclusion.* Therefore, it can be concluded that *preorthodontic trainer* is a valid treatment of choice in mixed dentition where transverse expansion is a part of the treatment plan, as the results obtained are within short period of time and have less chances of relapse, because the correction of a malocclusion is by elimination of soft tissue dysfunction.

1. Introduction

The use of functional appliances has been reported since early times to produce skeletal and dentoalveolar changes [1–5]. These appliances are known to produce neuromuscular changes which lead to morphological modifications in the craniofacial complex [6–9]. A treatment based on only moving teeth is like treating only part of the problem and relapse could be expected. Thus, treatment plan intending to correct a malocclusion must include appliances which eliminate soft tissue dysfunction acting on the muscles of the cheeks, lips, and tongue, at the same time, correcting teeth and jaws position [10]. Furthermore, a two-phase orthodontic treatment, where a functional appliance is used to treat the functional problems and then brackets are used to align teeth, has been reported to improve relapse frequently occurring after orthodontic treatment with brackets [11]. During the last decades, better functional appliances have been developed and have been reported to produce significant changes in oral function as well as to stimulate mandibular growth [12]. The Trainer for Kids (T4K, Myofunctional Research Co, Australia) is a prefabricated functional appliance which is claimed to correct malocclusions at an early age by acting on muscular dysfunction and repositioning the mandible in forward direction and it stimulates the transverse development as well [13]. By initiating treatment at the mixed dentition stage, more treatment options are available and the need for complex orthodontic treatment involving permanent tooth extraction or orthognathic surgery is also minimized. They are also simple and economical. But the cases need to be carefully selected, and the operator should be well trained in their use.

Abundant information is available on preorthodontic trainer but less case reports have been reported in the literature that actually demonstrate the benefits of the trainer especially in mixed dentition. There is no literature published yet on the effect of trainer on end-on-molar relation in mixed dentition. The purpose of this paper is to present a clinical case where a patient with end on molar relation and proclination of teeth was successfully treated during the mixed dentition with preorthodontic trainer in a short period of time. Thus, this case report substantiates the importance of proper case selection and the use of preorthodontic trainer as a treatment modality in the correction of malocclusion in mixed dentition in children.

2. Case Report

An eleven-year-old female child of Asian origin was reported to the Department of Pedodontics, College of Dental Sciences, Davangere, Karnataka, India. The chief complaint of the patient was forwardly placed upper front teeth and

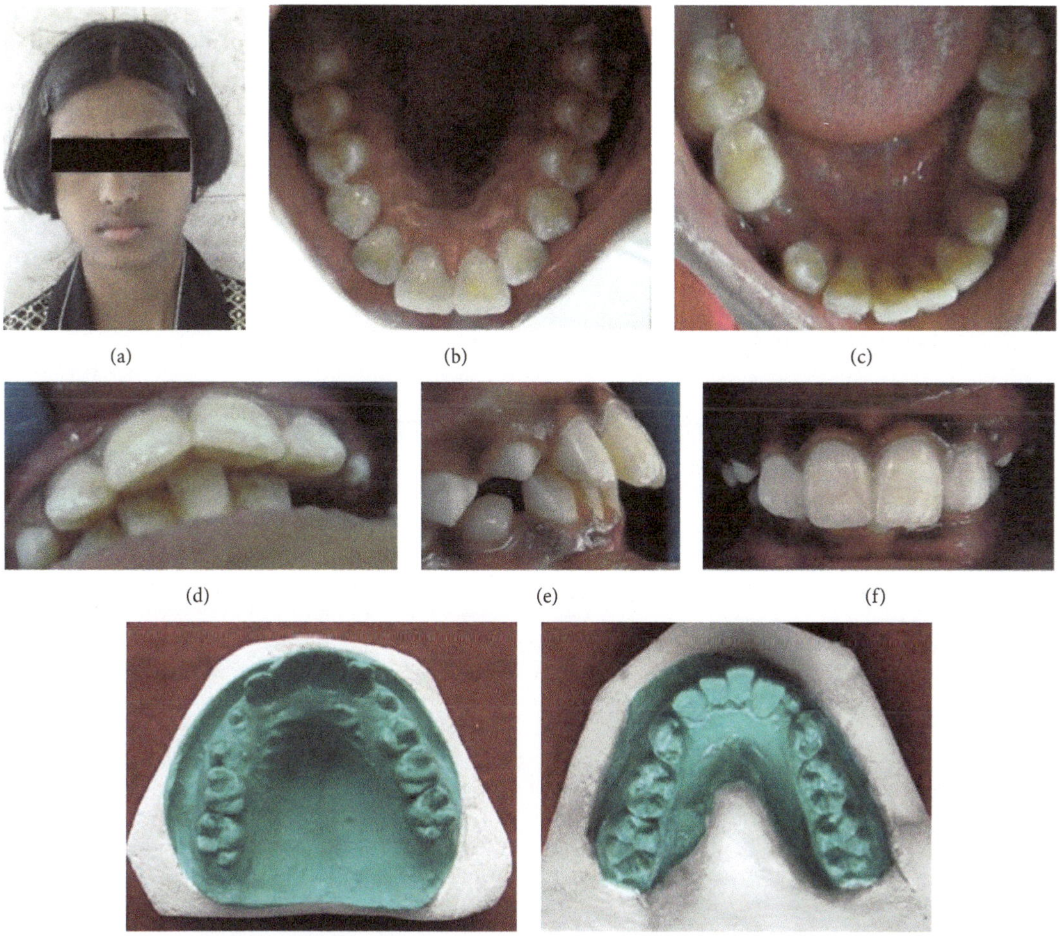

FIGURE 1: (a) Preoperative profile photograph. (b) Preoperative clinical photograph of maxillary arch. (c) Preoperative clinical photograph of mandibular arch. (d) Preoperative clinical photograph showing the upper and lower incisors in occlusion. (e) Preoperative clinical photograph showing the overjet. (f) Preoperative clinical photograph showing the overbite. (g) Preoperative study model of maxillary arch. (h) Preoperative study model of mandibular arch.

irregular lower front teeth. The patient did not give any history of deleterious oral habits.

3. Diagnosis and Etiology

Extraoral examination revealed a convex profile, hyperactivity of the mentalis musculature, and potentially competent lips (Figure 1(a)). On intraoral examination, V-shaped upper arch (Figure 1(b)) and lower arch were seen (Figure 1(c)). Bilateral end on molar relation was present (Figures 3(a) and 3(b)). Proclination of the upper and lower teeth with 5.5 mm of overjet (Figure 1(e)) and overbite of 95% was present (Figure 1(f)). Crowding was seen in the lower anterior teeth and less space for the eruption of lower premolar and permanent canines (Figure 1(h)). Fluorosis stains were seen with anterior teeth. The mixed dentition analysis revealed that there was optimum space for the eruption of the maxillary premolars and for the mandibular arch there was deficiency of 2.5 mm of space. Steiner's cephalometric analysis was performed. Skeletal analysis showed values within normal range. Dental analysis showed increased upper incisor to NA (linear and angle), increased lower incisor to NB (linear and angle), and reduced interincisal angle (Figure 5(a)). There was no skeletal discrepancy; but dental analysis revealed proclination of upper and lower incisors. There were multiple problems to be corrected in this patient. Since the child was in mixed dentition, an appliance would redirect the growth as well as correct the existing problems.

4. Treatment Objectives

Treatment objective would include correcting the proclination of the maxillary teeth and relieving crowding in the mandible anterior teeth. Arch expansion was also desired to accommodate the erupting permanent teeth, correct the resting position of the tongue and improve the arch forms. Since dental and muscular problems were involved and the patient was in growing age, myofunctional appliance was planned for the patient. Preorthodontic trainer (Figure 6) was suggested to the patient as the child was in mixed dentition and there were no obvious skeletal discrepancies and she was found to be cooperative. The advantages, the amount of cooperation required, and the importance of regular use for the success of the treatment were explained to both the patient and the parents.

5. Treatment Progress

The patient was asked to wear the appliance for 1-2 hours in the day for two weeks and then overnight also. The patient was followed up for every 15 days for first two months and later once in every month.

6. Treatment Results

Six months later, there were reduced mentalis activity and less convexity of the profile as the proclination of the teeth was reduced. The lips became competent (Figure 2(a)). There was an improvement in the upper and lower arches (Figures 2(b) and 2(c)). There was an increase in the intercanine distance which was evident by accommodating the erupting canine in the arch (Figures 2(g) and 2(h)). Crowding was relieved in the mandibular anterior teeth (Figure 2(h)). The molar relation changed from end on molar relation to Angle's class I molar relation (Figures 4(a) and 4(b)). The overjet was reduced from 5.5 mm to 2 mm (Figures 2(d) and 2(e)). There was reduction in the deep bite (Figure 2(f)). The interincisal angle increase was positively modified (Figure 5(b)). All these changes were seen just in a span of 6 months. The patient was asked to wear the same appliance for two more months as retention appliance. The patient was happy with the results of the treatment and did not opt for any fixed appliance therapy which was suggested to her for further fine detailing of the positions of the teeth. The parents of the patient also denied the treatment of the fluorosis stains that was suggested to them.

7. Discussion

Since there were no skeletal discrepancies, trainer was selected as a treatment of choice. Case selection is an important criterion for the success of the treatment with this appliance. The case presented here required the retraction of the anterior teeth, correction of the molar relation to Angle's class I, decrowding of the lower anterior teeth, transverse expansion of the maxillary and the mandibular arches, correction of muscular imbalances, and reduction of deep bite. According to model analysis, there was no space deficiency in the maxillary arch, but the retraction of the anterior teeth would require space and the decrowding of the lower teeth would also require space. The patient was in late mixed dentition with no skeletal discrepancies. All these corrections were expected out of use of single appliance. The trainer is often not able to offset major jaw discrepancies such as those at 11 years of age but the other dental effects of trainer were still desirable. The parents and the patient were cooperative and followed the instructions correctly. Hence the patient was put on preorthodontic trainer.

The clinical case presented showed that the preorthodontic trainer successfully treated an end on molar relation along with the proclination of the anterior teeth and deep bite in less than a year. The postoperative study models demonstrated well-aligned upper and lower arches (Figures 2(g) and 2(h)). The cephalometry demonstrated a positive modification in upper incisor to NA (linear and angle), lower incisor to NB (linear and angle), and interincisal angles within 6 months of treatment. The soft tissue dysfunction was eliminated and resting position of the tongue was also corrected. The treatment goals were achieved within half a year and further treatment became unnecessary.

The three effects of the trainer are tooth guidance, myofunctional training, and jaw positioning. It aligns the teeth and provides functional advantage. *Tooth guidance* in a trainer is made from a nonthermoplastic silicone or polyurethane which has both flexibility and inherent memory. The premoulded upper and lower labial bows have a similar effect to that of orthodontic arch wire. That is, they are premoulded to the parabolic shape of the natural arches and they adapt to any arch size, large or small. The labial bows combined with anterior tooth channels afford a constant force on misaligned anterior teeth to assist in the correction of their position. These components of the trainer might have caused the alignment of the teeth and hence the improvement in the arch forms in the clinical case presented here.

Myofunctional training effects of the trainer are correcting the incorrect tongue position and function, tongue thrusting, and oral habits which are the cause of many malocclusions. The design incorporates a tongue tag for proprioceptive location of the tongue tip. The raised section on the tag trains the child to place the tongue tip in the correct position with the trainer in place. This also acts as a "reminder" to place the tongue tip correctly without the trainer. The tongue guard prevents a tongue thrust swallow when being in place, which is a "position training" process for the tongue. Correction of these soft tissue problems has been shown to greatly influence growth, development, and long-term stability [10]. Lip bumpers or mentalis stretchers are incorporated to stretch and deactivate overactive mentalis contraction. Lip bumpers have been shown to gain arch length in mild to moderately crowded cases. This component of the trainer might have helped relieve the crowding in the lower arch in the present clinical case. The soft tissue problems were also taken care of by the tongue tag, tongue guard, and lip bumpers in the appliance.

The *jaw positioning* is by producing maxillary expansion which is accompanied by a spontaneous mandibular response, which increases the dental arch perimeter [14, 15] and rotates the mandible posteriorly [16–18]. The edge-to-edge class I jaw positioning of the appliance might have produced Angle's class I molar relation in the present clinical case.

In the present clinical case, the growth of the jaws might have also caused the desired effects but according to results of study by Ramirez and coworkers both maxillary

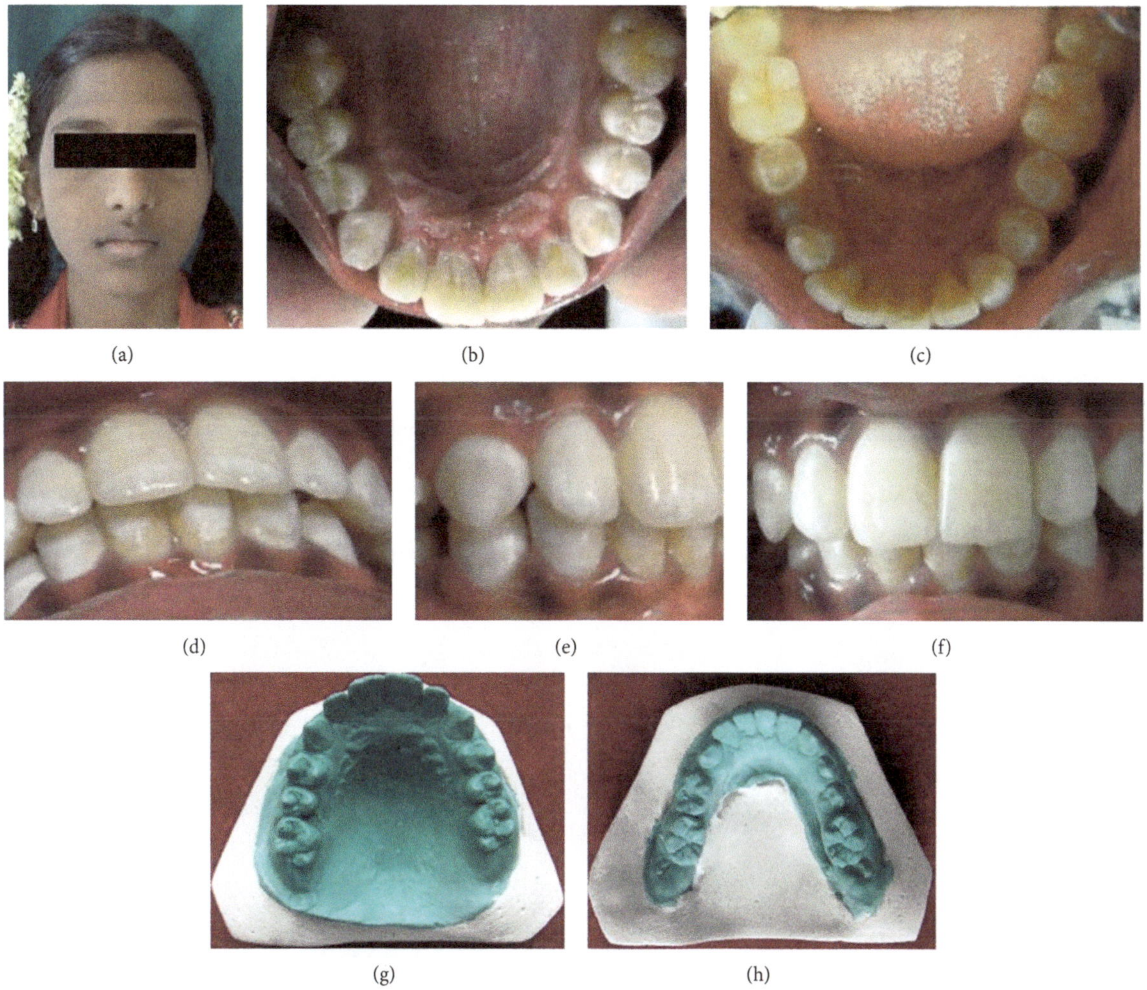

Figure 2: (a) Postoperative profile photograph. (b) Postoperative clinical photograph of maxillary arch. (c) Postoperative clinical photograph of mandibular arch. (d) Postoperative clinical photograph showing the upper and lower incisors in occlusion. (e) Postoperative clinical photograph showing the overjet. (f) Postoperative clinical photograph showing the overbite. (g) Postoperative study model of maxillary arch. (h) Postoperative study model of mandibular arch.

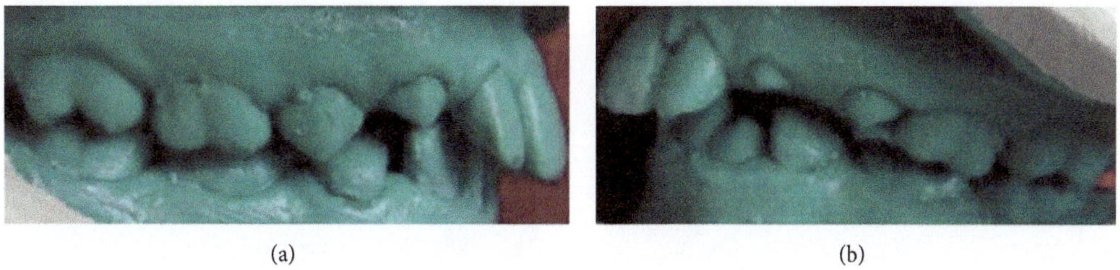

Figure 3: (a) Preoperative molar relation on the right side of the study model. (b) Preoperative molar relation on the left side of the study model.

and mandibular interpremolar and intermolar distances are significantly increased by the T4K, thus the arch perimeter providing more room for tooth alignment. It thus appears that the prefabricated functional appliance stimulates further transverse development overlapping that produced by natural growth, which may be an asset when treating patients with crowding caused by decreased maxillary or mandibular transverse development [19]. Thus, it may be inferred that most of the effects seen were because of the use of the preorthodontic trainer.

Another interesting finding in the present case is the reduction of the deep bite. Deep bite was diagnosed before the

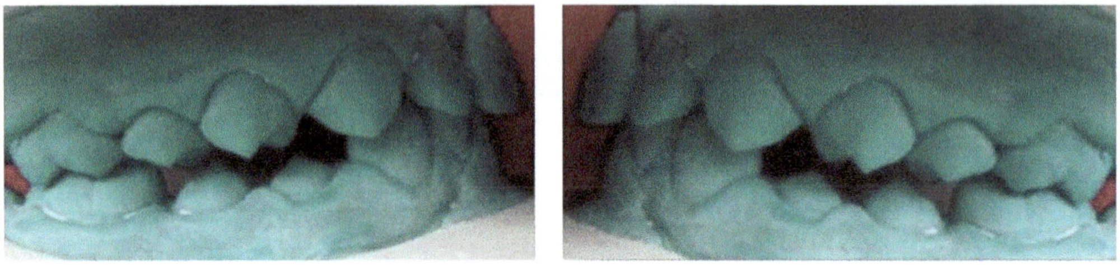

(a) (b)

FIGURE 4: (a) Postoperative molar relation on the right side of the study model. (b) Postoperative molar relation on the left side of the study model.

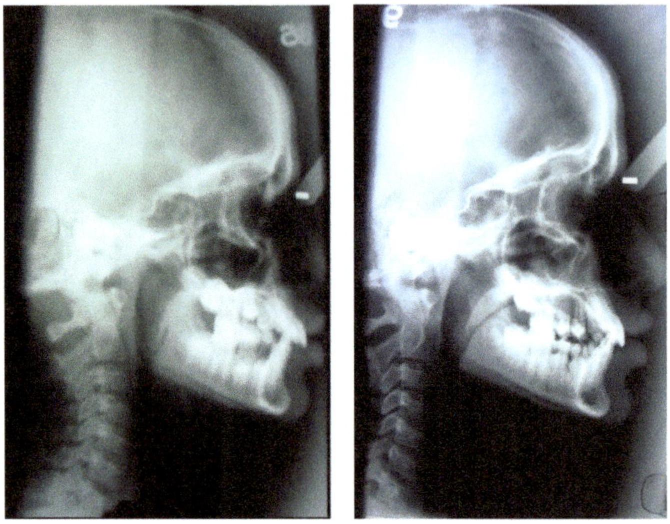

(a) (b)

FIGURE 5: (a) Preoperative lateral cephalogram. (b) Postoperative lateral cephalogram.

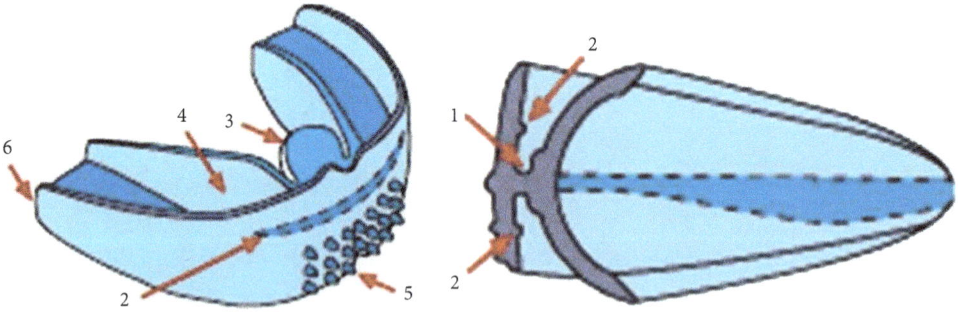

(a) (b)

FIGURE 6: *Tooth guidance*: molded into the anterior section (similar to orthodontic archwire). 1—tooth channels. 2—labial bows (impart a light force on misaligned anterior teeth). *Myofunctional training*: 3—tongue tag (for the proprioceptive positioning of the tongue tip as in myofunctional and speech therapies). 4—tongue guard (stops tongue thrusting when being in place and forces child to breathe through the nose). 5—Lip bumpers (discourage overactive mentalis muscle activity). *Jaw positioning*: 6—edge-to-edge class I jaw position (is produced when in place (same as most functional appliances). Combined with prevention of tongue thrusting and forcing the child to nose breathe is how the class II corrections are achieved in the cases shown (a big assistance to the orthodontist in future treatment)).

treatment which clinically got improved. This was a skeletal change and was confirmed with the McNamara analysis in which increase in the ANS-Me distance was observed (Figure 5(b)). This suggests that there was increase in the lower facial height. This result was mainly due to increase in maxillary arch dimensions which in turn caused mandibular growth. The mandible is relocated anteriorly and inferiorly by the remodeling at the condyle which clinically manifests as increase in the lower facial height and reduction in deep bite [13]. It can be inferred that skeletal changes can be a possibility in the late mixed dentition which was doubtful as mentioned in the earlier part of the discussion.

This paper only reports one patient. Controlled studies with an optimum sample have to be performed to confirm the actions of the T4K on various types of malocclusions. It is difficult to determine the reasons of the quick treatment success because the treatment is given in periods of accelerated growth [20]. But it can be inferred that the growth of the jaws as well as the position of the teeth can be guided to more favorable positions with the use of this appliance and the operator can be more certain of the results instead of waiting for the growth of the jaws to take place which may or may not take place.

8. Conclusion

It can be concluded that preorthodontic trainer permits treating several problems that are participating in the malocclusions development and thus permits treating the problem at different points. Case selection must be done with utmost care. The key to success of this appliance is *daily use* and there is no other substitute for the better results of this appliance.

References

[1] C. Nelson, M. Harkness, and P. Herbison, "Mandibular changes during functional appliance treatment," *American Journal of Orthodontics and Dentofacial Orthopedics*, vol. 104, no. 2, pp. 153–161, 1993.

[2] J. F. Tulloch, C. Phillips, G. Koch, and W. R. Proffit, "The effect of early intervention on skeletal pattern in Class II malocclusion: a randomized clinical trial," *American Journal of Orthodontics and Dentofacial Orthopedics*, vol. 111, no. 4, pp. 391–400, 1997.

[3] J. F. Tulloch, W. R. Proffit, and C. Phillips, "Influences on the outcome of early treatment for Class II malocclusion," *American Journal of Orthodontics and Dentofacial Orthopedics*, vol. 111, no. 5, pp. 533–542, 1997.

[4] L. R. Toth and J. A. McNamara Jr., "Treatment effects produced by the twin-block appliance and the FR-2 appliance of Fränkel compared with an untreated Class II sample," *American Journal of Orthodontics and Dentofacial Orthopedics*, vol. 116, no. 6, pp. 597–609, 1999.

[5] V. Pangrazio Kulbersh, J. L. Berger, D. S. Chermark, R. Kaczynski, E. S. Simon, and A. Haerian, "Treatment effects of themandibular anterior repositioning appliance on patients with Class II malocclusion," *American Journal of Orthodontics and Dentofacial Orthopedics*, vol. 123, pp. 286–295, 2003.

[6] G. S. Antonarakis and S. Kiliaridis, "Short-term anteroposterior treatment effects of functional appliances and extraoral traction on class II malocclusion: a meta-analysis," *Angle Orthodontist*, vol. 77, no. 5, pp. 907–914, 2007.

[7] P. Cozza, T. Baccetti, L. Franchi, L. de Toffol, and J. A. McNamara Jr., "Mandibular changes produced by functional appliances in Class II malocclusion:a systematic review," *American Journal of Orthodontics and Dentofacial Orthopedics*, vol. 129, pp. 118–122, 2006.

[8] S. Hiyama, T. Ono, Y. Ishiwata, T. Kuroda, and J. A. McNamara Jr., "Neuromuscular and skeletal adaptations following mandibular forward positioning induced by the herbst appliance," *Angle Orthodontist*, vol. 70, no. 6, pp. 442–453, 2000.

[9] X. Du and U. Hägg, "Muscular adaptation to gradual advancement of the mandible," *Angle Orthodontist*, vol. 73, no. 5, pp. 525–531, 2003.

[10] G. O. Ramirez-Yañez and C. Farrel, "Soft tissue dysfunction: a missing clue treating malocclusions," *Revista Internacional de Ortopedia Funcional*, vol. 1, no. 5/6, pp. 483–494, 2005.

[11] D. Mahony, "Combining functional appliances in the straight-wire system," *The Journal of Clinical Pediatric Dentistry*, vol. 26, no. 2, pp. 137–140, 2002.

[12] G. O. Ramirez-Yañez, "In to Orthodontic Treatment," Dental Asia, July-August 2006.

[13] C. Quadrelli, M. Gheorgiu, C. Marcheti, and V. Ghiglione, "Early myofunctional approach to skeletal Class II.," *Mondo Ortodontico*, vol. 2, pp. 109–122, 2002.

[14] A. C. Lima, A. L. Lima, R. M. A. L. Filho, and O. J. Oyen, "Spontaneous mandibular arch response after rapid palatal expansion: a long-term study on Class I malocclusion," *American Journal of Orthodontics and Dentofacial Orthopedics*, vol. 126, no. 5, pp. 576–582, 2004.

[15] J. A. McNamara Jr., T. Baccetti, L. Franchi, and T. A. Herberger, "Rapid maxillary expansion followed by fixed appliances: a long-term evaluation of changes in arch dimensions," *Angle Orthodontist*, vol. 73, no. 4, pp. 344–353, 2003.

[16] Z. Sari, T. Uysal, S. Usumez, and F. A. Basciftci, "Rapid maxillary expansion. Is it better in the mixed or in the permanent dentition?" *Angle Orthodontist*, vol. 73, no. 6, pp. 654–661, 2003.

[17] C.-H. Chung and B. Font, "Skeletal and dental changes in the sagittal, vertical, and transverse dimensions after rapid palatal expansion," *American Journal of Orthodontics and Dentofacial Orthopedics*, vol. 126, no. 5, pp. 569–575, 2004.

[18] S. Usumez, T. Uysal, Z. Sari, F. A. Basciftci, A. I. Karaman, and E. Guray, "The effects of early preorthodontic trainer treatment on class II, division 1 patients," *Angle Orthodontist*, vol. 74, no. 5, pp. 605–609, 2004.

[19] G. O. Ramirez-Yañez, A. Sidlauskas, E. Junior, and J. Fluter, "Dimensional changes in dental arches after treatment with a prefabricated functional appliance," *Journal of Clinical Pediatric Dentistry*, vol. 31, no. 4, pp. 279–283, 2007.

[20] G. O. Ramirez-Yañez and P. Faria, "Early treatment of a class II, division 2 malocclusion with the trainer for kids (T4K): a case report," *Journal of Clinical Pediatric Dentistry*, vol. 32, no. 4, pp. 325–329, 2008.

5

Intraoral Adult Rhabdomyoma: A Case Report

Ana Amelia Souza,[1] Vera Cavalcanti de Araújo,[1] Fabricio Passador Santos,[1] Elizabeth Ferreira Martinez,[1] Jose Ferreira de Menezes Filho,[2] Ney Soares de Araujo,[1] and Andresa Borges Soares[1]

[1] *Department of Oral Pathology, São Leopoldo Mandic Institute and Research Center, Rua José Rocha Junqueira 13 Ponte Preta, 13045-755 Campinas, SP, Brazil*
[2] *Instituto Tocatinense Presidente Antonio Carlos-Araguaína, Avenida Filadélfia 568, 77816-540 Araguaína, TO, Brazil*

Correspondence should be addressed to Andresa Borges Soares; andresabs@hotmail.com

Academic Editors: A. I. Abdalla and M. Dündar

A case of adult rhabdomyoma is reported. The lesion is a rare benign tumor of skeletal muscle origin which occurs predominantly in the head and neck region. In the present case, the clinical diagnosis favored a benign salivary gland tumor. Histologically, the tumor was composed of large round, oval, and polygonal cells of varying size with abundant pale, eosinophilic, fine, granular cytoplasm with peripherally located nuclei. Immunohistochemically, the lesion was positive for muscle-specific actin, smooth muscle actin, desmin, S100 protein, and Masson's trichrome. Electron microscopic examination confirmed the presence of numerous myofibrils. The lesion was treated by surgical resection. The clinical, histological, immunohistochemical, and ultrastructural features are discussed in this study.

1. Introduction

Rhabdomyomas are rare benign tumors derived from striated muscle, and can be classified generally into two types: cardiac type and extracardiac type. Cardiac rhabdomyoma occurs almost exclusively in the pediatric age group and may be associated with tuberous sclerosis, neurofibromatosis, and sebaceous adenomas. Current opinion is that the cardiac type represents a hamartomatous growth [1].

Extracardiac rhabdomyoma can be divided into three groups (adult, fetal, and genital types) with regards to clinical and morphological differences. The adult type is characterized by a slowly growing mass typically seen in the head and neck of elderly patients. In the fetal type, the lesion also typically involves the head and neck region and tends to occur at younger ages. The genital type is almost always found in the vulvovaginal region of middle-aged women [2]. The fetal and vaginal types are morphologically similar [3]. Seventy-seven percent of all extracardiac rhabdomyomas occur in the head and neck and 14% in the genital region [4].

The adult rhabdomyoma is the most common form of extracardiac rhabdomyoma. The tumor arises mainly within the head and neck region where it is believed to originate from the skeletal musculature of the third and fourth branchial arches. It is so called because of the histological resemblance to mature skeletal muscle cells [5]. These tumors are usually solitary; however, several authors have reported cases of adult multifocal extracardiac rhabdomyomas [6, 7]. In this paper we report a rare case of an adult rhabdomyoma originating in the floor of the mouth.

2. Case Report

The patient, a 40-year-old white woman, came to dentistry complaining of a painless swelling in the left floor of mouth that had been present for 6 months. The patient's medical history and extraoral examination did not show significant alteration.

Intraoral examination revealed a soft, painless, nontender mass in the left floor of the mouth, with extension posteriorly into the supraglotic region (Figure 1(a)). A computerized tomography examination confirmed the existence of hyperdense lesion. The lesion appeared as a single homogenous

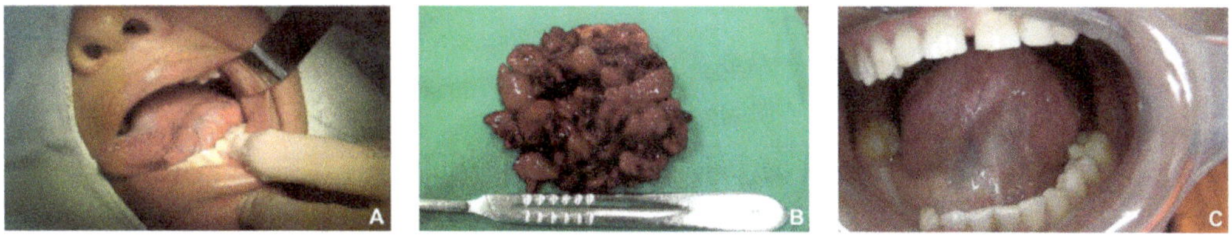

(a) (b) (c)

FIGURE 1: Clinical appearance of the lesion. Extensive soft tissue mass in the left floor of the mouth (a). Gross specimen revealed lobules of tumor tissue (b). Clinical aspect after surgery (c).

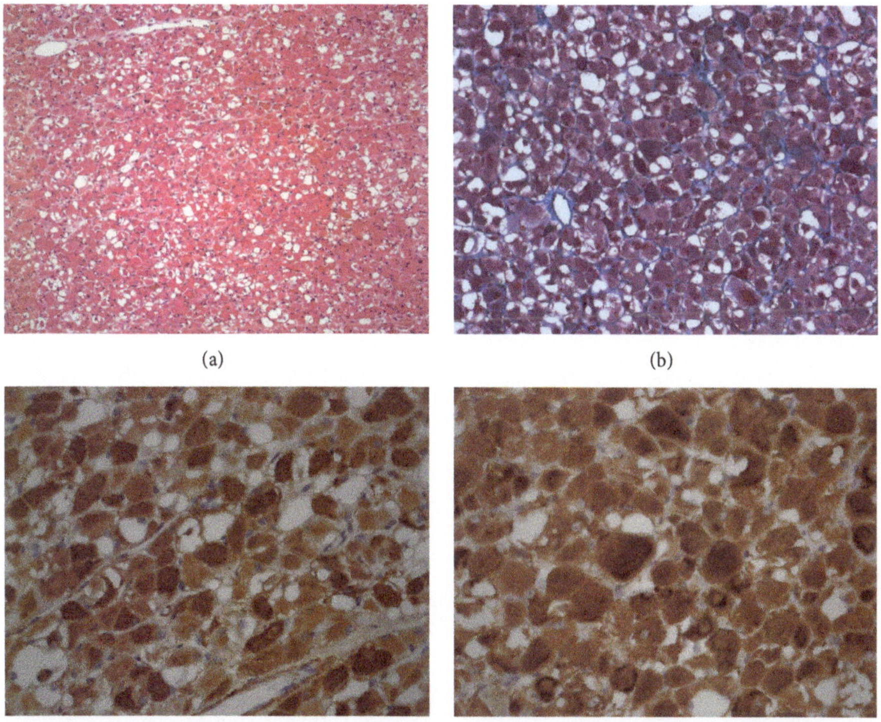

(a) (b) (c) (d)

FIGURE 2: Histopathology and immunohistochemistry of the lesion. Microscopic examination showing large polygonal cells with eosinophilic and vacuolated cytoplasm (hematoxylin and eosin stain; original magnification: 20x) (a), Masson's trichrome staining demonstrating red round, oval, and polygonal cells (original magnification 20x) (b), immunohistochemical stain showing strong positivity against muscle-specific actin (c), and desmin antigens (d) (original magnification, 40x).

mass in the lower middle portion in the floor of the mouth. The clinical diagnosis was a benign salivary gland tumor and an incisional biopsy was performed.

The specimen was fixed with 10% formalin, and paraffin sections were prepared for light microscopy using routine procedures. The initial sections were stained with hematoxylin and eosin (H&E). Microscopic examination revealed a tumor composed of large round, oval, and polygonal cells of varying sizes with abundant, pale, eosinophilic, fine, granular cytoplasm with peripherally located nuclei. Many tumor cells were vacuolated, with the extent of vacuolization varying from one cell to another. In most cells the vacuoles were located in the periphery, and in a few cells the extensive cytoplasmic vacuolization resulted in a spider web appearance. Mitoses and necrosis were absent. Masson's trichrome staining demonstrated red round, oval, and polygonal cells (Figures 2(a) and 2(b)).

Immunohistochemistry demonstrated tumor cells with strong reactivity to antibodies directed against muscle-specific actin (clone HHF35, Dako Cytomation) and desmin (clone D33, Dako Cytomation) as well as focal reactivity for smooth muscle actin (clone 1A4, Dako Cytomation) (Figures 2(c) and 2(d)).

The ultrastructural morphological examination revealed numerous myofibrils displayed in a longitudinal and transversal pattern. In addition, some glycogen inclusions and mitochondria were identified (Figures 3(a) and 3(b)).

Based on these features, a final diagnosis adult rhabdomyoma was rendered and the treatment of choice was local excision.

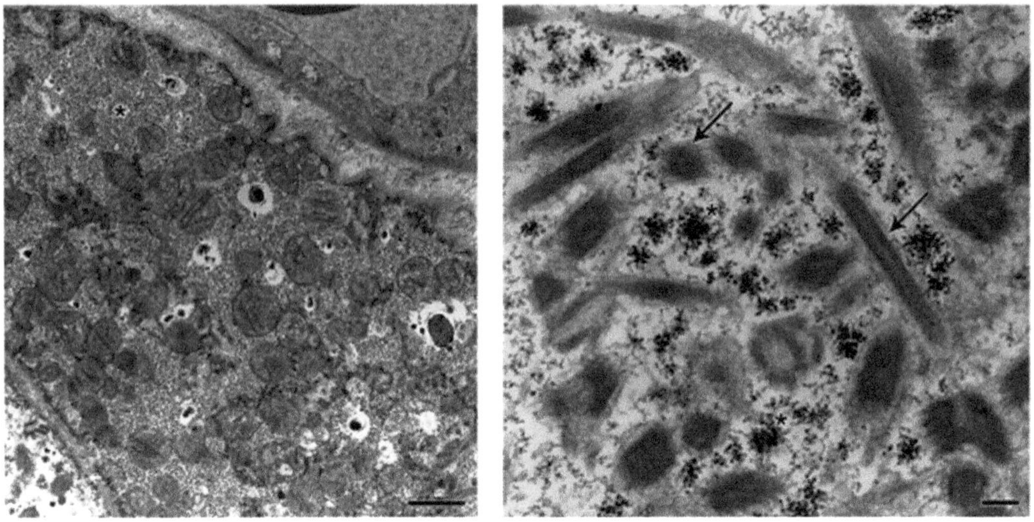

(a) (b)

FIGURE 3: Transmission electron micrograph of rhabdomyoma. Numerous mitochondria and glycogen inclusions (asterisk) are seen (a) among the myofibrils (arrows) (b). Bars: A = 2,5 μm; B = 1 μm.

The tumor was successfully removed en bloc under general anesthesia (Figure 1(b)). Surgical margins were tumor-free. No signs of local recurrence were observed two years after the surgical procedure (Figure 1(c)).

3. Discussion

The case reported fulfills the clinical, histological, immunohistochemical, and ultrastructural criteria for the diagnoses of adult rhabdomyoma, which is a rare benign tumor. The term rhabdomyoma was introduced by Zenker in 1864 [2, 5, 8–10].

In the present case, the lesion was presented in a 40 year-old woman, located in the floor of the mouth. The neoplasm has a predilection for the head and neck. The most commonly affected site is the neck and other sites include the oral cavity (base of the tongue and floor of mouth), pharynx, and larynx [6, 10]. A review of the literature suggests that these tumors are most frequently found in muscles derived from the pharyngeal arches [11].

The mean age of adult rhabdomyomas is 50 years (reported age range from 2 to 80 years); it occurs more commonly in males than females (ratio 4 : 1), and there is no predilection for any particular race [12].

The lesion usually presents as a smooth, movable, solitary (but occasionally multifocal), asymptomatic, round, or polypoid nodule in the head and neck region, or as a circumscribed intramuscular mass in the tongue, the sublingual region, lips, cheek, orbit, or submandibular region that is neither tender nor painful [13]. However, it may compress or displace the tongue or may protrude and partially obstruct the pharynx or larynx. As a consequence, it may cause hoarseness or progressive difficulty in breathing or swallowing. Multifocal rhabdomyomas may occur simultaneously, or the lesions may develop several years apart. Rhabdomyomas are slowly growing, and the lesions vary in size from a few millimeters to 15 cm [5, 14]. In our case, the patient presented with a painless solitary nodule; however, the nodule did make swallowing difficult for her.

Tissue specimens from the current case showed histological features typical to adult rhabdomyoma. Histologically, the adult rhabdomyoma type is characterized by a sheet-like proliferation of tightly packed, large polygonal to round cells with abundant, deeply eosinophilic, granular cytoplasm with one or two peripherally placed vesicular nuclei; prominent nucleoli may occasionally be identified. Many cells show cytoplasmic vacuolization due to intracytoplasmic glycogen accumulation. Some cells have a small central acidophilic cytoplasmic mass connected by thin strands of cytoplasm to a condensed rim of cytoplasm at the periphery. These so-called "spider-cells" are more prevalent in cardiac rhabdomyomas than in extracardiac rhabdomyomas. Cross-striations are usually readily identifiable. Mitoses and necrosis are absent [1, 6, 15]. PAS staining with diastase digestion reveals large numbers of tumor cells rich in glycogen particles. This likely reflects the degree of maturation of the tumor cells because fetal rhabdomyomas are composed predominantly of immature skeletal muscle cells with little or no glycogen [5].

The results of our immunohistochemical studies are in agreement with previously published data that show positive immunoreactivity against desmin and muscle-specific actin. These findings are consistent with the known staining properties of muscle cells but are not specific for neoplasia. Desmin is present in muscle cells of all types but has a greater staining reliability for skeletal muscle. HHF35 is a specific and sensitive marker for tumors of muscle origin [16]. The adult rhabdomyoma showed variable immunoreactivity for vimentin, S100, and smooth muscle actin [4, 6].

Transmission electron microscope examination revealed features of rhabdomyoma. Thick and thin myofilaments were found in varying proportions, as well as degrees of organization disposable among numerous mitochondria, as well as glycogen inclusions. Although immunocytochemistry may provide evidence to support the pathologist's impression in many cases; electron microscopy is especially important in undifferentiated tumors when immunocytochemistry is noncontributory or when there is aberrant, confusing immunoreactivity with several different, unrelated antibodies [6, 17–22].

The main consideration of the histological differential diagnosis of this tumor includes lesions consisting of cells having abundant eosinophilic cytoplasm. One such entity is the granular cell tumor; both granular cell tumor and rhabdomyoma can form syncytial cell clusters with abundant eosinophilic cytoplasm. Immunohistochemistry can also be helpful in distinguishing the two lesions. Granular cell tumors show diffuse S-100 positivity and desmin negativity. Other entities that should be considered are salivary gland tumors, namely, acinic cell carcinoma or oncocytoma [2, 23]. Malignant tumors showing rhabdoid differentiation such as rhabdomyosarcoma and malignant rhabdoid tumor may also be included. Generally, the nuclear atypia and pleomorphism present allow for separation of these malignant tumors from rhabdomyoma [13].

The treatment of choice for rhabdomyoma is surgical excision. Recurrence occurred in 16% of cases reported in the literature, but most were caused by incomplete removal. Recurrence may develop after many years because the tumor grows extremely slowly. There is also the possibility that a recurrence actually represents a new lesion. Malignant transformation or locally aggressive behavior has yet to be reported with any of these lesions. Patients after resection require regular follow-up visits [5, 23–25].

Conflict of Interests

The authors declare that there is no conflict of interests regarding the publication of this paper.

Acknowledgments

The authors wish to thank Jeruza Pinheiro da Silveira Bossonaro and Nadir Freitas for their excellent technical expertise and assistance.

References

[1] C. O. Reid and C. J. Smith, "Rhabdomyoma of the floor of the mouth: a new case and review of recently reported intraoral rhabdomyomas," *British Journal of Oral and Maxillofacial Surgery*, vol. 23, no. 4, pp. 284–291, 1985.

[2] D. Etit, U. Bayol, S. Cumurcu, I. Erdogan, and A. Tan, "Cytology of a giant adult-type rhabdomyoma of the tongue," *Diagnostic Cytopathology*, vol. 39, no. 9, pp. 686–688, 2011.

[3] H. Kawaba, J. Kawada, K. Iwahara, S. Kawai, S. Ikeda, and H. Ogawa, "Multiple cutaneous rhabdomyomas in a child," *European Journal of Dermatology*, vol. 14, no. 6, pp. 418–420, 2004.

[4] S. S. Napier, C. G. Pagni, and J. G. McGimpsey, "Sublingual adult rhabdomyoma. Report of a case," *International Journal of Oral and Maxillofacial Surgery*, vol. 20, no. 4, pp. 201–203, 1991.

[5] N. Zachariades, C. Skoura, A. Sourmelis, and G. Liapi-Avgeri, "Recurrent twin adult rhabdomyoma of the cheek," *Journal of Oral and Maxillofacial Surgery*, vol. 52, no. 12, pp. 1324–1328, 1994.

[6] B. Wenig, "Neoplasms of the oral cavity, nasopharynx, oropharynx, and neck," in *Atlas of Head and Neck Pathology*, B. Wenig, Ed., pp. 254–389, Elsevier, London, UK, 2nd edition, 2007.

[7] R. L. Corio and D. M. Lewis, "Intraoral rhabdomyomas," *Oral Surgery Oral Medicine and Oral Pathology*, vol. 48, no. 6, pp. 525–531, 1979.

[8] J. K. Jones and D. W. Buntine, "Benign rhabdomyoma of the submandibular region," *Journal of Otolaryngology*, vol. 6, no. 3, pp. 215–218, 1977.

[9] S. Weitzner, M. W. Lockey, and V. G. Lockard, "Adult rhabdomomyoma of soft palate," *Oral Surgery Oral Medicine and Oral Pathology*, vol. 47, no. 1, pp. 70–73, 1979.

[10] J. G. Batsakis and J. T. Manning, "Soft tissue tumors: unusual forms," *Otolaryngologic Clinics of North America*, vol. 19, no. 4, pp. 659–683, 1986.

[11] D. K. McGregor, B. Krishnan, and L. Green, "Fine-needle aspiration of adult rhabdomyoma: a case report with review of the literature," *Diagnostic Cytopathology*, vol. 28, no. 2, pp. 92–95, 2003.

[12] D. B. Cleveland, S.-Y. Chen, C. M. Allen, S. I. Ahing, and J. A. Svirsky, "Adult rhabdomyoma. A light microscopic, ultrastructural, virologic, and immunologic analysis," *Oral Surgery, Oral Medicine, Oral Pathology*, vol. 77, no. 2, pp. 147–153, 1994.

[13] G. Favia, L. Lo Muzio, R. Serpico, and E. Maiorano, "Rhabdomyoma of the head and neck: clinicopathologic features of two cases," *Head and Neck*, vol. 25, no. 8, pp. 700–704, 2003.

[14] Y. Fukuda, H.-O. Okamura, T. Nemoto, and S. Kishimoto, "Rhabdomyoma of the base of the tongue," *Journal of Laryngology and Otology*, vol. 117, no. 6, pp. 503–507, 2003.

[15] T. Thomas Zacharia and P. M. Som, "Multiple adult rhabdomyomas of the oropharynx, base of the tongue, and floor of the mouth: magnetic resonance findings," *Archives of Otolaryngology*, vol. 134, no. 8, pp. 892–894, 2008.

[16] J. De Medts, C. Dick, J. Casselman, and I. Van Den Berghe, "Intraoral multifocal adult rhabdomyoma: a case report," *B-ENT*, vol. 3, no. 4, pp. 205–208, 2007.

[17] A. Delides, N. Petrides, and K. Banis, "Multifocal adult rhabdomyoma of the head and neck: a case report and literature review," *European Archives of Oto-Rhino-Laryngology*, vol. 262, no. 6, pp. 504–506, 2005.

[18] J. S. Sidhu, M. M. Nicolas, and W. Taylor, "Mediastinal rhabdomyoma: a case report and review of the literature," *International Journal of Surgical Pathology*, vol. 10, no. 4, pp. 313–318, 2002.

[19] B. W. Neville, D. D. Damm, C. M. Allen, and J. E. Bouquout, "Soft tissue tumors," in *Oral and Maxillofacial Pathology*, pp. 552–554, Elsevier, Philadelphia, Pa, USA, 3nd edition, 2009.

[20] G. W. Mierau, "Electron microscopy for tumour diagnosis: is it redundant?" *Histopathology*, vol. 35, no. 2, pp. 99–108, 1999.

[21] G. W. Mierau, P. J. Berry, R. L. Malott, and D. A. Weeks, "Appraisal of the comparative utility of immunohistochemistry and electron microscopy in the diagnosis of childhood round cell tumors," *Ultrastructural Pathology*, vol. 20, no. 6, pp. 507–517, 1996.

[22] E. A. Konrad and G. Hubner, "Rhabdomyoma of the eyebrow region: a light- and electron microscopic study of a recurrent rhabdomyoma of fetal type," *Graefe's Archive for Clinical and Experimental Ophthalmology*, vol. 220, no. 4, pp. 187–192, 1983.

[23] E. Parara, P. Christopoulos, K. Tosios, I. Paravalou, C. Vourlakou, and K. Alexandridis, "A swelling of the floor of the mouth," *Oral Surgery, Oral Medicine, Oral Pathology, Oral Radiology and Endodontology*, vol. 109, no. 1, pp. 12–16, 2010.

[24] G. Z. Zhang, G. Q. Zhang, J. M. Xiu, and X. M. Wang, "Intraoral multifocal and multinodular adult rhabdomyoma: report of a case," *Journal of Oral and Maxillofacial Surgery*, vol. 70, no. 10, pp. 2480–2485, 2012.

[25] X. Huang, X. Yang, Z. Wang et al., "Adult rhabdomyoma of the tongue in a child," *Pathology*, vol. 44, no. 1, pp. 51–53, 2012.

6

Autotransplantation of Mandibular Third Molar: A Case Report

Pabbati Ravi kumar, Mandava Jyothi, Kantheti Sirisha, Khushboo Racca, and Chalasani Uma

Department of Conservative Dentistry and Endodontics, GITAM Dental College and Hospital, Visakhapatnam 530045, Andhra Pradesh, India

Correspondence should be addressed to Pabbati Ravi kumar, drpabbati@yahoo.co.in

Academic Editors: C. Farah and M. J. Wahl

Autogenous transplantation is a feasible, fast, and economical option for the treatment of nonsalvageable teeth when a suitable donor tooth is available. This paper presents successful autotransplantation of a mature mandibular left third molar (38) without anatomical variances is used to replace a mandibular left second molar (37). The mandibular second molar was nonrestorable due to extensive root caries and resorption of distal root. After extraction of mandibular second and third molars, root canal therapy was done for the third molar extraorally, and the tooth was reimplanted into the extracted socket of second molar site. After one year, clinical and radiographic examination revealed satisfactory outcome with no signs or symptoms suggestive of pathology. In selected cases, autogenous tooth transplantation, even after complete root formation of the donor tooth, may be considered as a practical treatment alternative to conventional prosthetic rehabilitation or implant treatment.

1. Introduction

The earliest report of tooth transplantation involves slaves in ancient Egypt, who were forced to give their teeth to their pharaohs [1]. This type of dental surgical intervention was documented first by Abulcassis, in 1050; however, only in 1564, the French dentist Ambroise Paré performed the first recorded surgery with details about tooth bud transplantation. In 1956, a transplantation technique for molars was described, and until today, the general guidelines of this surgical technique are practically the same. Not withstanding, some techniques have been developed aiming to improve the prognosis, such as two-stage transplantation and prototyping [2].

Tooth transplantation can be classified into autogenous (where a tooth/tooth bud from one socket is inserted into another socket in the same person), homogenous (if the donation is performed by a person of the same specie of the receptor), and heterogeneous (if the donor is from a different specie of the receptor) [2]. Autogenous tooth transplantation or autotransplantation is the surgical transplantation of a vital or endodontically treated tooth from its original location in the mouth to another site in the same individual [1].

Tooth transplantation is a possible treatment option for the replacement of extracted permanent tooth that is malformed or involved with carious destruction or traumatic injury. Despite the widespread use of dental implants, autogenous tooth transplantation is frequently performed to replace missing mature teeth [3]. The main advantages of this procedure are alterations in the development of the maxilla and mandibular alveolar bone can be avoided, and it constitutes a viable method due to high success rate and relatively low cost compared to the traditional methods of rehabilitation such as osseointegrated implants [2]. Successful transplantation depends on specific requirements of the patient, the donor tooth, and the recipient site.

1.1. Case Selection Criteria. Candidates must be in good health, able to follow postoperative instructions and should be available for follow-up visits. They should also demonstrate an acceptable level of oral hygiene and be amenable

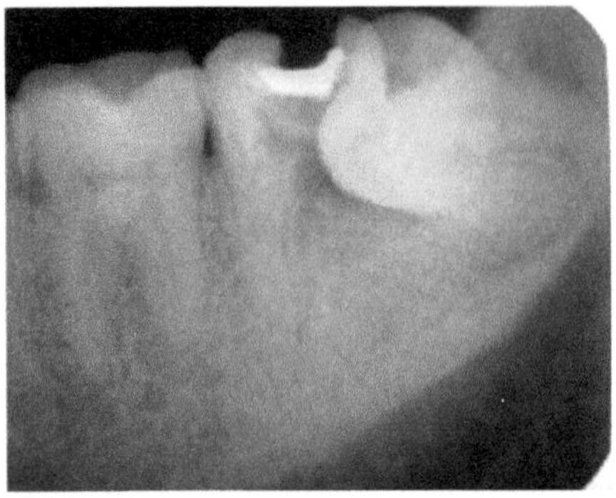

FIGURE 1: Preoperative radiograph showing 36, 37 and 38.

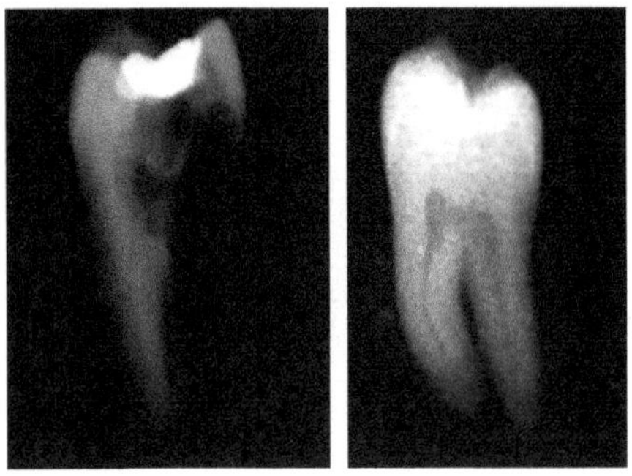

FIGURE 2: Extracted teeth 37, 38.

to regular dental care. Most importantly, the patients must have a suitable recipient site and donor tooth. Patient cooperation and comprehension are extremely important to ensure predictable results.

1.2. Recipient Site Criteria. The most important criteria for success involving the recipient site is adequacy of bone support. There must be sufficient alveolar bone support in all dimensions with adequate attached keratinized tissue to allow for stabilization of the transplanted tooth. In addition, the recipient site should be free from acute infection and chronic inflammation.

1.3. Donor Tooth Criteria. The donor tooth should be positioned such that extraction will be as atraumatic as possible. Abnormal root morphology, which makes the tooth removal difficult and may involve tooth sectioning, is contraindicated for this surgery. Teeth with either open or closed apices may be donors; however, the most predictable results are obtained with teeth showing one-half to two-thirds of root development. Surgical manipulation of teeth with less than one-half root formation may be too traumatic and could compromise further root development causing incomplete maturation or alteration in morphology. When root development is greater than two-thirds, the increased length may cause encroachment on vital structures such as the maxillary sinus or the inferior alveolar nerve. Furthermore, a tooth with complete or near complete root formation will generally require root canal therapy, while a tooth with an open apex will remain vital and should continue root development after transplantation. In the latter case, successful transplantation without the need for further endodontic therapy is usually seen [4].

The donor tooth chosen for autotransplantation should be of limited value in the dentition, for example, a third molar. This case report presents successful transplantation of a mandibular third molar with complete root formation.

2. Case Report

A 36-year-old male patient reported to the Department of Conservative Dentistry with a chief complaint of caries with 37 and food impaction in relation to 37 and 38. Clinical and radiographic examination (Figure 1) revealed caries on the distal aspect of 37 encroaching into the pulp space with resorbed distal root and a mesioangular impaction of 38. Involved second molar tooth (37) was nonrestorable and was indicated for extraction. Impacted third molar 38 was a sound, mature tooth without caries and was found to be ideal for transplantation. The mesiodistal dimensions of 37 and 38 were suitable for transplantation.

After taking the complete medical history and explaining the risks and benefits of the procedure to the patient, an informed consent was taken. Patient was prescribed 1000 mg Amoxycillin one hour before surgery to prevent infection and 400 mg of Ibuprofen was prescribed to prevent post-treatment pain. 37 and 38 were extracted atraumatically (Figure 2) without damaging the buccal and lingual cortical plates. Root canal therapy for 38 was completed extra-orally within 30 minutes using ProTaper NiTi rotary files. Care was taken to prevent any damage to periodontal ligament (PDL) cells by holding the tooth at cementoenamel junction, and the roots were kept moist with sterile gauze soaked in coconut water during access cavity preparation. During biomechanical preparation and obturation of the root canals, the roots were wrapped with sterile gauze and were submerged in coconut water in a sterile dappen dish. Access cavity was restored with high copper silver amalgam. Alveolar socket of 37 was widened using surgical bur in a slow speed hand piece, under copious saline irrigation and 38 was transplanted into 37 socket. Suturing was performed with silk thread to stabilize the soft tissues and the transplanted tooth. Nonrigid intraradicular occlusal splinting with malleable orthodontic wire and composite resin was done from 35 to 37 (Figure 3). Postoperative IOPA radiograph revealed radioopaque object in the interdental area of 36 and transplanted tooth. This could be a fragment of amalgam restoration of 37 that may got impregnated into the tissues during intraradicular groove preparation for splinting. The patient was instructed to perform daily mouth rinsing with 0.12% Chlorhexidine gluconate, twice a day for seven days, Amoxicillin 500 mg thrice daily, Metronidazole 400 mg thrice a day, and Etrobax 120 mg twice daily for 5 days were prescribed.

Sutures were removed after a week and healing appeared satisfactory. The patient was reviewed after 1 week, 1 month, 2 months, 6 months, and 1 year. Non rigid splinting was

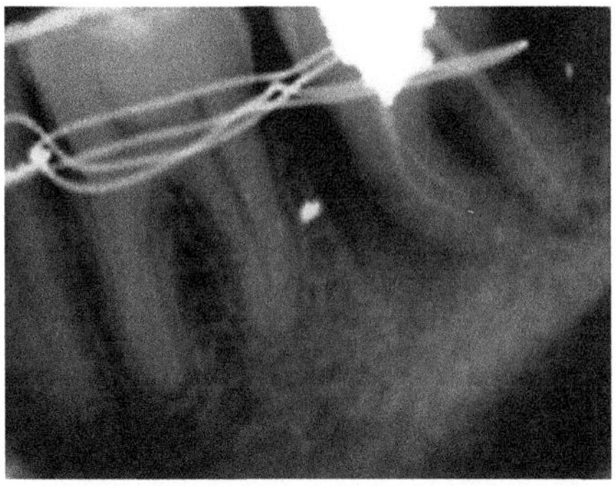

FIGURE 3: After transplantation and splinting.

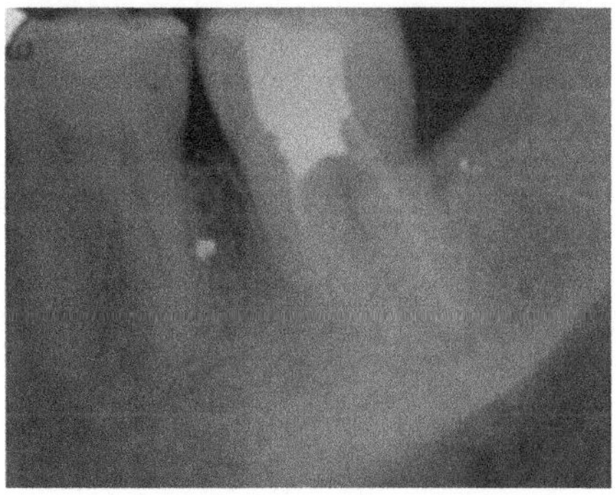

FIGURE 4: 1-year recall radiograph.

removed after 2 months. Patient was asymptomatic during recall visits. Clinical examination demonstrated absence of mobility and masticatory dysfunction.The occlusion was found to be normal. There were no signs of loss of attachment. Percussion test did not produce the characteristic metallic sound of ankylosis. At the 1-year followup, radiographic examination revealed healing of the site (Figure 4). There were no signs suggestive of root resorption or other pathological processes and revealed normal periodontal attachment. At the end of 1 year, bone growth around the transplanted tooth was considered satisfactory.

3. Discussion

Patient was insistent on maintaining the number of teeth in his arch as he is a diver by profession in navy. Other treatment option for this case was to extract 37 and 38 followed by the placement of an implant. But due to the expenses of implant therapy, and due to local limitations like the remaining bone support and close proximity to the anatomical structure, autotransplantation was selected as treatment option.

The success rate of autogenous tooth transplantation in the 1950s was approximately 50% because of the difficulty in predicting root development after transplantation and dental root resorption [5, 6]. Because too little was known of the causes and prevention of root resorption of transplanted autogenous teeth, the procedure was used infrequently. Since 1990, many studies have evaluated the healing of periodontal tissues and the incidence of dental root resorption after transplantation and the transplant success rate has increased rapidly, drawing new clinical interest [7–9]. Tsukiboshi [7] reported a 90% survival rate and an 82% success rate in 250 cases observed for 6 years. Lundberg and Isaksson [8] reported a success rate of 94% in cases with incompletely formed roots and 84% in cases with completely formed roots, whereas Mejàre et al. [9] reported a high success rate for cases with mature teeth.

Like other surgical procedures, careful case selection and treatment planning is essential for successful autotransplantation. The donor tooth and recipient site should be both examined meticulously for suitability and appropriate dimensions [4, 10]. The recipient site should have adequate bone support with sufficient attached keratinized tissue to allow tooth stabilization and be free of infection and/or inflammation [4].

Insufficient buccolingual width in the recipient site or excessive preparation of the site may result in resorption of the alveolar ridge, loss of buccal bone coverage, and consequent loss of periodontal integrity. An extensive study that evaluated autotransplantation of 53 molar teeth with developed roots reported that lack of buccal bone plate was the only significant predictor for transplant failure [9].

In the present case, occlusal reduction of the transplanted tooth was done to protect the tooth from any occlusal trauma and to allow proper healing of the periradicular tissues. As the bone support in the recipient site was poor, a physiological splint was kept in place for 2 months without having the risk of ankylosis.

Preservation of the periodontal ligament (PDL) cells is critical for the success of a tooth transplant [11–14]. Accordingly, teeth which have sharp root curvatures are not good candidates for transplantation because there is an increased risk of PDL damage and cemental tear during extraction [1, 10]. Extraction procedure was carried out with special care and to preserve periodontal ligament cells of third molar, the roots were wrapped with gauze soaked in coconut water.

The periodontal ligament cells are extremely sensitive, and their survival ability is significantly reduced if the extraoral dry time is prolonged [15]; this effect has been demonstrated to be significant after 18 minutes [12, 16]. The increased length of the extra-alveolar time increases the possibility of inflammatory replacement resorption, reduces the healing capability of the periodontal ligament cells which in turn induces unfavourable consequences such as inflammatory external root resorption. In the present case, inspite of keeping 30 minutes of extra alveolar time, there was no external root resorption that may be due to coconut water used for maintaining the viability of the cells. Coconut water is an excellent storage media for avulsed teeth, as it has a P^H and osmolality compatible to PDL cells [14].

After autotransplantation of permanent teeth with fully developed roots pulpal revascularization or revitalization is not expected [17, 18]. Previous studies have shown a high incidence of pulp necrosis in mature teeth. Therefore, root canal therapy or root resection with retrograde filling has been advised to prevent pulpal infection and/or inflammation and subsequent root resorption [19–21], Routinely, root canal therapy is performed a few weeks after transplantation [21]. However, Bae et al. recommend that if the donor tooth is easily accessed, root canal therapy should be performed before transplantation [15]. In this case, root canal therapy was done extraorally due to limited accessibility and presence of mesial root curvature of the donor tooth that may hamper the effective endodontic treatment.

Effective and successful transplantation requires approximation between shape and size of the donor tooth and the receptor site. It also has been postulated that maxillary transplants have greater risk of failure due to the wide variation in the size and shape of the teeth and the proximity of the maxillary antrum to the molar sockets [15]. However in this case, the tooth to be transplanted fitted the recipient site; thus, the procedure caused minimal trauma. In addition, the favorable cervical adaptation between the tooth and bone decreased the chance of infection and increased the likelihood of an uneventful healing and periodontal reattachment. The healing was satisfactory inspite of presence of amalgam fragment between 36 and the transplanted tooth.

It can be assumed that the physiologic mobility of the transplanted tooth stimulated the activation of periodontal ligament cells (i.e., fibroblasts, cementoblasts and osteoblasts) and bone repair [5]. The transplanted molar tooth in the present case had complete developed roots, that encouraged transplantation in these teeth. Both clinical, and radiographic outcomes were considered satisfactory after 1 year.

Complications of autogenous tooth transplant include root resorption and attachment loss, and its success rate is lower than implant prosthesis. Nonetheless, autogenous teeth transplantation results in good utilization, the maintenance and regeneration of alveolar bone, and the maintenance of attached gingiva with a natural shape.

4. Conclusions

There is obvious limitation in terms of versatility in the application of transplantation versus implantation in replacing missing teeth. The availability of suitable size and morphology of donor tooth are the major constraint. The success rate of implant is also higher than that of transplant. Reported survival rates of autotransplantation vary from 74–100%, artificially drilled recipient sockets tend to be at the lower range of success rate. With appropriate patient selection, and presence of a suitable donor tooth and recipient site, autogenous transplantation should be considered as a viable option for avoiding/prevention of an edentulous space.

References

[1] A. S. Cohen, T. C. Shen, and M. A. Pogrel, "Transplanting teeth successfully: autografts and allografts that work," *The Journal of the American Dental Association*, vol. 126, no. 4, pp. 481–500, 1995.

[2] P. P. Reich, "Autogenous Transplantation of Maxillary and Mandibular Molars," *Journal of Oral and Maxillofacial Surgery*, vol. 66, no. 11, pp. 2314–2317, 2008.

[3] S. Asgary and S. Ehsani, "Autotransplantation of a third molar with complete root development: a case report," *International Journal of Surgical Research*, vol. 1, no. 1, pp. 1–6, 2012.

[4] C. M. L. Clokie, D. M. Yau, and L. Chano, "Autogenous tooth transplantation: an alternative to dental implant placement?" *Journal of the Canadian Dental Association*, vol. 67, no. 2, pp. 92–96, 2001.

[5] H. Apfel, "Autoplasty of enucleated prefunctional third molars," *Journal of Oral Surgery, Anesthesia, and Hospital Dental Service*, vol. 8, no. 4, pp. 289–296, 1950.

[6] H. M. Miller, "Transplantation, a case report," *The Journal of the American Dental Association*, vol. 40, article 237, 1950.

[7] M. Tsukiboshi, "Autotransplantation of teeth: requirements for predictable success," *Dental Traumatology*, vol. 18, no. 4, pp. 157–180, 2002.

[8] T. Lundberg and S. Isaksson, "A clinical follow-up study of 278 autotransplanted teeth," *British Journal of Oral and Maxillofacial Surgery*, vol. 34, no. 2, pp. 181–185, 1996.

[9] B. Mejàre, K. Wannfors, and L. Jansson, "A prospective study on transplantation of third molars with complete root formation," *Oral Surgery, Oral Medicine, Oral Pathology, Oral Radiology, and Endodontics*, vol. 97, no. 2, pp. 231–238, 2004.

[10] C. S. Teixeira, B. Pasternak Jr., L. P. Vansan, and M. D. Sousa-Neto, "Autogenous transplantation of teeth with complete root formation: two case reports," *International Endodontic Journal*, vol. 39, no. 12, pp. 977–985, 2006.

[11] E. Kim, J. Y. Jung, I. H. Cha, K. Y. Kum, and S. J. Lee, "Evaluation of the prognosis and causes of failure in 182 cases of autogenous tooth transplantation," *Oral Surgery, Oral Medicine, Oral Pathology, Oral Radiology and Endodontology*, vol. 100, no. 1, pp. 112–119, 2005.

[12] J. O. Andreasen, "Periodontal healing after replantation and autotransplantation of incisors in monkeys," *International Journal of Oral Surgery*, vol. 10, no. 1, pp. 54–61, 1981.

[13] G. Nethander, "Periodontal conditions of teeth autogenously transplanted by a two-stage technique," *Journal of Periodontal Research*, vol. 29, no. 4, pp. 250–258, 1994.

[14] V. Gopikrishna, T. Thomas, and D. Kandaswamy, "A quantitative analysis of coconut water: a new storage media for avulsed teeth," *Oral Surgery, Oral Medicine, Oral Pathology, Oral Radiology and Endodontology*, vol. 105, no. 2, pp. e61–e65, 2008.

[15] J. H. Bae, Y. H. Choi, B. H. Cho, Y. K. Kim, and S. G. Kim, "Autotransplantation of teeth with complete root formation: a case series," *Journal of Endodontics*, vol. 36, no. 8, pp. 1422–1426, 2010.

[16] J. O. Andreasen, "Effect of extra-alveolar period and storage media upon periodontal and pulpal healing after replantation of mature permanent incisors in monkeys," *International Journal of Oral Surgery*, vol. 10, no. 1, pp. 43–53, 1981.

[17] A. Skoglund, "Pulpal changes in replanted and autotransplanted apicoectomized mature teeth of dogs," *International Journal of Oral Surgery*, vol. 10, no. 2, pp. 111–121, 1981.

[18] A. Skoglund, "Vascular changes in replanted and autotransplanted apicoectomized mature teeth of dogs," *International Journal of Oral Surgery*, vol. 10, no. 2, pp. 100–110, 1981.

[19] P. C. Azevedo, C. C. G. Moura, D. Zanetta-Barbosa, and N. Bernadineli, "Time of endodontic treatment in autogenic transplants of mature teeth: histological study in dogs," *Oral Surgery, Oral Medicine, Oral Pathology, Oral Radiology and Endodontology*, vol. 104, no. 2, pp. 287–293, 2007.

[20] R. A. Mendes and G. Rocha, "Mandibular third molar autotransplantation—literature review with clinical cases," *Journal*

of the Canadian Dental Association, vol. 70, no. 11, pp. 761–766, 2004.
[21] S. Asgary, "Autogenous transplantation of mandibular third molar to replace vertical root fractured tooth," *Iranian Endodontic Journal*, vol. 4, no. 3, pp. 118–122, 2009.

7

Role of Cone Beam Computed Tomography in Rehabilitation of a Traumatised Deficient Maxillary Alveolar Ridge Using Symphyseal Block Graft Placement

Shipra Arora, Arundeep Kaur Lamba, Farrukh Faraz, Shruti Tandon, and Abdul Ahad

Department of Periodontics and Oral Implantology, Maulana Azad Institute of Dental Sciences, New Delhi 110002, India

Correspondence should be addressed to Shipra Arora; dr.shipraarora09@gmail.com

Academic Editors: J. J. Segura-Egea and K. Seymour

Deficiencies in the alveolar ridges cause multiple problems in achieving aesthetic and functional outcome of implant therapy and are commonly restored by using onlay graft from intraoral source. Careful assessment of the recipient as well as the donor site using cone beam computed tomography (CBCT) is a prerequisite to ideal treatment planning. This paper highlights the critical role of CBCT in planning a successful rehabilitation of traumatised deficient anterior maxillary alveolar ridge using autogenous block graft from mandibular symphysis, followed by implant placement. A 21-year-old male reported with missing right maxillary lateral incisor due to traumatic avulsion 6 months back. A concavity was found on the labial aspect of edentulous area. Serial transplanar images on CBCT revealed gross irregular radiolucency in place of labial cortical plate. Using CBCT, size of the required block was estimated, and mandibular symphyseal area was evaluated for the feasibility of harvesting a graft of suitable dimension. Onlay block graft was harvested from mandibular symphysis and placed at the edentulous site to augment the alveolar ridge. Implants were placed 5 months later and loaded successfully after osseointegration. After 1 year of followup, implant-based prosthesis is working well, without any complications.

1. Introduction

Edentulous sites with insufficient bone volume present a challenge to many clinicians planning an implant based prosthetic rehabilitation. A successful implant therapy with restoration of aesthetics and functions requires sufficient alveolar bone, with acceptable maxillary-mandibular relationship.

In cases of tooth loss due to dentoalveolar fracture, generally, the quantity and quality of the existing ridge are grossly compromised. Thickness of the facial bone wall may directly influence the convexity of the tissues at the emerging implant crown. In anterior maxilla, detailed assessment of the existing bone is required to ensure the satisfactory outcome in terms of aesthetics as well as function. Intraoral periapical (IOPA) and panoramic radiographs often fail to reveal the true morphology of the ridge, particularly a defect in labial cortical plate. Cone beam computed tomography (CBCT) is now a preferred technique for 3-dimensional assessment of alveolar bone anatomy [1]. It offers axial, reformatted panoramic and serial transplanar images at the desired location. CBCT of the jaws helps in detecting the bone morphology at the edentulous site and appropriately planning the augmentation procedure, size of the block required, and feasibility of the donor site at symphysis of the mandible. The technique offers high image resolution of 0.123 mm in addition to improved image quality and much lower radiation exposure compared to conventional computed tomography (CT) [1].

The ideal solution for the problem of deficient alveolar ridge lies in the careful assessment and planning reestablishment of the lost bone volume for a favourable anatomy with suitable lamellar bone for implant stability and aesthetics.

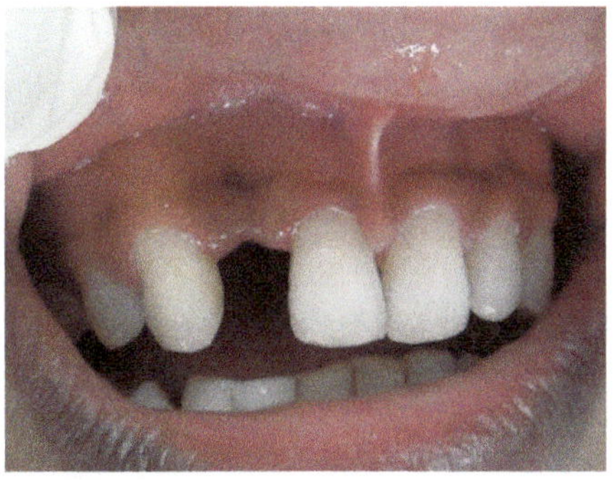

FIGURE 1: Preoperative view of the edentulous area showing concavity on the labial surface.

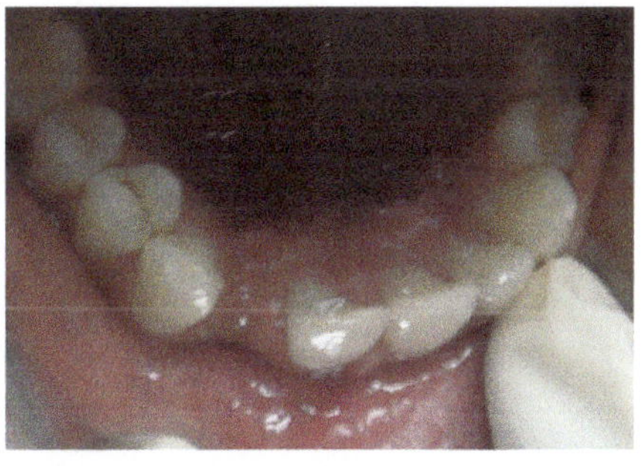

FIGURE 2: Preoperative occlusal view of the edentulous area.

Bone grafting materials and techniques that have been developed to cope with this challenge show promising outcomes. An ideal bone grafting material should be biocompatible, have no rejection response, pose no risk of disease transmission, provide a scaffold promoting bone regeneration, and afford initial mechanical stability maintained throughout the entire treatment time.

Autogenous bone grafting remains the most predictable and best documented method till date and is considered the gold standard for bone augmentation [2, 3]. The purported osteogenic potential of autogenous block grafts is one of the major considerations in promoting it as the gold standard. However, osteogenic potential may vary among patients, and it decreases with increasing age. The successful healing of block grafts, as with all grafts, depends primarily on the establishment of graft vascularisation. Osteogenesis cannot occur until the graft is vascularised [2].

Gains of 4-5 mm in width and height of alveolar ridge have been reported with autogenous onlay grafts with associated implant success rates [2, 4]. Although the various case reports document the successful placement of implants following ridge augmentation with onlay allografts, the effectiveness and predictability of these procedures for ridge augmentation remain unclear.

This paper reports a case of CBCT assisted diagnosis and treatment planning of severely deficient maxillary anterior edentulous site and successful augmentation using an onlay block graft from mandibular symphysis followed by prosthetic rehabilitation after implant placement.

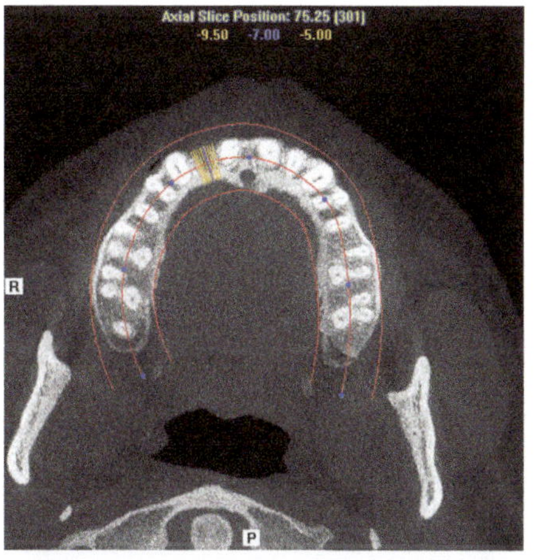

FIGURE 3: Preoperative axial section on CBCT. Decreased labio-palatal thickness of edentulous area may be noted.

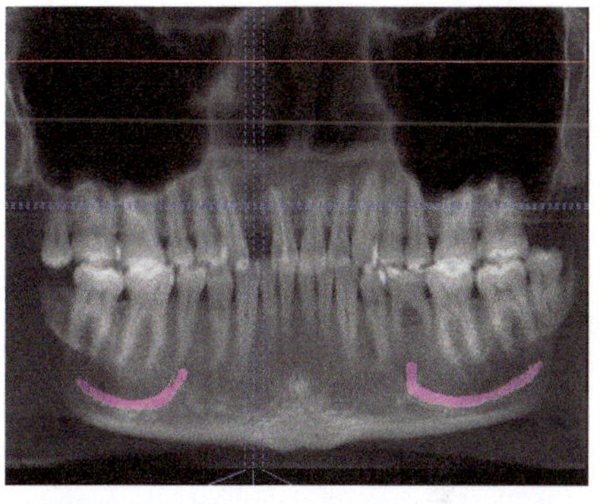

FIGURE 4: Preoperative CBCT with reformatted panoramic view. Gross radiolucency may be noted at the edentulous site.

2. Case Presentation

A 21-year-old male reported to the Maulana Azad Institute of Dental Sciences, New Delhi, India, with the chief complaint of missing upper front tooth for the last 6 months. Past history revealed that the tooth got avulsed due to contact sports 6 months back. However, patient reported no history of any fracture of the jaw bone. He was a nonsmoker, and there was no significant history of any chronic systemic disease. Intraoral examination showed that his oral hygiene was good. As per his chief complaint, tooth number 12 was missing. The tooth number 11 had a restoration on palatal surface. Due to the trauma, substantial hard and soft tissue loss had occurred, and an "hour glass" concavity could be noted on the labial surface of edentulous site (Figure 1). On ridge mapping the width of the bone at the centre of concavity was found to be only 3.7 mm which was insufficient for implant placement (Figure 2). To get a precise view, a CBCT of maxilla and mandible was obtained (Figures 3 and 4). On cross-sectional slice through middle of edentulous area, using a software (iCATVision—Imaging Sciences International), gross radiolucency was observed in place of labial cortical

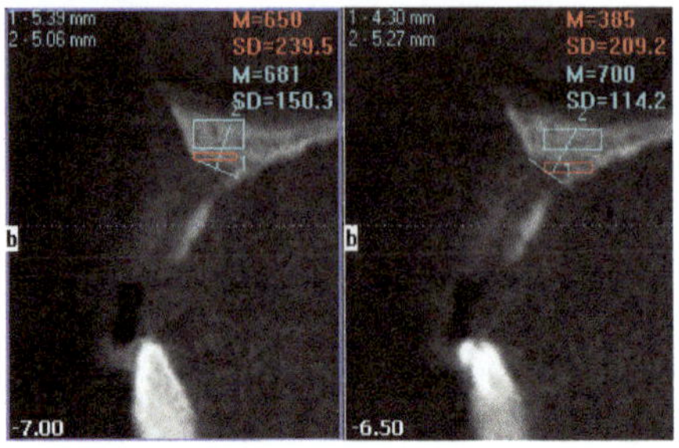

FIGURE 5: Transplanar images of of edentulous area on CBCT. Gross deficiency in dimensions of alveolar ridge is evident.

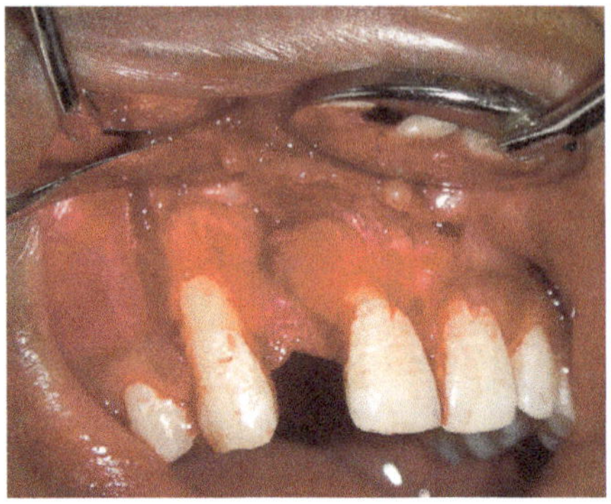

FIGURE 6: Defect at the edentulous site as viewed on surgical exposure.

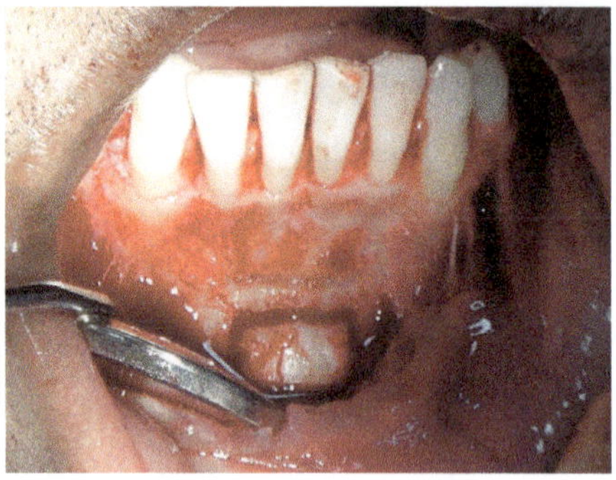

FIGURE 7: Outline of the block graft harvested from mandibular symphysis.

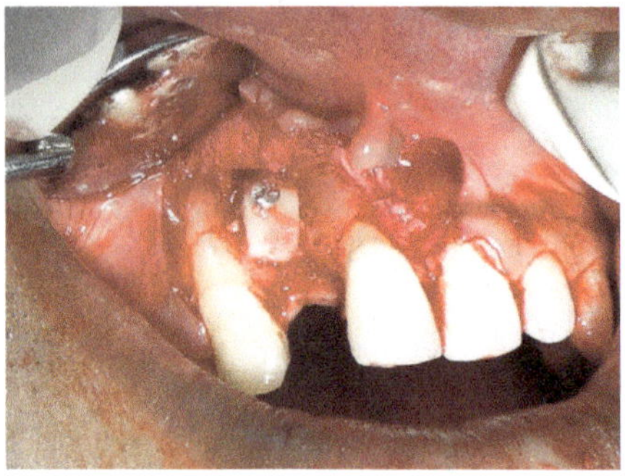

FIGURE 8: Block graft fixed at the recipient site.

plate (Figure 5). Amount of alveolar bone at the edentulous site was clearly insufficient for successful placement of an implant of appropriate dimension.

Transplanar images of mandibular symphysis were evaluated to assess the feasibility of harvesting the required block. Labiolingual thickness, length of roots of mandibular incisors, and position of incisive nerve were found to be favourable.

2.1. Management of the Case. A surgical procedure was planned under local anaesthesia, after obtaining a written informed consent from the patient. Since the labiopalatal dimension was insufficient for correct placement of implant, onlay block grafting was planned. Mandibular symphysis was chosen as the donor site.

2.1.1. Preparation of the Recipient Site. After administering infraorbital nerve block using Lignocaine 2% (with Adrenaline 1 : 80,000), midcrestal incision on the edentulous area and two releasing incisions were given to reflect the mucoperiosteal flap. On reflection of flap, concavity was observed on the labial aspect of edentulous ridge (Figure 6). Width of the ridge was found to be 3.6 mm, 3 mm apical to the alveolar crest.

2.1.2. Harvesting of Block Graft from Mandibular Symphysis. Bilateral mental nerve blocks (Lignocaine 2% with Adrenaline 1 : 80,000) were given, followed by sulcular incision on labial aspect of mandibular anterior teeth, extending from mesial of right first premolar to the left one. Two releasing incisions were given to reflect the mucoperiosteal flap. Flap was extended up to 2 cm apically from the alveolar crest. A 5 mm × 7 mm outline was marked at 12 mm apical to alveolar crest to avoid iatrogenic trauma to root apices of mandibular incisors (Figure 7). A piezo surgical unit (Italia Medica, Milano, Italy) was then used to harvest the bone block with a thickness of 4 mm. Osteotomy site was filled with Decalcified Freeze Dried Bone Allograft (DFDBA) of particle size 500–1000 μm (Tata Memorial Hospital Tissue Bank, Mumbai), and flap was sutured with 3-0 silk (Ethicon, Johnson & Johnson Ltd.)

2.1.3. Placement of Block Graft at the Recipient Site. The recipient site was perforated with a fissure bur to induce bleeding and promote revascularization of the graft. The harvested block was adapted to the recipient site and held in position with a self-tapping screw (Figure 8). Edges of the graft were smoothened to avoid trauma to overlying flap. A chorion membrane (Tata Memorial Hospital Tissue Bank, Mumbai) was used to cover the area after DFDBA was placed on the periphery of the block (Figure 9). Interrupted 3-0 silk sutures were placed to close the site. Analgesics were prescribed, and postoperative instructions were given to patient.

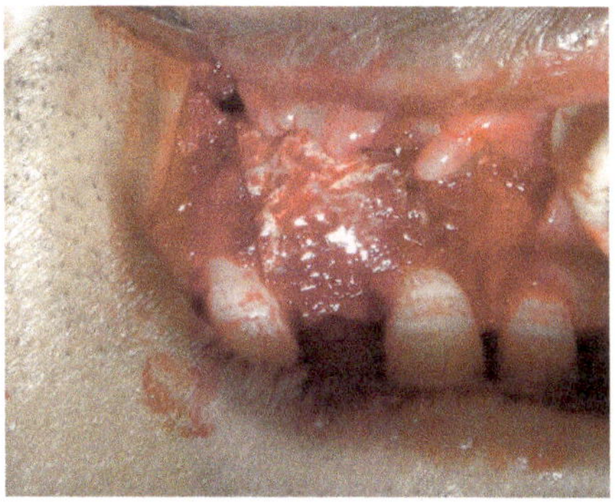

FIGURE 9: Chorion membrane placed over graft.

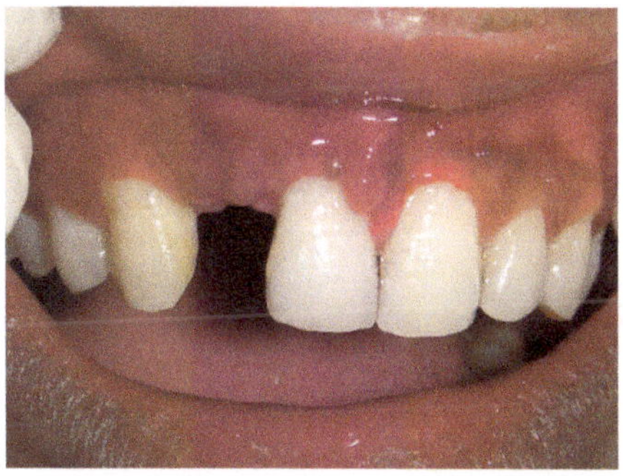

FIGURE 10: Edentulous area 3 weeks after graft placement.

Soft tissue healing at both sites was uneventful (Figure 10). Sutures were removed after 15 days.

5 months later, ridge mapping showed buccolingual width as 7.3 mm, 3 mm apical to the alveolar crest. A panoramic radiograph was obtained to evaluate the grafted area. A surgical reentry with implant placement in a single visit was planned.

2.1.4. Surgical Reentry and Implant Placement. A crestal incision was given after administering infraorbital nerve block (Lignocaine 2% with Adrenaline 1 : 80,000), followed by mucoperiosteal flap elevation to expose the grafted site. Buccolingual width of the ridge was found to be 6.9 mm. Fixation screw was removed, and osteotomy was done for implant placement. A 3.3 × 11.5 mm implant (Alpha-Bio Tec Ltd., Israel) was inserted (Figure 11). Primary stability was measured using Osstell device that showed Implant Stability Quotient (ISQ) value as 70. Interrupted sutures were given after placing cover screws and adaptation of flap. Postoperative period was uneventful. Sutures were removed on the 7th day.

2.1.5. Implant Exposure and Prosthesis Placement. Second stage implant surgery was done 6 months later. After topical application of anaesthetic gel (Lignocaine 2%) the mucosa overlying implant was removed with Er, Cr:YSGG laser (Waterlase YSGG C 100, Biolase Technology, USA), followed by placement of healing cap for 15 days. Impressions were made for prosthesis fabrication, followed by metal ceramic crown placement, completing the prosthetic rehabilitation.

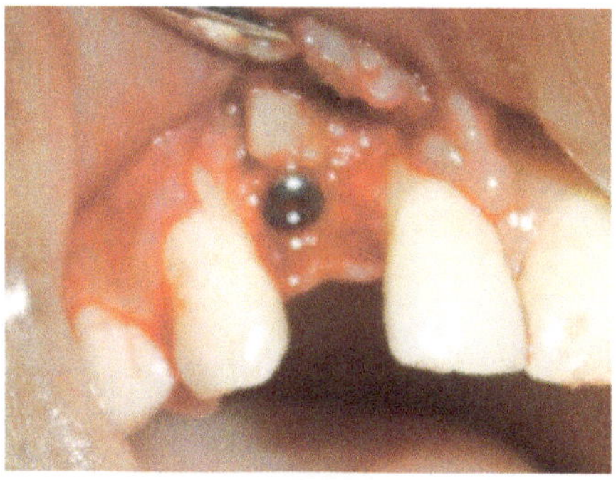

FIGURE 11: Implant placed in the augmented site.

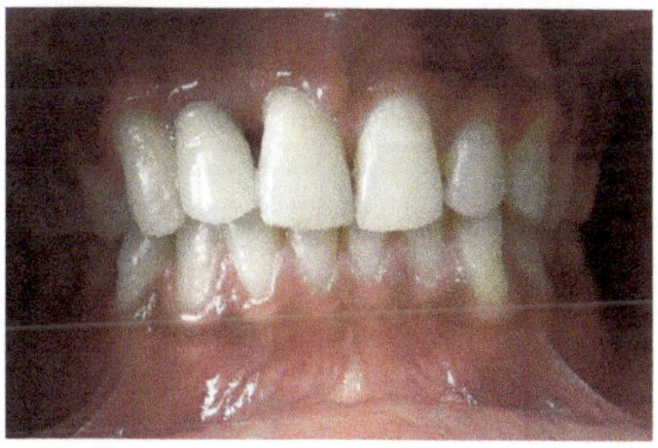

FIGURE 12: Restored implant 1 year after loading.

2.2. Clinical Outcome. This case is being followed regularly for last 1 year after crown placement, and no complication has been reported till now (Figures 12 and 13). The prosthesis is functioning without any discomfort to the patient. IOPA radiograph taken 1 year after loading shows no evidence of bone loss around the implant.

3. Discussion

Adequate bone volume at the future implant site is a prerequisite for good aesthetic outcome and sound biomechanical support of the osseointegrated implant. However, alveolar deficiencies due to trauma and subsequent unpredictable patterns of bone resorption may prevent an ideal implant therapy for prosthodontic rehabilitation. Identification of the exact anatomy of the edentulous site is essential before planning an implant placement. As in the present case, it was difficult to predict the morphology of underlying bone, since the only information we got through clinical examination was a concavity on the labial aspect of edentulous area. Radiographic evaluation thus became necessary to get an idea of the size and shape of underlying defect. Two-dimensional radiographs, such as Intraoral Periapical (IOPA) or panoramic views, could not reveal the exact condition of labial cortical plate. To get a cross-sectional view of the site, a 3-dimensional technique was required. Conventional computed tomography (CT) fulfils this requirement very

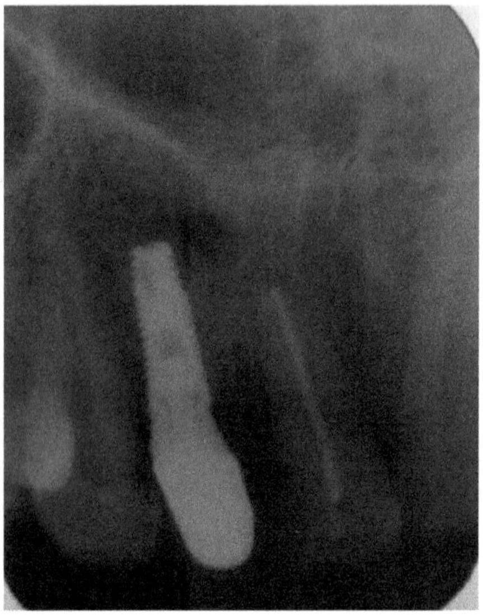

Figure 13: IOPA radiograph of the restored site 1 year after loading.

well, but the radiation dose is much higher than cone beam computed tomography (CBCT) which gives better view with 40 to 60 times less radiation [5]. A slight concavity on the labial aspect of the ridge found on clinical examination, turned out to be a gross defect on CBCT evaluation.

Various modalities have been reported to successfully augment the alveolar ridge in such cases. These include inlay or onlay block grafts and guided bone regeneration.

As compared to onlay grafts, particulate grafts require additional materials to ensure space maintenance and graft containment such as barrier membranes, tenting screws, and/or graft binders, while onlay grafts are self-contained and provide an inherent ability to support the soft tissue [4]. Therefore, onlay autografts are the best grafting material for ridge augmentation procedure. Iliac crest graft was first to be used to increase mandibular alveolar bone height in 1951. More recently developed procedures harvested cortico-cancellous bone grafts from the mandibular symphysis and the buccal ramus areas [3, 6–8].

Because of high risk associated with harvesting iliac crest bone and life-threatening complications with calvarial bone, intraoral source has been suggested to be a safer and easier option when amount of bone is not a concern. Additionally, harvesting graft from extraoral sources requires general anaesthesia and hospital admission with a longer healing period which can be avoided when an intraoral site is chosen [3, 4]. Several studies have shown that intraoral autogenous grafts have a lower rate of resorption and better revascularization compared to iliac crest grafts [4].

In this case, mandibular symphysis was chosen to be the donor site, as it is easily accessible for harvesting block grafts, and we needed a small block of bone. It has advantages of considerably less discomfort, no visible scar formation, no need of general anaesthesia, and faster healing. When planning a block graft harvesting from mandibular symphysis, CBCT has another important role to play. Labiolingual width of the mandible and depth of the lingual concavity have to be accurately assessed, which is not possible with two-dimensional imaging modalities. We found CBCT an invaluable tool for treatment planning in this case.

The surgical procedure was easily done under local anaesthesia with a short recovery period and uneventful healing at the donor site as in majority of the reported cases [4, 7].

Piezoelectric unit was used for harvesting of block, as it is a minimally invasive technique with lesser risk of damage to surrounding mucosa, nerves, or vessels. Rapid cutting by piezoelectric unit prevents increase in temperature at surgical site, thus maintaining osteogenic potential of bone cells. It requires much less hand pressure than rotary instruments for its cutting action, providing more tactile sensitivity and accuracy to the operator. When used under local anaesthesia, it is more acceptable to patients compared to conventional surgical burs or saws [8, 9].

Using a particulate graft such as DFDBA helps bridging the minute gaps between cortical block and native bone, thus resulting in a more uniform and aesthetic alveolar ridge, in addition to providing osteoinductive effect [10, 11]. Particulate grafts also have the advantage of rapid vascularization; however, they must be protected by a membrane to reduce the risk of resorption.

As it has been suggested that block and particulate grafts show less resorption when covered with a barrier membrane through the healing period [12], a chorion membrane was placed in the present case. It is composed of immunoprivileged tissues and offers various advantages over alloplastic membranes. These membranes possess antibacterial and antimicrobial properties, reduce inflammation at the wound site, and provide a protein enriched matrix to facilitate cell migration [13].

Surgical reentry and implant placement was done 5 months after placement of block graft as Pikos suggested that block grafts can be reentered at 3-4 months in the mandible and at 4-5 months in the maxilla [14].

Primary stability of the implants placed in the grafted bone can be easily assessed at the time of placement using resonance frequency analysis (RFA). In the present case, ISQ value was found to be 70 which indicates good primary stability.

In this case, the implant has been free of any complications after one year of placement in accordance with several studies reporting high success rates of implants placed in onlay grafts. Clementini et al. [7] reported that success rate of implants placed in onlay graft regenerated ridges ranged from 72.8% to 97% after follow-up periods ranging from 6 months to 10 years, very similar to those obtained in case of implants placed in pristine bone, and suggested that onlay graft augmentation is a quite predictable technique to allow the placement of implants in severely atrophic areas. In a systematic review, Aghaloo and Moy [6] reported implant survival rate as 95.5% for guided bone regeneration, 90.4% for onlay/veneer grafting, 94.7% for distraction osteogenesis, and 83.8% for combinations of onlay, veneer, and interpositional inlay grafting.

4. Conclusion

Well-functioning implant after 1-year followup indicates that bone lost to trauma in maxillary anterior region can be successfully restored with an onlay block graft from mandibular symphysis, without much morbidity and complications. Cone beam computed tomography (CBCT) is invaluable tool in diagnosis and treatment planning of such cases.

Conflict of Interests

The authors report no conflict of interests related to this paper.

References

[1] V. Braut, M. M. Bornstein, U. Belser, and D. Buser, "Thickness of the anterior maxillary facial bone wall-a retrospective radiographic study using cone beam computed tomography," *The International Journal of Periodontics and Restorative Dentistry*, vol. 31, no. 2, pp. 125–131, 2011.

[2] P. J. Louis, "Bone grafting the mandible," *Oral and Maxillofacial Surgery Clinics of North America*, vol. 23, no. 2, pp. 209–227, 2011.

[3] L. M. E. Scheerlinck, M. S. M. Muradin, A. van der Bilt, G. J. Meijer, R. Koole, and E. M. V. Cann, "Donor site complications in bone grafting: comparison of iliac crest, calvarial, and mandibular ramus bone," *International Journal of Oral and Maxillofacial Implants*, vol. 28, pp. 222–227, 2013.

[4] N. Toscano, D. Holtzclaw, Z. Mazor, P. Rosen, R. Horowitz, and M. Toffler, "Horizontal ridge augmentation utilizing a composite graft of demineralized freeze-dried allograft, mineralized cortical cancellous chips, and a biologically degradable thermoplastic carrier combined with a resorbable membrane: a retrospective evaluation of 73 consecutively treated cases from private practices," *The Journal of Oral Implantology*, vol. 36, no. 6, pp. 467–474, 2010.

[5] D. E. Clark, R. A. Danforth, R. W. Barnes, and M. L. Burtch, "Radiation absorbed from dental implant radiography: a comparison of linear tomography, CT scan, and panoramic and intra-oral techniques," *The Journal of Oral Implantology*, vol. 16, no. 3, pp. 156–164, 1990.

[6] T. L. Aghaloo and P. K. Moy, "Which hard tissue augmentation techniques are the most successful in furnishing bony support for implant placement?" *International Journal of Oral and Maxillofacial Implants*, vol. 22, pp. 49–70, 2007.

[7] M. Clementini, A. Morlupi, C. Agrestini, and L. Ottria, "Success rate of dental implants inserted in autologous bone graft regenerated areas: a systematic review," *Oral & Implantology*, vol. 4, no. 3-4, pp. 3–10, 2011.

[8] P. Felice, G. Iezzi, G. Lizio, A. Piattelli, and C. Marchetti, "Reconstruction of atrophied posterior mandible with inlay technique and mandibular ramus block graft for implant prosthetic rehabilitation," *Journal of Oral and Maxillofacial Surgery*, vol. 67, no. 2, pp. 372–380, 2009.

[9] D. S. Sohn, M. R. Ahn, W. H. Lee, D. S. Yeo, and S. Y. Lim, "Piezoelectric osteotomy for intraoral harvesting of bone blocks," *International Journal of Periodontics and Restorative Dentistry*, vol. 27, no. 2, pp. 127–131, 2007.

[10] A. R. G. Cortes, D. N. Cortes, and E. S. Arita, "Cone beam computed tomographic evaluation of a maxillary alveolar ridge reconstruction with iliac crest grafts and implants," *Journal of Craniofacial Surgery*, vol. 23, no. 1, pp. e12–e13, 2012.

[11] B. Le, J. Burstein, and P. P. Sedghizadeh, "Cortical tenting grafting technique in the severely atrophic alveolar ridge for implant site preparation," *Implant Dentistry*, vol. 17, no. 1, pp. 40–50, 2008.

[12] E. Nyström, J. Ahlqvist, P. E. Legrell, and K. E. Kahnberg, "Bone graft remodelling and implant success rate in the treatment of the severely resorbed maxilla: a 5-year longitudinal study," *International Journal of Oral and Maxillofacial Surgery*, vol. 31, no. 2, pp. 158–164, 2002.

[13] E. H. Chen and A. J. Tofe, "A literature review of the safety and biocompatibility of amnion tissue," *Journal of Implant & Advance Clinical Dentistry*, vol. 2, no. 3, pp. 67–75, 2010.

[14] M. A. Pikos, "Mandibular block autografts for alveolar ridge augmentation," *Atlas of the Oral and Maxillofacial Surgery Clinics of North America*, vol. 13, no. 2, pp. 91–107, 2005.

8

Maxillary and Mandibular First Premolars Showing Three-Cusp Pattern: An Unusual Presentation

Ramakant Nayak,[1] Vijayalakshmi Kotrashetti,[1] Aarati Nayak,[2] Viraj Patil,[3] Mayuri Kulkarni,[1] Pradeep Somannavar,[1] and Jagadish Hosmani[1]

[1] *Department of Oral Pathology and Microbiology, Maratha Mandal's NGH Institute of Dental Sciences and Research Centre, Belgaum, Karnataka 590010, India*
[2] *Department of Periodontology, Maratha Mandal's NGH Institute of Dental Sciences and Research Centre, Belgaum, Karnataka 590010, India*
[3] *Department of Prosthodontics, Maratha Mandal's NGH Institute of Dental Sciences and Research Centre, Belgaum, Karnataka 590010, India*

Correspondence should be addressed to Vijayalakshmi Kotrashetti; drviju18@yahoo.com

Academic Editors: J. Asaumi, D. W. Boston, and J. C. de la Macorra

Dental anatomy is the study of morphology of various teeth in human dentitions. The application of dental anatomy in clinical practice is important, and dentist should have a thorough knowledge regarding the morphology of the teeth. At times as a result of genetic variation, environmental factors, diet of an individual and race, variations in the morphology of the teeth can be observed. These variations have been extensively studied by the researcher in the field of anthropology to define a particular race. The most commonly observed changes include peg-shaped laterals, shovel-shaped incisors, and extra cusp on molar. Common variations documented with regard to maxillary and mandibular first premolars are the variation in the number of roots. But the variations with respect to crown morphology are few. We report a first documented unusual presentation of maxillary and mandibular first premolars with three-cusps pattern in a female patient.

1. Introduction

Dental anthropology is the study of the origin and variations in the human dentitions. These structural variations are used to determine a population or a race. Dental anthropologic structures useful in identification include metric and nonmetric traits. The study of dental morphology (nonmetric trait) is easily observed and documented. Nonmetric dental traits (NDTs) are of value because they possess high taxonomic value and have been used to estimate biological relationships among diverse population which allows comparative analysis of the historical, cultural, biological development of primitive and modern human groups. NDT can be used to evaluate population differences according to microevolutionary processes which in turn give information about racial variations among the population. Thus it is important to describe systematically the morphological variation in each person's clinical dental history. The most commonly studied traits include study of cusp size, number and location, occlusal pattern, root configuration, and number of roots [1, 2].

Maxillary first premolars are described morphologically as showing two cusps and two roots, whereas the mandibular first premolars shows presence of two cusps and one root, with lingual cusp being rudimentary in most cases. Superimposed on these basic shapes of teeth are minor morphological variations that affect both deciduous and permanent teeth [3, 4]. Such variations are inherited and dependent on many genes, culture, conditions of life, diet, and adaptation processes [4]. The common variation documented in the morphology of maxillary first premolar is presence of three root canals with the incidence of 5-6% [5]. Donald HM found morphological variations in maxillary first premolar in two girls and one boy of Papago Indians. He observed that buccolingual dimension of the crown was increased when compared to second maxillary premolar. The buccal cusp was affected in the study population, which showed presence of hypertrophied medial occlusal paracone ridge. Similarly Brabant et al. noted increased buccolingual dimension of maxillary first premolars due to the presence of supernumerary cusp on the buccal surface of the paracone [6]. Apart from these reports which were documented in late 1960s, no other cases have been documented reporting variation in the crown morphology of maxillary first premolar. Presence of three-cusp pattern in mandibular second premolar is a normal phenomenon [3, 4]. Common variation in the crown morphology observed in this tooth is presence of four cusps [4] and tubercle [1]. The reported variation in the crown morphology of mandibular first premolar varies from no lingual cusp to as many as four lingual cusplets [7].

In this paper we report first unusual case showing three cusp crown pattern in the maxillary and mandibular first premolars in a female patient.

2. Case Report

A 46-year-old female patient reported with a chief complaint of draining sinus in the alveolar mucosa of 16. On examination, 16 showed presence of metal crown restoration which was root canal treated about 5 years back. Silver amalgam filling restoration with 17 and 37 was present. Porcelain fused to metal bridges was present with 45, 46, 47 and 24, 25, 26, 27 and porcelain fused to metal crown on 34.

We also noticed an unusual variation in the crown morphology of 14 (right maxillary first premolar) and 44 (right mandibular first premolar). Both the crowns showed three-cusp pattern showing "Y" shaped occlusal groove. There was presence of one buccal cusp and two lingual cusps, that is, mesiolingual and distolingual separated by the groove which was extending on to the lingual surface and appeared as lingual developmental groove. On the contralateral side, we examined whether the same phenomenon exists but 34 was root canal treated with porcelain fused metal crown and 24 had crown which was an abutment for bridge. In case of mandibular first premolar the possibility of transposition could not be ascertained as 45 was an abutment for a bridge. Of the two lingual cusps in 44, the mesiolingual cusp was more prominent (Figures 1(a) and 1(b)) and in case of 14, the mesiolingual cusp was marginally larger than the distolingual cusp (Figures 2(a) and 2(b)). Occlusal aspect of 14 and 44 showed well developed marginal ridges and prominent mesial and distal fossa. The mesial and distal occlusal developmental groove was prominent and was extended till the marginal ridge in 14, whereas it was less prominent in 44. Occlusion was class I, and there was no interference in the occlusion with opposing teeth with respect to 14 and 44. The buccal cusp of 44 occluded in the central pit of 14 (at the junction of occlusal and palatal groove). The distolingual cusps of both the teeth were not in contact with the opposing teeth, as they were small in size. The emerging pattern and timing of teeth were normal. The intraoral periapical radiograph of 14 did not show any root variations (Figures 3(a) and 3(b)). The thickness of enamel and dentin appeared to be normal. The crown size of the teeth was measured using digital vernier caliper on dental cast. The mesiodistal dimension of 14 was 6.62 mm and buccolingual was 7.84 mm. The mesiodistal dimension of 44 was 5.85 mm and buccolingual was 7.86 mm.

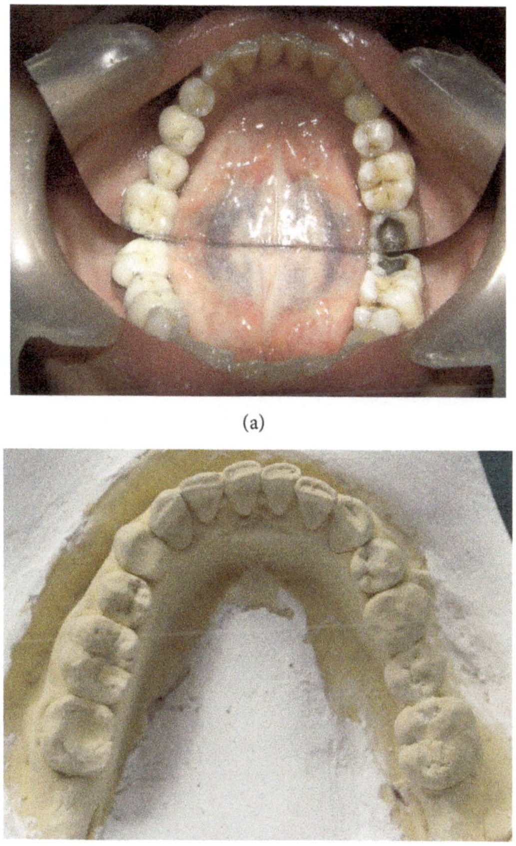

(a)

(b)

FIGURE 1: (a) Mirror image photograph showing 44 with mesiolingual and distolingual cusp. (b) Photograph of mandibular cast showing 44 with typical "Y" shaped occlusal groove with 3 cusps resembling mandibular second premolar.

3. Discussion

The commonest morphological variations described in dental anatomy include presence of shovel-shaped maxillary central incisor, peg-shaped maxillary lateral incisor, accessory cusp on the maxillary first permanent molar, additional cusp on the mandibular second premolar giving a total of four cusps to the tooth, reduced size or absence of a distopalatal cusp on the maxillary second molar [4]. "At times certain of these changes go unnoticed and will not be documented in routine dental practice."

Knowing some common variations occurring in tooth morphology about each individual tooth can help in performing dental treatment and also can be used for anthropological research for identification of population [2].

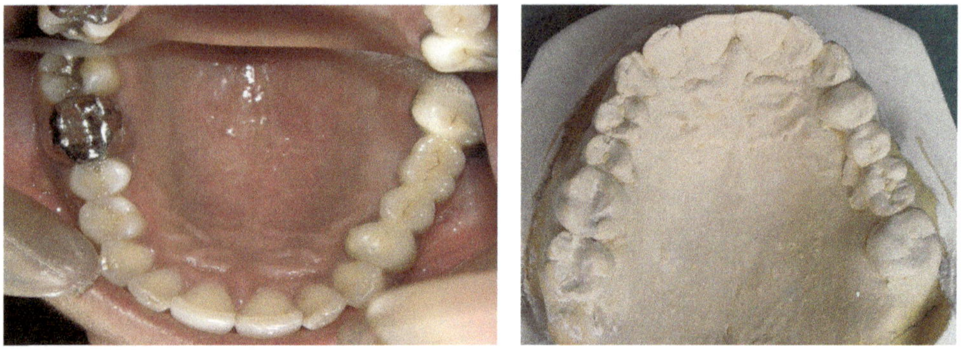

(a) (b)

Figure 2: (a) Mirror image photograph showing 14 with mesiolingual and distolingual cusp. (b) Photograph of maxillary cast showing 14 with typical “Y” shaped occlusal groove, 3 cusps and a prominent lingual groove.

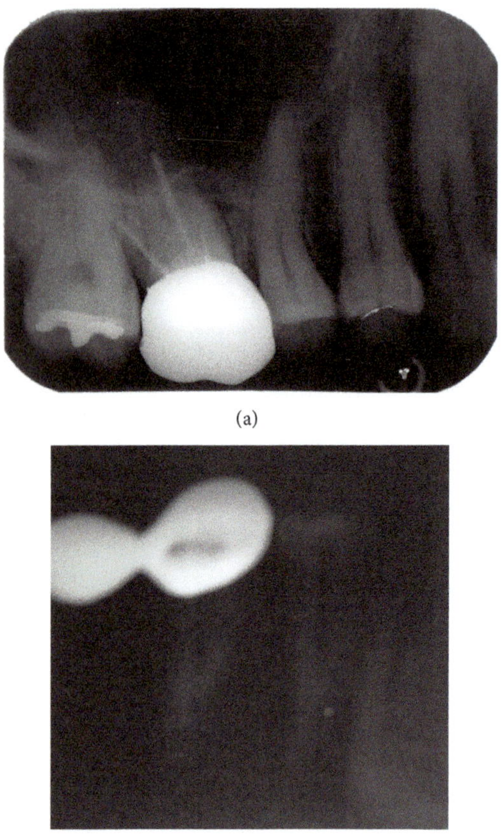

(a)

(b)

Figure 3: (a) Photograph of intraoral periapical radiograph of 14 showing normal root morphology. (b) Photograph of intraoral periapical radiograph of 44 showing normal root morphology.

We report a first ever documented case of maxillary first premolar and mandibular first premolar showing three cusps. It is one of the rare variations observed. Both the teeth showed classic presence of mesiolingual and distolingual cusp. Probably the same morphology of crown was present on the contralateral side but we could not confirm as patient had porcelain fused to metal crowns on 34 and 24 was an abutment for bridge. The size of the teeth appeared larger mesiodistally when compared to normal average dimension [3].

The etiology for extra cusp formation is unknown. However, earlier it was thought to be due to over-activity of the dental lamina. But now it is believed that PAX and MSX genes are responsible for variation in shape of the teeth [8]. Extra cusps develop due to abnormal proliferation and folding of a portion of inner enamel epithelium (IEE) along with adjacent ectomesenchymal cells of the dental papilla into the stellate reticulum of the enamel organ during bell stage of tooth formation. The resultant formation is defined as either tubercle or supplemental solid elevation on some portion of the crown surface [9].

Current embryological evidence suggests that primary and secondary enamel knots direct the folding of IEE which determines the characteristic morphology of the crown. Enamel knots begin to form in the cap stage of tooth development and location of primary enamel knot coincides with the presumptive apex of the first-forming cusp, and subsequently secondary enamel knots develop during the bell stage, which coincides with the number and position of the other presumptive cusps [10].

Enamel knots are transitory condensations of IEE situated in the stellate reticulum atop the IEE projecting toward dental papilla. Enamel knot acts as a signaling center and consists of nondividing cells, and it stimulates rapid proliferation of adjacent dental epithelium though they themselves are nonproliferative. This relationship seems to be central to the formation of the tooth cusps [10, 11]. Localized differences in cell proliferation cause folding of the IEE, where the enamel knots define the number and position of the presumptive cusps tips. During this process, topographic difference in proliferation rates of the epithelium accounts for the angularity of the cusps and also for differences in cusp height. This indicates that activator from the primary enamel knot regulates the expression of secondary enamel knots. The resultant cusp morphogenesis and positions appear to be determined sequentially, and cusps that form late in development, after the main cusps, are typically small. The secondary enamel knots disperse after formation of the cusp tips, which indicates termination of crown morphogenesis. Furthermore, the actual number of cusps realized in each tooth is also determined by the initiation of root formation [10, 12]. This may be the probable reason for the presence of three cusps in our case.

It is also stated that maxillary premolars and mandibular first premolar develop from four lobes (mesial, distal, buccal, and palatal), whereas mandibular second premolar which often has two lingual cusps develop from five lobes (mesial, buccal, distal, mesiolingual, and distolingual lobes) [3]. Probably in the present case the maxillary first premolar and mandibular first premolar have developed from five lobes thus showing three cusps.

4. Conclusion

We present a first reported case of three-cusp pattern of maxillary and mandibular first premolar. This can be considered as one of the morphological variations which can be seen and is not suggestive of any kind of a developmental anomaly. They are normal morphological features of the dentition. As a dentist we should be aware of such morphological variations observed during routine dental examination and one should not be very dogmatic about the standard morphological features of the teeth. Proper documentation of these variations may help anthropologists in their study of a population.

References

[1] R. Carolina and M. Freddy, "Paramolar tubercle in the left maxillary second premolar: a case report," *Dental Anthropology*, vol. 19, no. 3, pp. 65–69, 2006.

[2] M. Ramin, E. Behnaz, Z. Ali, N. Akhlaghi, N. Shamashian, and L. Karimi, "Occlusal morphology of mandibular second molars in Iranian adolescents," *Indian Journal of Dental Research*, vol. 21, no. 1, pp. 16–19, 2010.

[3] M. M. Ash and J. N. Stanley, *Wheeler's Dental Anatomy, Physiology and Occlusion*, Elsevier, A Division of Reed Elsevier, Noida, India, 8th edition, 2003.

[4] B. K. B. Berkovitz, G. R. Holland, and B. J. Moxham, *Oral Anatomy, Histology and Embroyology*, Mosby International, Philadelphia, Pa, USA, 3rd edition, 2002.

[5] D. A. Hacer and A. Tayfun, "Diagnosis and treatment of three rooted maxillary premolars," *European Journal of Dentistry*, vol. 3, pp. 62–65, 2009.

[6] D. H. Morris, "Maxillary premolar variation among the Papago Indians," *Journal of Dental Research*, vol. 46, no. 4, pp. 736–738, 1967.

[7] C. S. Rickne and W. Gabriela, *Woelfel's Denatl Anatomy. Its Relevance to dentistry*, Williams and Wilkins, Philadelphia, Pa, USA, 8th edition, 2011.

[8] H. O. Sedano, F. Ocampo-Acosta, R. I. Naranjo-Corona, and M. E. Torres-Arellano, "Multiple dens invaginatus, mulberry molar and conical teeth. Case report and genetic considerations," *Medicina Oral, Patologia Oral y Cirugia Bucal*, vol. 14, no. 2, Article ID 5123658801, pp. E69–E72, 2009.

[9] S. V. S. G. Nirmala, R. C. Ramasubba, V. Lalitha, and N. Sivakumar, "Unusual occurrence of accessory cusp in the maxillary second primary molar," *Contemporary Clinical Dentistry*, vol. 2, no. 2, pp. 127–130, 2011.

[10] J. Jernvall, P. Kettunen, I. Karavanova, L. B. Martin, and I. Thesleff, "Evidence for the role of the enamel knot as a control center in mammalian tooth cusp formation: non-dividing cells express growth stimulating Fgf-4 gene," *International Journal of Developmental Biology*, vol. 38, no. 3, pp. 463–469, 1994.

[11] N. Antonio, *Tencate's Oral Histology Development, Structure and Function*, Elsevier, New Delhi, India, 6th edition, 2006.

[12] I. Thesleff, S. Keranen, and J. Jernvall, "Enamel knots as signaling centers linking tooth morphogenesis and odontoblast differentiation," *Advances in Dental Research*, vol. 15, pp. 14–18, 2001.

Provisional Crown Dislodgement during Scuba Diving: A Case of Barotrauma

Meenal Nitin Gulve[1] and Nitin Dilip Gulve[2]

[1] *Department of Conservative Dentistry and Endodontics, M.G.V.'s K.B.H. Dental College and Hospital, Mumbai Agra Road, Panchavati, Nashik 422002, India*
[2] *Department of Orthodontics, Dentofacial Orthopedics and Dental Materials, M.G.V.'s K.B.H. Dental College and Hospital, Nashik 422002, India*

Correspondence should be addressed to Meenal Nitin Gulve; gulve_meenal@hotmail.com

Academic Editors: D. W. Boston and T. Lombardi

Changes in ambient pressure, for example, during flying, diving, or hyperbaric oxygen therapy, can lead to barotrauma. Although it may seem that this issue was neglected in dental education and research in recent decades, familiarity with and understanding of these facts may be of importance for dental practitioners. We report the case of a patient who experienced barotrauma involving dislodgement of a provisional crown during scuba diving. Patients who are exposed to pressure changes as a part of their jobs or hobbies and their dentists should know the causes of barotrauma. In addition, the clinician must be aware of the possible influence of pressure changes on the retention of dental components.

1. Introduction

In recent years it has become increasingly common to go to a tropical destination for a holiday [1]. There is often an opportunity to dive. Diving with self-contained underwater breathing apparatus (SCUBA) has witnessed explosive growth in the past decade, as 8.5 million people are certified in the United States alone. Around three million Europeans are thought to be recreational scuba divers, diving to depths up to around 40 meters sea water (msw). Additionally, there are approximately 800 professional civilians and 700 military divers registered in Germany as well as some 500 compressed air (caisson) workers, for example, for tunnel or bridge construction work [2]. With the increasing number of professional and leisure divers, the dentist may encounter related oral conditions that require immediate treatment. Although rare, dental emergencies while diving have been recognized as a potential cause of a diver suddenly becoming incapacitated, jeopardizing the safety of the affected person as well as others [3]. It is inevitable that the dental practitioner will have patients who participate in diving and they should be aware of a number of problems that a diver can experience that are associated with the teeth and related structures.

An oral (dental or nondental) pain caused by change in barometric pressure in an otherwise asymptomatic organ is known as barodontalgia. The name of this dental pain was given the prefix "aero" (i.e., aerodontalgia) and was reported for the first time as an in-flight physiologic and pathologic phenomenon at the beginning of the 20th century. In the 1940s, with the appearance of SCUBA, many in-flight manifestations caused by barometric changes were found to be associated with diving as well. Consequently, the prefix was changed to "Baro" [4, 5]. Barodontalgia has been experienced on one or more occasions by 9.2% to 21.6% of American and Australian civilian scuba divers. Among military divers, an incidence of 17.3% was reported [6]. Barotrauma is defined as pressure induced damage that can occur both in high and low pressure [4]. Dental barotrauma can manifest itself as tooth fracture [7], restoration fracture, and dislodgement of the restoration [7, 8].

In this paper, we present a case in which a patient experienced barotrauma involving a provisional crown while diving.

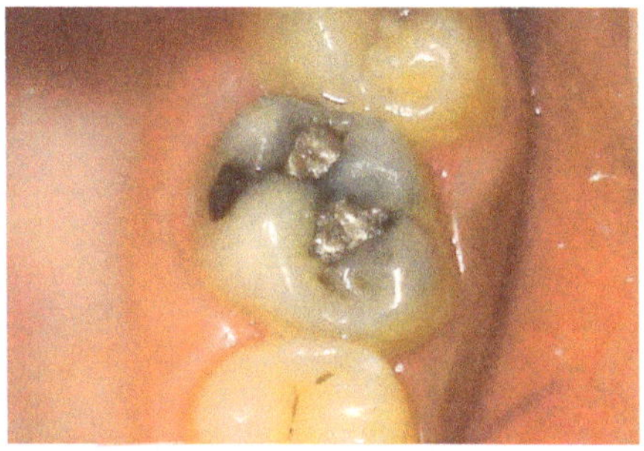

FIGURE 1: Amalgam restoration with secondary caries in the maxillary left first molar.

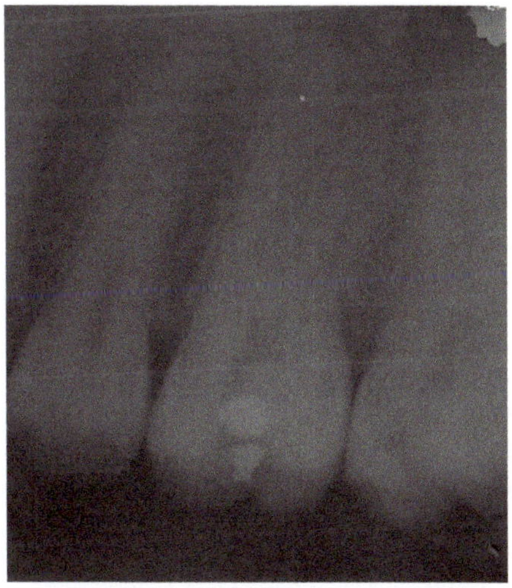

FIGURE 2: Radiolucent area approaching the pulp space with periodontal ligament space widening.

2. Diagnosis and Treatment

A 25-year-old man presented with a chief complaint of spontaneous pain on the left side of his face for the past 3 days. History revealed intermittent pain to hot and cold stimuli for the past 1 month. The medical history was noncontributory. Clinical examination revealed an amalgam restoration with secondary caries in the maxillary left first molar (Figure 1). The tooth was tender to vertical percussion. Tooth mobility was within physiologic limit, and the gingival attachment apparatus was normal. Vitality testing of the involved tooth with heated gutta-percha (Dentsply Maillefer, Ballaigues, Switzerland) and dry ice (RC Ice; Prime Dental Product, Mumbai, India) caused an intense lingering pain, whereas electric pulp stimulation (Parkel Electronics Division, Farmingdale, NY, USA) caused a premature response. The preoperative radiographic evaluation showed evidence of radiolucent area in relation to maxillary left first molar approaching the pulp space with periodontal ligament space widening in relation to the mesial root (Figure 2). A diagnosis of symptomatic irreversible pulpitis with symptomatic apical periodontitis was made, and endodontic treatment was suggested to the patient.

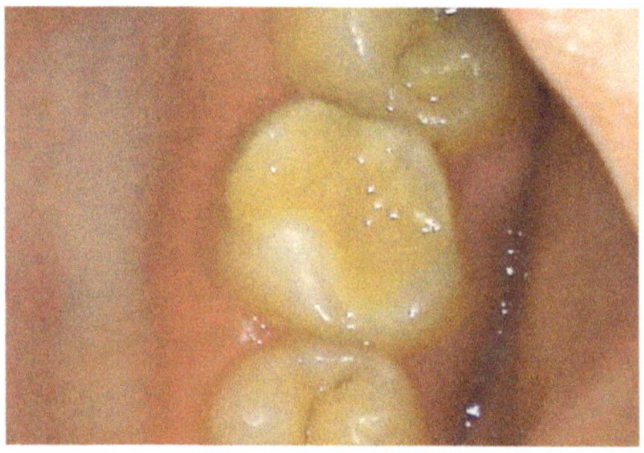

FIGURE 3: The tooth was restored with a posterior composite resin.

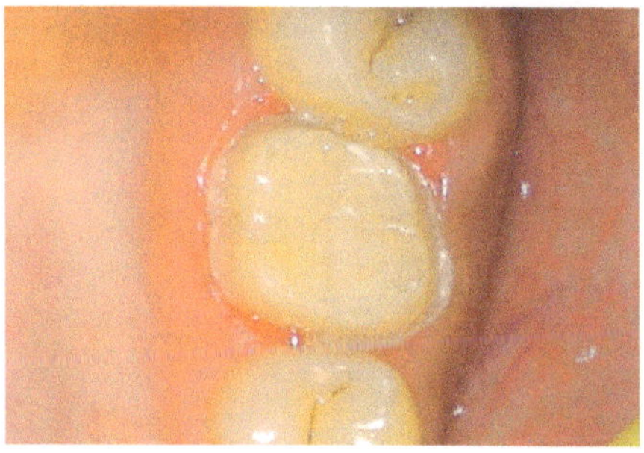

FIGURE 4: The tooth was prepared to receive metal-ceramic crown.

Informed consent was taken. The tooth was anesthetized by using 1.8 mL 2% lignocaine containing 1 : 200,000 epinephrine. Endodontic treatment was completed and the tooth was then restored with a posterior composite resin core (Z350; 3M ESPE Dental Products, St. Paul, MN, USA) (Figure 3).

The tooth was prepared 1 week after endodontic treatment to receive a metal-ceramic crown in a conventional manner with the aim of obtaining a 6-degree convergence between walls (Figure 4). Gingival displacement was done, and two impressions were made: an alginate impression to prepare a provisional crown and another with hydrophilic polyvinyl siloxane impression material (Virtual; Ivoclar Vivadent, Schaan, Liechtenstein) to prepare metal-ceramic crown, poured using type IV dental stone (Kalrock; Kalabhai, India). The shade was determined with a shade guide. The patient was given a provisional crown, which was made from a bis-acryl material (Integrity; Dentsply Caulk, Konstanz, Germany) and was cemented with zinc phosphate cement (DeTrey Zinc; Dentsply DeTrey GmbH, Konstanz, Germany) (Figure 5). Excess cement was removed with a scalpel. The patient was recalled after 7 days to receive the final crown.

However, the patient presented with dislodged provisional crown (Figure 6). He gave a history of SCUBA diving at a destination where he went for previously unplanned vacation. He reported that the provisional crown came out while he was diving at about 27 to 35 meters deep. After the crown dislodged, he had to keep it under his tongue until he returned to the surface to avoid aspiration or swallowing.

The tooth was cleaned of the temporary cement with a slurry of fine flour of pumice. The metal-ceramic crown

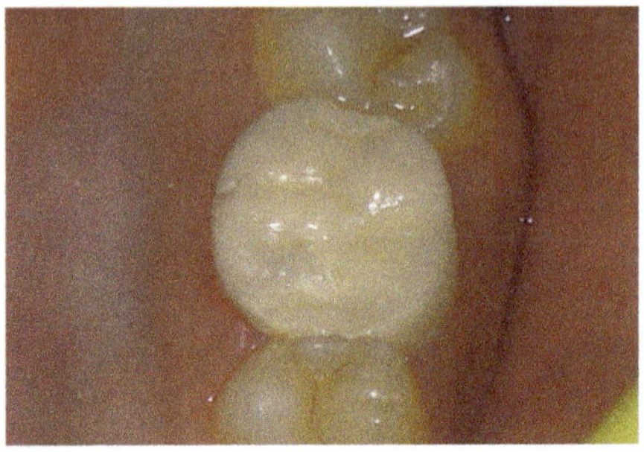

FIGURE 5: Provisional crown cemented with zinc phosphate cement.

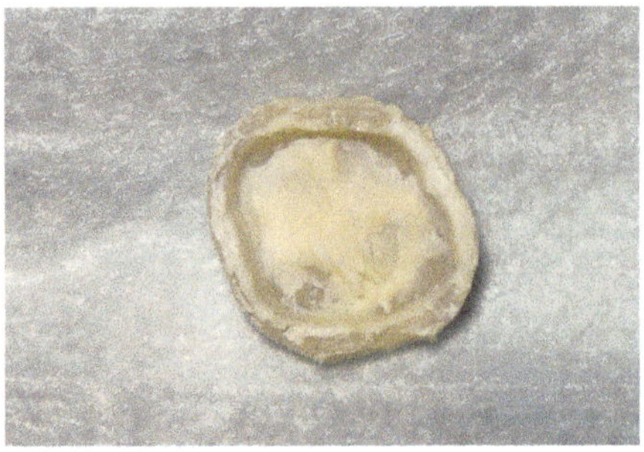

FIGURE 6: Dislodged provisional crown.

was tried in to assess the marginal fit and contacts. The patient previewed and approved the shape and the shade of the crowns. The crown was cemented with self-adhesive resin cement (Multilink Speed; Ivoclar Vivadent AG, Schaan, Liechtenstein) in accordance with the manufacturer's instructions (Figure 7). Postoperative care instructions were given to the patient and recall appointments were scheduled.

3. Discussion

In recent years it has become increasingly common to go to a tropical destination for a holiday. There is often an opportunity to dive. Also scuba diving is one of the fastest growing sports in the world [1]. In the case we presented, a leisure diver experienced barotrauma in which a provisional crown was dislodged while he was diving at about 27 to 35 meters deep under the surface of the sea. A diver at 30 m is subjected to four times the pressure encountered on the surface [9]. Although the exact mechanisms of barodontalgia and barotrauma are not known, the air trapped beneath a restoration or an endodontically treated tooth may be a factor [10].

The possible reason for dislodging of provisional crown cemented with zinc phosphate could be associated Boyle's law, which states that, at a constant temperature, the volume of a gas varies inversely with the surrounding pressure. As pressure increases, the volume of a confined gas decreases. Vice versa, volume increases as pressure decreases [9]. The problem arises when the enclosed spaces containing gases cannot expand or contract to adjust the internal pressure to correspond to the outer pressure. During the mixing process

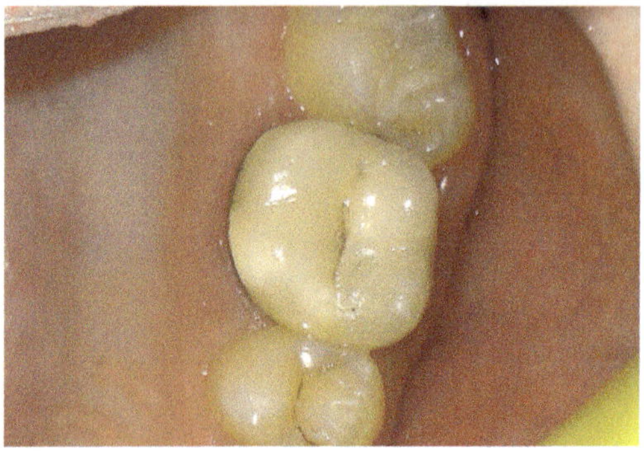

FIGURE 7: The metal-ceramic crown was cemented with self-adhesive resin cement.

of luting cement, air may become incorporated into the mixture, forming voids [11]. The expansion or contraction of these microbubbles during pressure cycling, which eventually led to disruption and weakening of cement layer, could affect the retention [12]. Davidson et al. [13] found that microcracks appear as a result of volumetric contraction in luting cements and, when subjected to the pressure cycling, may have produced tensile stresses that exceeded the cohesive and adhesive strength of the material, resulting in the significant reduction in tensile bond strength.

Lyons et al. [12] studied the effect of cycling environmental pressure changes on the retention of crowns on the extracted teeth. The crowns that were cemented with either zinc phosphate or glass ionomer cement had significantly reduced retention (in approximately 90% and 50%, resp.), whereas crowns that were cemented with resin cement were not subjected to reduced retention after pressure cycling. Moreover, microleakage was detected in the zinc phosphate and glass ionomer cements after pressure cycling, whereas no microleakage was detected in the resin cement. Musajo et al. [9] also reported similar results with crowns cemented with zinc phosphate cement. Gulve et. al [14] found that the pullout strength of orthodontic bands cemented with glass ionomer cement is reduced after pressure cycling.

It seems that, currently, the incidence of in-flight dental barotrauma is relatively low compared to reported incidences from the first half of the 20th century owing to the current inside compression of airplane chambers. The pressure inside the chamber fits pressure at altitudes of 5,000 to 10,000 feet, whereas cases of dental barotraumas were reported in pressure at altitudes of 18,000 feet and higher [15]. However, whereas in flight the theoretically possible pressure changes range from 1 atm (at ground level) to 0 atm (at outer space), in diving the changes are more significant, since each descent of 10 meters (32.8 feet) elevates the pressure by 1 atm. Thus, the barometric changes during diving may be more significant and responsible for more frequent and/or severe related pathogenesis than in-flight barometric changes. However, while aviators are obligated to be examined periodically, it is a rarity among divers [16].

Divers and aircrew medical examiners should recommend their aviator and diver patients to be periodically examined by a dental practitioner who is familiar with the subject. It is important for a dentist to be aware of the effect of pressure changes on dental components in terms of retentive strength, as danger resulting from dislodgement of component during a dive is obvious.

The dentist should advise patients not to dive while having a provisional crown or temporary cement in the mouth.

Consent

Written informed consent was obtained from the patient for publication of this paper and accompanying images.

Conflict of Interests

The authors declare that they have no conflict of interests.

References

[1] R. G. Jagger, S. J. Jackson, and D. C. Jagger, "In at the deep end—an insight into scuba diving and related dental problems for the GDP," *British Dental Journal*, vol. 183, no. 10, pp. 380–382, 1997.

[2] W. H. G. Goethe, H. Bäter, and C. Laban, "Barodontalgia and barotrauma in the human teeth: findings in navy divers, frogmen, and submariners of the Federal Republic of Germany," *Military Medicine*, vol. 154, no. 10, pp. 491–495, 1989.

[3] Y. Zadik, "Barodontalgia," *Journal of Endodontics*, vol. 35, no. 4, pp. 481–485, 2009.

[4] Y. Zadik, "Aviation dentistry: current concepts and practice," *British Dental Journal*, vol. 206, no. 1, pp. 11–16, 2009.

[5] R. Robichaud and M. E. McNally, "Barodontalgia as a differential diagnosis: symptoms and findings," *Journal of the Canadian Dental Association*, vol. 71, no. 1, pp. 39–42, 2005.

[6] Y. Zadik, "Barodontalgia: what have we learned in the past decade?" *Oral Surgery, Oral Medicine, Oral Pathology, Oral Radiology and Endodontology*, vol. 109, no. 4, pp. e65–e69, 2010.

[7] Y. Zadik, S. Einy, R. Pokroy, Y. B. Dayan, and L. Goldstein, "Dental fractures on acute exposure to high altitude," *Aviation Space and Environmental Medicine*, vol. 77, no. 6, pp. 654–657, 2006.

[8] I. Peker, H. Erten, and G. Kayaoglu, "Dental restoration dislodgment and fracture during scuba diving: a case of barotrauma," *Journal of the American Dental Association*, vol. 140, no. 9, pp. 1118-1121, 2009.

[9] F. Musajo, P. Passi, G. B. Girardello, and F. Rusca, "The influence of environmental pressure on retentiveness of prosthetic crowns: an experimental study," *Quintessence International*, vol. 23, no. 5, pp. 367–369, 1992.

[10] M. T. Brandt, "Oral and maxillofacial aspects of diving medicine," *Military Medicine*, vol. 169, no. 2, pp. 137–141, 2004.

[11] A. D. Milutinović-Nikolić, V. B. Medić, and Z. M. Vuković, "Porosity of different dental luting cements," *Dental Materials*, vol. 23, no. 6, pp. 674–678, 2007.

[12] K. M. Lyons, J. C. Rodda, and J. A. A. Hood, "The effect of environmental pressure changes during diving on the retentive strength of different luting agents for full cast crowns," *Journal of Prosthetic Dentistry*, vol. 78, no. 5, pp. 522–527, 1997.

[13] C. L. Davidson, L. Van Zeghbroeck, and A. J. Feilzer, "Destructive stresses in adhesive luting cements," *Journal of Dental Research*, vol. 70, no. 5, pp. 880–882, 1991.

[14] M. N. Gulve, N. D. Gulve, R. Shinde, and S. J. Kolhe, "The effect of environmental pressure changes on the retentive strength of cements for orthodontic bands," *Diving and Hyperbaric Medicine*, vol. 42, no. 2, pp. 78–81, 2012.

[15] M. Stoetzer, C. Kuehlhorn, M. Ruecker, D. Ziebolz, N. C. Gellrich, and C. V. See, "Pathophysiology of barodontalgia: a case report and review of the literature," *Case Report in Dentistry*, vol. 2012, Article ID 453415, 4 pages, 2012.

[16] Y. Zadik, "Dental barotrauma," *The International Journal of Prosthodontics*, vol. 22, no. 4, pp. 354–357, 2009.

10

Endodontic Treatment of Maxillary Premolar with Three Root Canals Using Optical Microscope and NiTi Rotatory Files System

João Bosco Formiga Relvas,[1] Fredsom Marcio Acris de Carvalho,[2] André Augusto Franco Marques,[3] Emílio Carlos Sponchiado Jr.,[1] and Lucas da Fonseca Roberti Garcia[4]

[1] *Department of Endodontics, School of Dentistry, Federal University of Amazonas, 69077-000 Manaus, AM, Brazil*
[2] *Department of Endodontics, School of Dentistry, Paulista University, 69050-010 Manaus, AM, Brazil*
[3] *Department of Endodontics, School of Dentistry, State University of Amazonas, 69050-030 Manaus, AM, Brazil*
[4] *Department of Dental Materials and Prosthodontics, Ribeirão Preto School of Dentistry, University of São Paulo, 14040-900 Ribeirão Preto, SP, Brazil*

Correspondence should be addressed to Lucas da Fonseca Roberti Garcia; drlucas.garcia@gmail.com

Academic Editors: M. B. D. Gaviao, M. M. Kassab, and A. Markopoulos

The aim of the study was to report a clinical case of endodontic treatment of a maxillary first premolar with three root canals using an optical microscope and rotary instrumentation technique. The main complaint of the patient, a 16-year-old girl, was pain in tooth 14. After clinical and radiographic examination, irreversible pulpitis was diagnosed. An alteration in the middle third of the pulp chamber radiographically observed suggested the presence of three root canals. Pulp chamber access and initial catheterization using size number 10 K-files were performed. The optical microscope and radiographic examination were used to confirm the presence of three root canals. PathFiles #13, #16, and #19 were used to perform catheterization and ProTaper files S1 and S2 for cervical preparation. Apical preparation was performed using F1 file in the buccal canals and F2 in the palatal canal up to the working length. The root canals were filled with Endofill sealer by thermal compaction technique using McSpadden #50. The case has been receiving follow-up for 12 months and no painful symptomatology or periapical lesions have been found. The use of technological tools was able to assist the endodontic treatment of teeth with complex internal anatomy, such as three-canal premolars.

1. Introduction

The constant development of equipment and instrumentation techniques has made it possible to solve several clinical cases in the field of Endodontics [1]. However, it is still imperative that professionals have a thorough knowledge of the internal anatomy of the pulp chamber and the entire root canal system in order to increase efficiency and, consequently, the rate of clinical success of endodontic treatment [2, 3].

Among permanent teeth, the roots of maxillary first premolars often have two conical roots, that is one buccal and one palatal root, which may present root fusion with a distinct line between them [4]. The buccal root may be further divided into two, an incidence of 1% to 5%, which causes the tooth to have three canals, a palatal, a distobuccal, and a mesiobuccal canal [4, 5].

Despite the low incidence, several studies have demonstrated the existence of three-canal maxillary first premolars, which considerably makes endodontic treatment difficult [5]. According to Gondim Jr. et al. [6], diagnosis and treatment of root canals represent an additional challenge for the professional. Thus, a careful examination of preoperative radiographs and the use of computed tomography as an additional diagnostic tool will be important to detect anatomical variations [7, 8].

On the other hand, the development of NiTi endodontic files used in rotatory systems allows biomechanical preparation in a shorter period of time than the conventional manual files, despite the difficulties due to the complex variation in the root canal anatomy [1]. Moreover, the use of optical microscope in Endodontics has been increased over the course of years [9]. The optical microscope offers many benefits, such as great lighting and better visualization of the operative field [10]. The high magnification is needed to assist in locating calcified canals, detect root microfractures, identify isthmuses, assist in the posts removal in the field and interpret the complexities of the root canal system [11].

Therefore, the aim of this paper was to report a clinical case of endodontic treatment of a three-canal premolar using the ProTaper system and optical microscope.

2. Case Report

The patient, a 16-year-old girl, presented at the Dental Clinic of the Federal University of Amazonas to undergo endodontic treatment of tooth 14, reporting persistent pain after cold stimulation. Considerable destruction by caries was visible in the distal surface of the tooth. In the anamnesis, the patient reported no systemic or heart diseases and no use of medications or drugs.

From the radiographic examination, an alteration in the radiopacity in the middle third of the pulp chamber of tooth 14 was observed, suggesting trifurcation of the root canal (Figure 1). The tooth was diagnosed as asymptomatic irreversible pulpitis and endodontic treatment was instituted. After local anesthesia (Xylestesin 2%, Cristália—Produtos Químicos Farmacêuticos Ltda., Itapira, SP, Brazil) and rubber dam isolation (Hygienic, Coltene/Whaledent AG, Alstatten, Switzerland) of the operative area, pulp chamber access was performed using a diamond spherical bur number 1013 (KG Sorensen, São Paulo, SP, Brazil). Next, the root canals orifices were located with number 10 K-file (Dentsply/Maillefer, Ballaigues, Switzerland), with the aid of an operative optical microscope (DF Vasconcelos, Valencia, RJ, Brazil) to facilitate visualization (Figure 2).

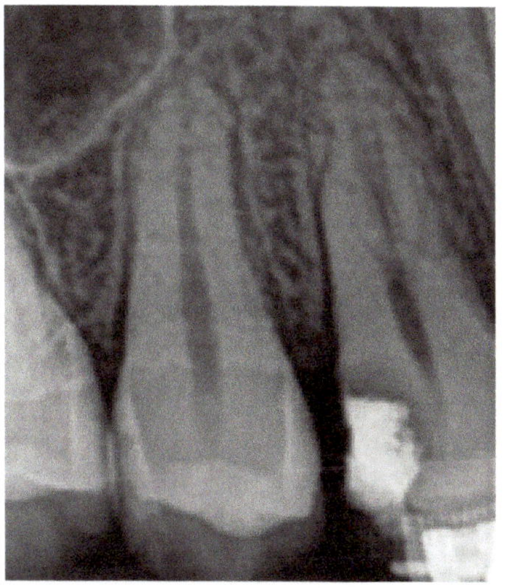

Figure 1: Initial periapical radiography. Radiopacity alteration in the middle third of the pulp chamber of tooth 14, suggesting trifurcation of the root canal.

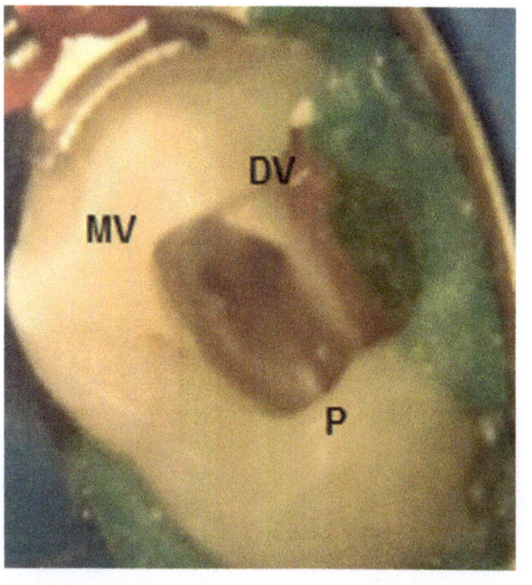

Figure 2: Root canal orifices located with operative optical microscope.

At each change of instrument, the canals were irrigated with 2.5 mL of 2.5% sodium hypochlorite solution (Biodinâmica, Ibiporã, PR, Brazil). During odontometry, the presence of three canals (Figure 3) was confirmed with the aid of an electronic apex locator (Joypex 5, Denjoy, China), two canals in the buccal root and one in the palatal root. The glide path was performed using PathFiles #13, #16, and #19 (Dentsply/Maillefer), cervical preparation with the ProTaper S1 and S2 instruments (Dentspy/Maillefer) and apical preparation with the ProTaper F1 and F2 instruments in the buccal canals and palatal canal up to the working length of 16 mm.

At the end of biomechanical preparation, 17% EDTA (Biodinâmica) was applied for 1 minute to remove smear layer and the final washing was performed with 2.5% sodium hypochlorite. Afterwards the root canals were dried with absorbent paper cones (Conetech, Manaus, AM, Brazil).

The root canals were filled with Endofill sealer (Dentsply, Petrópolis, RJ, Brazil) and gutta-percha points F1 and F2 (Dentsply) by thermal compaction technique using McSpadden #50 (Dentspy/Maillefer). Next, final radiography was performed (Figure 4).

The pulp chamber was cleaned to remove the excess of gutta-percha and sealer, and the tooth was temporarily restored with glass ionomer restorative cement (Ketac Molar, 3M ESPE, Sumaré, SP, Brazil). After 1 week, the tooth was definitely restored with composite resin (Z250, 3M ESPE, Sumaré, SP, Brazil). Follow-up over 12 months has shown a successful outcome from endodontic perspective. The tooth presented no painful symptomatology, and, radiographically, no signs of failure in root canal filling or periapical lesions were observed (Figure 5).

3. Discussion

An accurate diagnosis of the anatomy of the root canal system is a prerequisite for successful endodontic treatment [12].

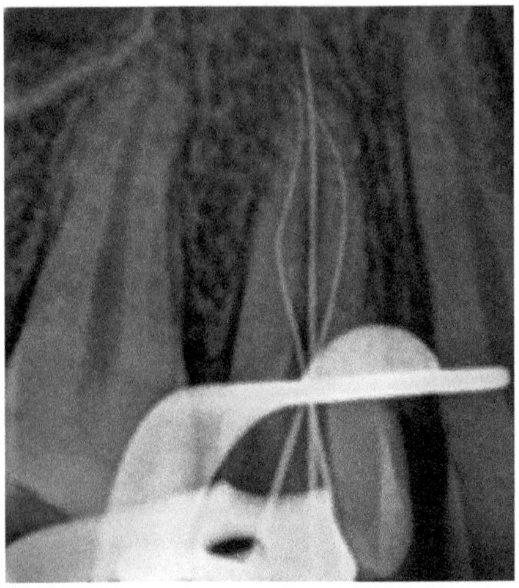

Figure 3: Odontometry confirming the presence of three root canals.

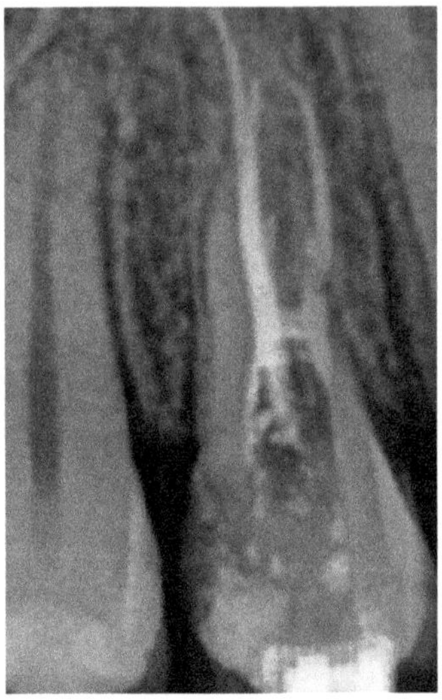

Figure 4: Final radiography after root canals filling.

Therefore, the radiographic signs that demonstrate the presence of anatomical variations must be considered an important condition when planning the tooth treatment [2].

Several studies have shown that the presence of three-rooted canals in maxillary first premolars is rare, ranging from 1.5% to 5% of the cases [2, 4, 5]. Although the frequency is low, the professional must be prepared to diagnose and plan a suitable treatment for this type of clinical event [2, 4, 5].

According to several case reports regarding the endodontic treatment of three-rooted maxillary premolars, it can be stated that, irrespective of the biomechanical preparation and filling technique used, the importance of early diagnosis of anatomical variations for satisfactory treatment outcome is imperative [13–16].

According to Vertucci [2], two radiographic signs indicate the presence of three-rooted maxillary first premolars. First, if it was radiographically detected that the middle third of the

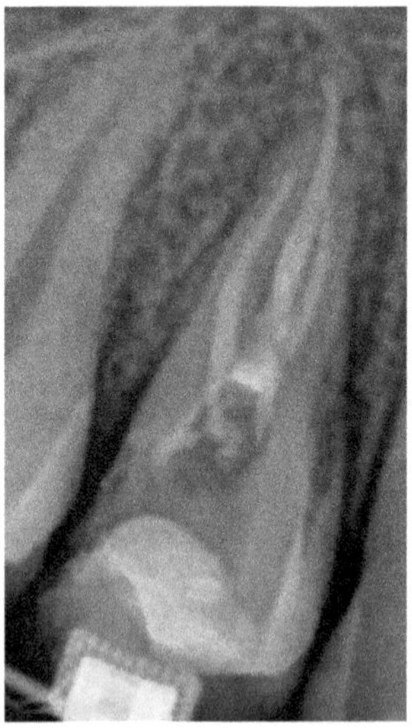

Figure 5: Periapical radiography of tooth 14 after 12 months, revealing no presence of failure in filling of root canals or periapical lesions.

root has a mesiodistal distance equal to or greater than the cervical third, this might indicate that there are two buccal roots or two root canals in a single-wide buccal root [2]. The second radiographic sign is the rapid disappearance of the continuity of radiolucent image of the root canal [2]. In this clinical case, the sudden disappearance of the continuity of the radiolucent image related to the root canal, as observed in the initial radiograph (Figure 1), was suggestive of a third root canal.

To confirm the presence of the third canal in the maxillary premolar in this case, the operative optical microscope was used for improved clinical visualization. According to Karapinar-Kazandag et al. [11], the optical microscope has many advantages because it provides better illumination and visualization of the operative field with a magnification up to twenty times. Therefore, high magnification helps the identification of the anatomical details of the pulp chamber floor and orifices of the root canal entrance [11].

The PathFile instruments were used in this case for initial catheterization because they maintain the trajectory of the root canal and perform preenlargement for the shaping files. Within the limits of the study conducted by Berutti et al. [1], the NiTi rotary PathFiles seem to be appropriate tools for creating secure and easy catheterization before using the NiTi rotatory instruments to shape the canal. These files presented better maintenance of the original canal anatomy causing less modification of canal curvature [1].

Moreover, the ProTaper Universal system was chosen to perform instrumentation of the root canal system in this case due to one of its main characteristics: the rate of taper varies along the cutting flutes, which significantly enhances flexibility, allowing instrumentation of difficult areas with cutting efficiency and safety [17].

Therefore, this case report demonstrated that the use of technological tools such as optical microscopy and rotatory instrumentation systems is capable of assisting the endodontic treatment of teeth with complex internal anatomy such as premolars with three root canals.

Conflict of Interests

The authors deny any conflict of interests related to this study.

References

[1] E. Berutti, G. Cantatore, A. Castellucci et al., "Use of nickel-titanium rotary PathFile to create the glide path: comparison with manual preflaring in simulated root canals," *Journal of Endodontics*, vol. 35, no. 3, pp. 408–412, 2009.

[2] F. J. Vertucci, "Root canal morphology and its relationship to endodontic procedures," *Endodontic Topics*, vol. 10, no. 1, pp. 3–29, 2005.

[3] F. Baratto Filho, S. Zaitter, G. A. Haragushiku, E. A. de Campos, A. Abuabara, and G. M. Correr, "Analysis of the internal anatomy of maxillary first molars by using different methods," *Journal of Endodontics*, vol. 35, no. 3, pp. 337–342, 2009.

[4] J. D. Pécora, P. C. Saquy, M. D. Sousa Neto, and J. B. Woelfel, "Root form and canal anatomy of maxillary first premolars," *Brazilian Dental Journal*, vol. 2, no. 2, pp. 87–94, 1992.

[5] L. Awawdeh, H. Abdullah, and A. Al-Qudah, "Root form and canal morphology of jordanian maxillary first premolars," *Journal of Endodontics*, vol. 34, no. 8, pp. 956–961, 2008.

[6] E. Gondim Jr., F. Setzer, P. Zingg, and B. Karabucak, "A maxillary central incisor with three root canals: a case report," *Journal of Endodontics*, vol. 35, no. 10, pp. 1445–1447, 2009.

[7] G. S. Sachdeva, S. Ballal, V. Gopikrishna, and D. Kandaswamy, "Endodontic management of a mandibular second premolar with four roots and four root canals with aid of spiral computed tomography: a case report," *Journal of Endodontics*, vol. 34, no. 1, pp. 104–107, 2008.

[8] A. F. de Paula, M. Brito-Júnior, A. C. Quintino, C. C. Camilo, A. M. Cruz-Filho, and M. D. Sousa-Neto, "Three independent mesial canals in a mandibular molar: four-year followup of a case using cone beam computed tomography," *Case Reports in Dentistry*, pp. 891–849, 20132013.

[9] K. S. Al-Fouzan, "The microscopic diagnosis and treatment of a mandibular second premolar with four canals," *International Endodontic Journal*, vol. 34, no. 5, pp. 406–410, 2001.

[10] D. D. Kersten, P. Mines, and M. Sweet, "Use of the microscope in endodontics: results of a questionnaire," *Journal of Endodontics*, vol. 34, no. 7, pp. 804–807, 2008.

[11] M. Karapinar-Kazandag, B. R. Basrani, and S. Friedman, "The operating microscope enhances detection and negotiation of accessory mesial canals in mandibular molars," *Journal of Endodontics*, vol. 36, no. 8, pp. 1289–1294, 2010.

[12] C. Aguiar, D. Mendes, A. Câmara, and J. Figueiredo, "Endodontic treatment of a mandibular second premolar with three root canals," *Journal of Contemporary Dental Practice*, vol. 11, no. 2, pp. 78–84, 2010.

[13] C. M. Ferreira, I. G. de Moraes, and N. Bernardineli, "Three-rooted maxillary second premolar," *Journal of Endodontics*, vol. 26, no. 2, pp. 105–106, 2000.

[14] J. A. Soares and R. T. Leonardo, "Root canal treatment of three-rooted maxillary first and second premolars—a case report," *International Endodontic Journal*, vol. 36, no. 10, pp. 705–710, 2003.

[15] N. Velmurugan, A. Parameswaran, D. Kandaswamy, A. Smitha, D. Vijayalakshmi, and N. Sowmya, "Maxillary second premolar with three roots and three separate root canals—case reports," *Australian Endodontic Journal*, vol. 31, no. 2, pp. 73–75, 2005.

[16] R. Chauhan and A. Chandra, "Endodotic management of three-rooted maxillary first and second premolars: a case report," *General Dentistry*, vol. 60, no. 5, pp. e288–e290, 2012.

[17] R. Grazziotin-Soares, F. Barato Filho, J. R. Vanni et al., "Flexibility of K3 and ProTaper universal instruments," *Brazilian Dental Journal*, vol. 22, no. 3, pp. 218–222, 2011.

11

Excision of Oral Submucous Fibrosis and Reconstruction with Full Thickness Skin Graft

Ahmad Alshadwi[1] and Ishwar Bhatia[2]

[1] *Department of Oral and Maxillofacial Surgery, Boston Medical Center, Boston University, 100 East Newton Street, Boston, MA 02118, USA*
[2] *Department of Oral and Maxillofacial Surgery, Henry Goldman School of Dental Medicine, Boston University, 100 East Newton Street, Boston, MA 02118, USA*

Correspondence should be addressed to Ahmad Alshadwi, alshadwi@bu.edu

Academic Editors: A. Kasaj and A. Loyola

Oral submucous fibrosis is a chronic debilitating disease characterized by gradually increasing fibrosis of the oral cavity and pharynx, mainly the buccal mucosa, resulting in trismus. The highest incidence of oral submucous fibrosis is seen in South India due to various deleterious habits. In spite of the numerous medical modalities employed in the management of oral submucous fibrosis, occasionally surgical intervention becomes inevitable. Various surgical approaches have been used to reconstruct the surgical defects following excision of fibrous bands. Full thickness skin grafts have been described in the literature with variable outcomes. In the present study a 38-year-old male presented with severe oral submucous fibrosis of the buccal mucosa, which was successfully treated and reconstructed using full thickness skin graft with stable functional result after one year of treatment. An integrated review of the literature regarding etiology, histopathology, diagnostic, and treatment modalities of the disease follows.

1. Introduction

Oral submucous fibrosis is commonly seen in the Indian subcontinent. The condition has a multifactorial origin but is commonly associated with chewing of areca nut (betal nut) habitually. This condition was first described by Schwartz in 1952 [1]. Oral submucous fibrosis is a chronic inflammatory reaction in the subepithelial tissue of the oral cavity. It results in increased fibroelastic changes by causing both increased collagen production and decreased collagen breakdown, accompanied by epithelial atrophy [2, 3]. The role of Arecoline and Tannis of areca nut causing juxtaepithelial hyalinization and muscle fibrosis is well described in the literature [4]. The clinical features such as excessive salivation, absent gustatory sensation, and limitation of mouth opening leads to difficulty in chewing, swallowing, articulation, and poor oral hygiene. The oral mucosa appears pale, dense, with vertical fibrotic bands extending to the anterior tonsillar pillars.

Various surgical techniques have been recommended to improve mouth opening in oral submucous fibrosis; we report a case of severe oral submucous fibrosis with limited mouth opening that has been released and reconstructed with full thickness skin graft.

2. Case Report

A 38-year-old Indian male was referred to the Oral and Maxillofacial Surgery Clinic, Boston University Goldman School of Dental Medicine for the evaluation and management of progressive trismus. Patient presented with main complaint of inability to chew food and limited mouth opening. He reported that this has been going on with him for the last few years but became more concern for

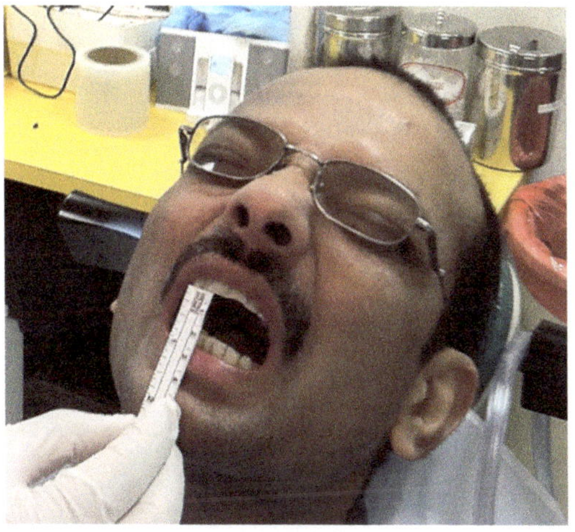

Figure 1: Preoperative view of the patient mouth opening.

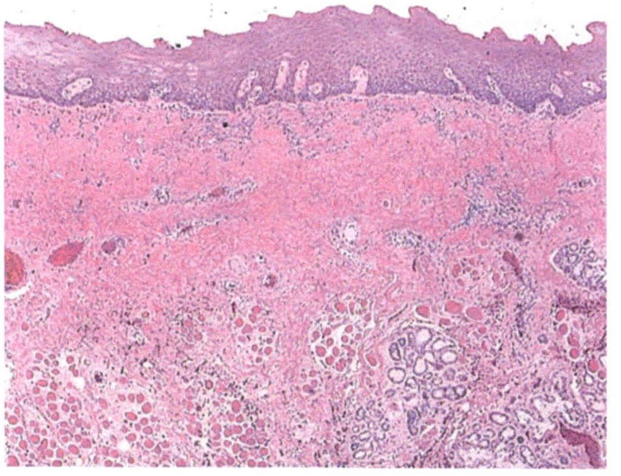

Figure 2: Low magnification H&E stained histopathological slide showing dense fibrosis of the stroma with infiltration to the skeletal muscular layer and minor salivary glands.

him just recently. His medical history was significant for hypertension, hypercholesterolemia, and benign prostatic hyperplasia which all are controlled by medications. Patient reported that he has been chewing pan of Indian tobacco for the last 15 years. Clinical exam showed no lymphadenopathy, swelling, or asymmetry. Limited mouth opening at 15 mm and cranial nerves exam is unremarkable except for alter sensation in the buccal branch of V 3 bilaterally (Figure 1). Intraoral exam showed poor oral hygiene, multiple carious teeth. Palpable severe fibrous bands in buccal mucosa from just inside the commeasure of the mouth up to the pterygomandibular raphe were felt bilaterally. Soft palate, tongue and floor of mouth were not involved. The fibrosis has resulted in pale-appearing mucosa. An incisional biopsy was taken for histopathological evaluation which confirmed the diagnosis of submucous fibrosis infiltrating the muscular layer (Figure 2), after discussion of the clinical findings and treatment options with the patient. The patient was taken to the operating room where he was placed on the surgical table hooked to the anesthesia, cardiac monitors, and pulse oximeter. Next patient was induced via intravenous general anesthesia and intubated with no complications. Local anesthesia was infiltrated in the intended surgical areas. Using a transoral approach a blade number 15 was utilized for the surgical excision of the fibrous bands and protecting underlying vital structures. Surgical dissection was carried out to the level of the buccinator muscle. After controlling bleeding the wound edges were prepared for the graft placement. Next attention was made toward the right thigh from which a 7 × 7 cm full thickness skin graft was harvested (Figure 3); using sharp dissection, was done to the level of the subcutaneous fat. Electrocautery was use to ensure homeostasis and appropriate pressure was placed on the donor site. After that the graft was cut to custom fit each defect and multiple perforations were done throughout the graft to ensure rapid revascularization and prevent hematomas from developing. Next the grafts were sutured into place using 3′0 Chromic Gut restorable sutures in simple interrupted fashion (Figure 4). Mouth opening was measured toward the end of the procedure and was recorded at 32 mm. After that the surgical area was irrigated and patient was extubated and transferred to the recovery room in stable condition. Postoperatively the patient was placed on full liquid diet for two weeks and one week supply of Motrin 400 mg, Percocet 5/325 mg, Keflex 250 mg, Medrol dose pack. Patient was followed regularly and on the second week his mouth opening was noted to decrease to 25 mm at which a course of total of 80 mg of Triamcinolone intramuscular injections were done with 40 mg in each side. Patient was placed on vigorous mouth opening exercises using Therabite devise. Patient responded well to the treatment regimen and maintained mouth opening at 30 mm after 12 months of treatment with good ability to have a satisfactory masticatory function (Figure 5).

3. Discussion

Oral submucous fibrosis is a well-recognized potentially premalignant lesion of the oral cavity. Oral submucous fibrosis is also a common disease in countries where betel nuts are chewed habitually. It is believed to have multiple causes. Local irritants (betel nuts, tobacco, and spicy food), general nutrition, and vitamin deficiencies are considered to risk factors for oral submucous fibrosis [5].

Clinically, the earliest sign of oral submucous fibrosis is mouth soreness with constant burning upon eating spicy foods. Oral submucous fibrosis is clinically divided into 3 stages: stomatitis, fibrosis, and sequelae [6]. During the stomatitis phase, the oral mucosa contains areas of erythema in which vesicles appear. These vesicles later rupture producing ulcers that heal via fibrosis. The primary presenting complaint in this disease is progressive trismus from fibrosis of the buccal submucosa.

Treatment is based on severity of disease. Typically, if the disease is noted before development of trismus, cessation of the betel habit will often resolve the disease. Once trismus has developed and disease is now considered mild to moderate, oral submucous fibrosis is irreversible disease, with the goal of medical and surgical therapy to maintain

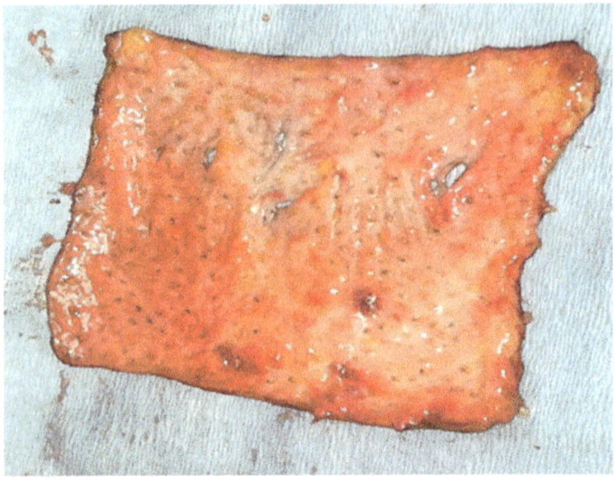

Figure 3: The harvested full skin graft measuring 7 × 7 cm.

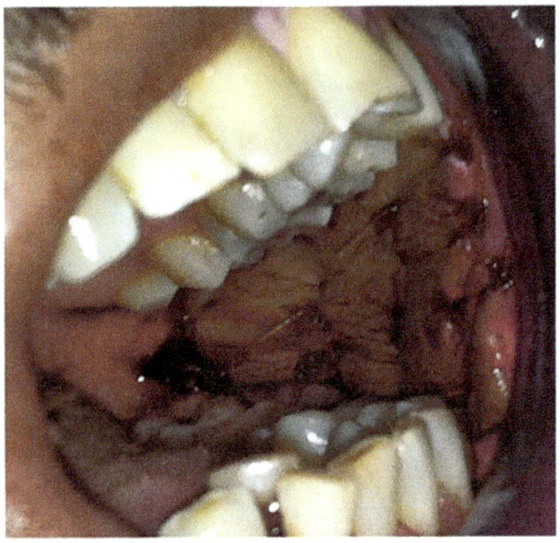

Figure 4: Intraoral views after suturing the graft to the buccal mucosa.

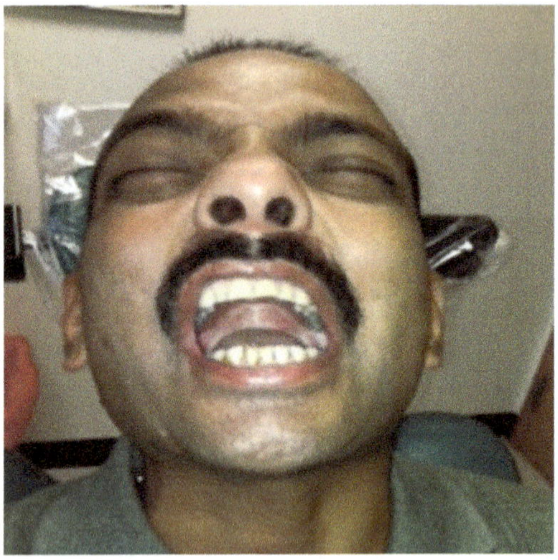

Figure 5: Sustained patient mouth opening at one year followup.

oral function and limit progression of disease. Treatment at this stage is focused on restoring mandibular range of motion, oral cancer surveillance, and cessation of betel nut habit. Physical therapy combined with medical treatment is often utilized. Medical therapy in the United States is limited to weekly submucosal injections of steroids to limit progression of oral submucous fibrosis [7]. For cases in which initial surgical intervention is unsuccessful resulting in recurrent trismus usually secondary to lack of compliance with physical therapy or less commonly from shrinkage of the skin graft or alloplastic graft a more aggressive surgical therapy is indicated. Again, through excision of any fibrous bands intraorally, repeated masticatory muscle myotomy is required. Often in this situation, a larger soft tissue buccal defect is created needing large soft tissue reconstruction. This can include a temporalis pedicled flap, superficial temporalis fascia pedicled flap, or a radial forearm free flap combined with split thickness skin graft coverage [8, 9].

Steroids and especially glucocorticoids were first used in the treatment of oral submucous fibrosis and were extensively used in the past several decades because of their anti-inflammatory property. Cytokines and growth factors produced by inflammatory cells can promote fibrosis by inducing a proliferation of fibroblasts, upregulating collagen synthesis and downregulating collagenase production. Several glucocorticoids were used such as short-acting drugs (hydrocortisone), intermediate-acting drugs (triamcinolone), and long-acting drugs (betamethasone and dexamethasone). Glucocorticoids exert their anti-inflammatory activity by inhibiting the generation of inflammatory factors and increasing the apoptosis of inflammatory cells. They partially relieved patients of their symptoms at an early stage of oral submucous fibrosis as confirmed in many studies [10, 11]. Steroids were less useful in reversing he abnormal deposition of fibrotic tissues and thus this treatment was always associated with a high incidence of relapse.

Several emerging advances were made past few years for the management of oral submucous fibrosis with promising results. Further studies recognized that proliferative fibroblasts, inactive collagenase, and the inhibited fibrinolytic system contributed to the initiation and development of oral submucous fibrosis [12, 13]. In a controlled clinical trial, H. J. Lin and J. C. Lin found that intralesional injections of collagenase resulted not only in significant improvement in mouth-opening but also in a striking reduction of hypersensitivity to spices, sour, cold, and heat. These results indicated that collagenase treatment was approximately fivefold more effective than triamcinolone diacetate [14]. Hyaluronidase also showed a much quicker effect in ameliorating the burning sensation and painful ulceration than did dexamethasone, though the effect was short-term [15]. Chymotrypsin, an endopeptidase, hydrolyzes ester and peptide bonds. It was also used as a proteolytic and anti-inflammatory agent in the treatment of oral submucous fibrosis [16].

Yen was the first to succeed in coveting the buccal defect with a split-thickness skin graft in treating a case of oral submucous fibrosis [17]. Kavarana and Bhathena filled the defect after sectioning of fibrous bands with 2 inferiorly based nasolabial flaps and division of the pedicle after 3 weeks they observed average mouth opening of 2.5 cm with acceptable external scars [18]. R. M. Borle and S. R. Borle reported disappointing results with skin grafting to cover the raw area and used tongue flap to cover the defect [19]. Khanna and Andrade reported the incidence of shrinkage, contraction, and rejection of split skin graft as very high leading to poor oral condition with recurrence in 12 cases [20]. Mehrotra et al. present a case series of 100 patients where they compared buccal fat pad graft, tongue flap, nasolabial fold flap, and split skin graft for correction of mucosal defect created after incising the fibrous bands. Esthetics and function achieved with split skin graft were good but showed some degree of relapse due to contracture of the graft. They found that buccal fat pad rotation was superior to other procedures [21].

Microscopically diffuse fibrosis in the submucosa with a chronic inflammatory infiltrate is the hallmark of oral submucous fibrosis. Atrophic changes in the mucosal layer include thinning of the epithelium, loss of rete ridges, sawtoothing, and liquefaction degeneration of the basal layer. Pigmentation is incontinence; Isaac et al. found that pigmentation was present in 62% of the 35 specimens they studied [22]. Areas of ulceration are usually seen replaced by granulation tissue. Fibrosis in the submucosa can be classified as mild if early fibrosis was present, moderate if diffuse fibrosis was seen, and severe if there was diffuse fibrosis with hyalinization and atrophic changes in minor salivary glands and skeletal muscle. Chronic inflammatory cells (i.e., lymphocytes, plasma cells, and macrophages) are also seen. As reported in the literature, the risk of oral cancer developing in oral submucous fibrosis is 7.6% over a period of 10 years [23]. Daftary reported that on followup, one third of his patients suffering from oral submucous fibrosis ultimately developing oral cancer [24].

In summary all available treatments for oral submucous fibrosis are basically palliative in nature. Surgical procedures are indicated only in cases with advanced disease. A safe and simple mode of treatment such as steroid or enzymes injection along with proper habit restriction should be selected in the earlier stages of the disease. Early detection is key toward better prognosis and outcome.

Conflict of Interests

The authors declare no conflict of interests.

References

[1] J. Schwartz, "Atrophia idiopathica mucosa oris," in *Proceedings of the 11th International Dental Congress*, London, UK, 1952.

[2] W. G. Shafer, M. K. Hine, and B. M. Levy, "Benign and malignant tumors of the oral cavity," in *A Textbook of Oral Pathology*, W. G. Shafer, M. K. Hine, and B. M. Levy, Eds., pp. 86–229, WB Saunders, Philadelphia, Pa, USA, 4th edition, 1983.

[3] B. W. Neville, D. D. Damm, C. M. Allen et al., "Epithelial pathology," in *Oral and Maxillofacial Pathology*, B. W. Neville, D. D. Damm, C. M. Allen et al., Eds., pp. 315–387, WB Saunders, Philadelphia, Pa, USA, 2nd edition, 2002.

[4] R. Pillai, P. Balaram, and K. S. Reddiar, "Pathogenesis of oral submucous fibrosis: relationship to risk factors associated with oral cancer," *Cancer*, vol. 69, no. 8, pp. 2011–2020, 1992.

[5] R. Maher, P. Aga, N. W. Johnson, R. Sankaranarayanan, and S. Warnakulasuriya, "Evaluation of multiple micronutrient supplementation in the management of oral submucous fibrosis in Karachi, Pakistan," *Nutrition and Cancer*, vol. 27, no. 1, pp. 41–47, 1997.

[6] J. J. Pindborg, "Oral submucous fibrosis—a review," *Annals of the Academy of Medicine*, vol. 18, no. 5, pp. 603–607, 1989.

[7] S. R. Aziz, "Oral submucous fibrosis: case report and review of diagnosis and treatment," *Journal of Oral and Maxillofacial Surgery*, vol. 66, no. 11, pp. 2386–2389, 2008.

[8] J. T. Lee, L. F. Cheng, P. R. Chen et al., "Bipaddled radial forearm flap for the reconstruction of bilateral buccal defects in oral submucous fibrosis," *International Journal of Oral and Maxillofacial Surgery*, vol. 36, no. 7, pp. 615–619, 2007.

[9] N. J. Mokal, R. S. Raje, S. V. Ranade, J. S. R. Prasad, and R. L. Thatte, "Release of oral submucous fibrosis and reconstruction using superficial temporal fascia flap and split skin graft—a new technique," *British Journal of Plastic Surgery*, vol. 58, no. 8, pp. 1055–1060, 2005.

[10] D. R. Lai, H. R. Chen, L. M. Lin, Y. L. Huang, and C. C. Tsai, "Clinical evaluation of different treatment methods for oral submucous fibrosis. A 10-year experience with 150 cases," *Journal of Oral Pathology & Medicine*, vol. 24, no. 9, pp. 402–406, 1995.

[11] P. K. Kakar, R. K. Puri, and V. P. Venkatachalam, "Oral submucous fibrosis—treatment with hyalase," *Journal of Laryngology and Otology*, vol. 99, no. 1, pp. 57–59, 1985.

[12] S. F. Yang, Y. S. Hsieh, C. H. Tsai, M. Y. Chou, and Y. C. Chang, "The upregulation of type I plasminogen activator inhibitor in oral submucous fibrosis," *Oral Oncology*, vol. 39, no. 4, pp. 367–372, 2003.

[13] T. Y. Shieh and J. F. Yang, "Collagenase activity in oral submucous fibrosis," *Proceedings of the National Science Council, Republic of China. Part B*, vol. 16, no. 2, pp. 106–110, 1992.

[14] H. J. Lin and J. C. Lin, "Treatment of oral submucous fibrosis by collagenase: effects on oral opening and eating function," *Oral Diseases*, vol. 13, no. 4, pp. 407–413, 2007.

[15] X. Jiang and J. Hu, "Drug treatment of oral submucous fibrosis: a review of the literature," *Journal of Oral and Maxillofacial Surgery*, vol. 67, no. 7, pp. 1510–1515, 2009.

[16] D. Gupta and S. C. Sharma, "Oral submucous fibrosis—a new treatment regimen," *Journal of Oral and Maxillofacial Surgery*, vol. 46, no. 10, pp. 830–833, 1988.

[17] D. J. C. Yen, "Surgical treatment of submucous fibrosis," *Oral Surgery, Oral Medicine, and Oral Pathology*, vol. 54, no. 3, pp. 269–272, 1982.

[18] N. M. Kavarana and H. M. Bhathena, "Surgery for severe trismus in submucous fibrosis," *British Journal of Plastic Surgery*, vol. 40, no. 4, pp. 407–409, 1987.

[19] R. M. Borle and S. R. Borle, "Management of oral submucous fibrosis: a conservative approach," *Journal of Oral and Maxillofacial Surgery*, vol. 49, no. 8, pp. 788–791, 1991.

[20] J. N. Khanna and N. N. Andrade, "Oral submucous fibrosis: a new concept in surgical management. Report of 100 cases," *International Journal of Oral and Maxillofacial Surgery*, vol. 24, no. 6, pp. 433–439, 1995.

[21] D. Mehrotra, R. Pradhan, and S. Gupta, "Retrospective comparison of surgical treatment modalities in 100 patients

with oral submucous fibrosis," *Oral Surgery, Oral Medicine, Oral Pathology, Oral Radiology and Endodontology*, vol. 107, no. 3, pp. e1–e10, 2009.

[22] U. Isaac, J. S. Issac, and N. Ahmed Khoso, "Histopathologic features of oral submucous fibrosis: a study of 35 biopsy specimens," *Oral Surgery, Oral Medicine, Oral Pathology, Oral Radiology and Endodontology*, vol. 106, no. 4, pp. 556–560, 2008.

[23] S. C. Cox and D. M. Walker, "Oral submucous fibrosis. A review," *Australian Dental Journal*, vol. 41, no. 5, pp. 294–299, 1996.

[24] D. K. Daftary, "Oral precancerous lesions and conditions of tropical interest," in *Oral Diseases in the Tropics*, S. R. Prabhu, D. F. Wilson, D. K. Daftary, and N. W. Johnson, Eds., p. 119, Oxford University Press, Oxford, UK, 1992.

12

Molariform Mesiodens in Primary Dentition

Sachin B. Mangalekar,[1] Tajammul Ahmed,[2] M. Zakirulla,[3]
Halawar Sangmesh Shivappa,[4] F. B. Bheemappa,[5] and Chandrashekar Yavagal[6]

[1] *Department of Periodontology, Maitri Dental College, Chattisgarh, India*
[2] *Department of Prosthodontics, Al Jabal Al Gharbi University, Gharyan, Libya*
[3] *Department of Pediatric Dentistry, College of Dentistry, King Khalid University, Abha, Saudi Arabia*
[4] *Vasant Dada Dental College, Kavalapur, Sangli, Maharashtra, India*
[5] *P.M.N.M. Dental College and Hospital, Bagalkot, Karnataka, India*
[6] *Department of Pediatric Dentistry, Dr. Hedgewar Dental College, Hingoli, Maharashtra, India*

Correspondence should be addressed to Sachin B. Mangalekar; drsachinbm@gmail.com

Academic Editors: I. Anic, P. G. Arduino, N. Brezniak, Y.-K. Chen, and E. F. Wright

Mesiodens is a midline supernumerary tooth commonly seen in the maxillary arch, and incidence of molariform mesiodens in the maxillary midline is rare in permanent dentition and extremely uncommon in primary dentition. A midline supernumerary tooth in the primary dentition can cause ectopic or delayed eruption of permanent central incisors which will further alter occlusion and may compromise esthetics and formation of dentigerous cysts. This paper reports a rare case of the presence of a molariform mesiodens in the primary dentition. On clinical and radiographic examination, flaring of the primary central incisors was seen, with a molariform mesiodens consisting of multiple lobes or tubercles on the occlusal surface with the well-formed root. The treatment plan consisted of the extraction of the supernumerary tooth and regular observation of permanent central incisors for proper eruption and alignment.

1. Introduction

The term mesiodens refers to a supernumerary tooth present in the midline of the maxilla between the two maxillary central incisors. The occurrence of mesiodens in primary dentition is quite rare despite the fact that in permanent dentition it has even been considered as the most common dental abnormality [1]. The reported prevalence in general population ranges between 0.15% and 3.8% in the permanent dentition whereas in the primary dentition, it ranges between 0% and 1.9% [2, 3]. No significant sex distribution is noted in the primary supernumerary teeth [4]. It has been believed that environmental factors along with hereditary factors are combined to cause the condition [5]. However, the presence of multilobed or tuberculate form of mesiodens in the deciduous dentition is extremely rare and is mentioned only once or twice in the literature [6].

2. A Case Report

A six-year-old girl along with her mother reported to the department with the complaint of a tooth with an unusual appearance in the upper front teeth area. On intraoral examination, a mesiodens was noticed in the maxillary arch with multiple lobes or tubercles on the occlusal surface. Patient had full complement of deciduous teeth with no other anomalies. Medical and family history was not relevant and noncontributory. Luten's criteria [7] and Howard's classification [8] were used to carefully evaluate the supernumerary tooth which revealed four separate lobes with well-formed developmental grooves on the occlusal surface of the mesiodens which could be clearly distinguished. The presence of the tuberculate mesiodens resulted in reduced space in arch between the central incisors causing flaring of them (Figure 1). On examination of the central incisors, they exhibited grade-II

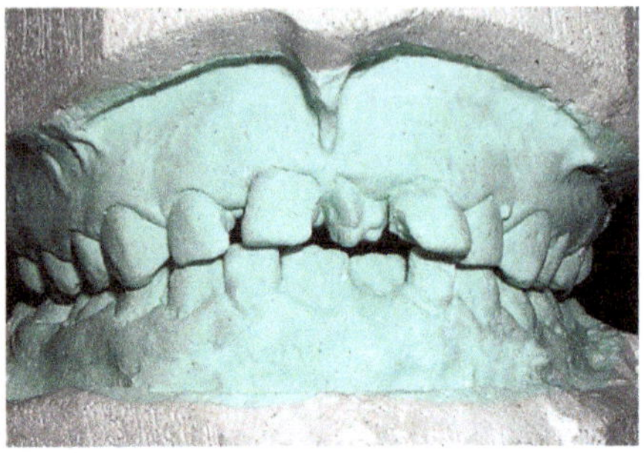

FIGURE 1: Model showing multilobulated mesiodens between maxillary primary central incisors.

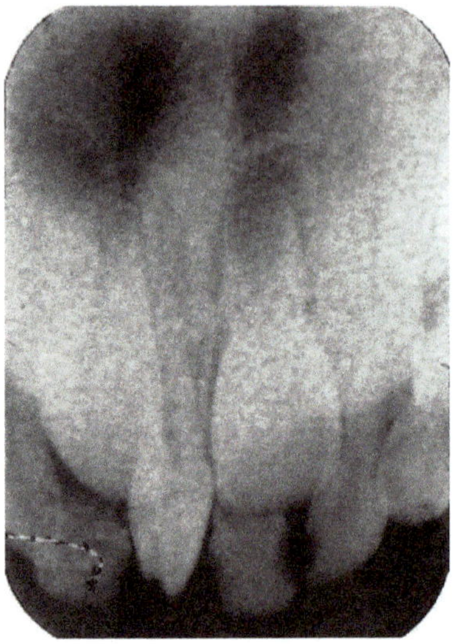

FIGURE 2: IOPA radiograph showing multilobulated mesiodens between maxillary primary central incisors.

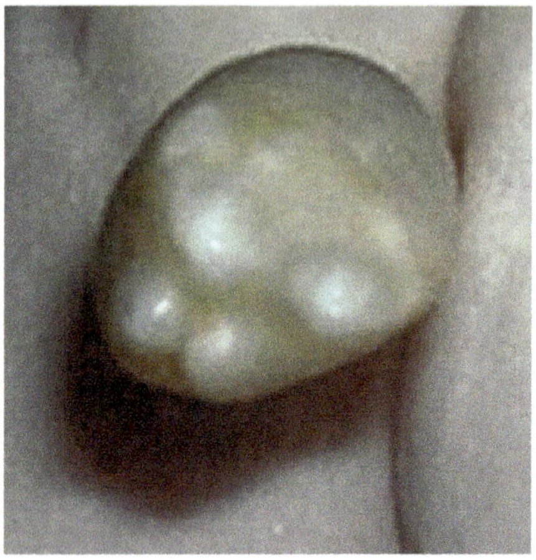

FIGURE 3: Molariform mesiodens after extraction.

mobility and neared exfoliation. There was no interference of the mesiodens in occlusion. Radiographic examination with periapical radiograph revealed completely formed root and the presence of multiple cusps that were well demarcated on the radiograph with resorption of incisors roots (Figure 2).

Based on the clinical and radiographic examinations, the supernumerary tooth was diagnosed as a multilobed tuberculate mesiodens in the deciduous dentition. A comprehensive treatment plan was formulated, which included extraction of the deciduous central incisors and the tuberculate mesiodens under local anaesthesia (Figure 3). Their presence would have significant impact on the eruption and position of the permanent central incisors and possibility of future malocclusion.

3. Discussion

The presence of the mesiodens in the permanent dentition is well documented. Mesiodens in the permanent dentition show great variation and are classified accordingly.

Possible explanation for the less frequent reporting of deciduous supernumerary teeth includes infrequent detection by parents, as the spacing frequently encountered in the deciduous dentition may be utilized to allow the supernumerary tooth or teeth to erupt with reasonable alignment. Also, many children have an initial dental examination following the eruption of the permanent anterior teeth so anterior deciduous teeth which have erupted and exfoliated normally would not be detected [9].

Numerous classifications have been proposed in the literature to classify supernumerary with varied acceptance. No single classification is adequate and is used according to the convenience.

The classifications are based on location; morphology, axial inclination, and other criterion are used for classification of such teeth. Sometimes the presence of supernumerary teeth is seen in developmental syndromic cases such as cleft lip, and palate, cleidocranial dysostosis, Down's syndrome and Gardener's syndrome. Other cases where syndromic involvement is seen are enumerated in Box 1.

The aetiology of the supernumerary teeth is not clearly understood despite its regular presentation. Various theories have been postulated to explain the same. Atavistic theory states that mesiodens represented a phylogenetic relic of extinct ancestors who exhibited three central incisors [10]. Another theory suggests that the supernumerary tooth is a result of dichotomy of the tooth bud; others suggest that they are the result of local independent conditioned hyperactivity of dental lamina. Heredity can also play a pivotal role in the formation of the supernumerary teeth sometimes associated with or without syndromes. Association of supernumerary teeth is also seen with cysts like dentigerous cysts and odontomes [11]. The presence of multilobed mesiodens with palatal talon cusp is also reported in the literature [12].

Management of patients with supernumerary teeth may vary from simple extractions coupled with orthodontic therapy to attain a good occlusion as well as aesthetics. Occasionally, retaining such teeth would be prudent where space considerations impacted supernumerary without any problems; in such cases simple routine followup is required.

Multiple lobulated mesiodens with developmental grooves can present with a problem in terms of maintaining a proper oral hygiene which would invariably lead to

(i) Cleidocranial dysplasia
(ii) Apert syndrome
(iii) Angio osteohypertrophy
(iv) Cranial metaphyseal dysplasia
(v) The Crouzon disease
(vi) The Curtis disease
(vii) The Ehler-Danlos syndrome
(viii) The Fabry-Anderson disease
(ix) The Fucosidosis
(x) The Hallermann-Streiff syndrome
(xi) The Klippel-Trénaunay-Weber syndrome
(xii) Laband syndrome
(xiii) Nance-Horan's syndrome
(xiv) Treacher-Collins's syndrome
(xv) Oral-facial-digital syndrome, type I and II
(xvi) The Sturge-Weber disease
(xvii) The Tricho-rhino-phalangeal syndrome.
(xviii) The Zimmermann-Laband syndrome

Box 1: Supernumerary teeth associated with syndromes.

(i) Delayed eruption of permanent teeth
(ii) Displacement of permanent teeth
(iii) Crowding
(iv) Aesthetic problem in the maxillary anterior region
(v) Abnormal formation of roots of permanent teeth.
(vi) Resulting in dilacerations
(vii) Diastema or spacing.
(viii) Impacted mesiodens may interfere with the eruption of permanent teeth causing malocclusion.
(ix) Failure of eruption or impaction of permanent teeth
(x) Resorption of roots of adjacent teeth
(xi) Loss of tooth vitality of adjacent teeth
(xii) Cystic lesions
(xiii) Ectopic eruption into nasal cavity and in other anatomical spaces
(xiv) Development of dental caries

Box 2: Complications that are associated with mesiodens.

development of caries. Complications that are associated with mesiodens are enumerated in Box 2.

In the present case, the erupted multilobulated mesiodens in the 6-year-old girl was a great aesthetic concern to the patient and their family members; however, the presence of the multilobulated mesiodens in the primary dentition is extremely rare. Only one case in the literature was reported by Sharma [13]. In the present case, the crown of the mesiodens presented with unusual crown morphology with 4 separately well-formed lobes with developmental grooves and full formed root. Failure to identify or not treating would have resulted in a deep impact on the child causing psychological trauma and imitate malocclusion.

4. Conclusion

A careful examination by clinical and radiographic methods can reveal a rare manifestation of the presence of hyperdontia, and they can cause and increase the incidence of malocclusion. No single tailored treatment is available. Treatment planning can be done based on the clinical case. In the present case, the presence of such teeth would have created a different path of eruption of the permanent central incisors and would have resulted in deranging the occlusion and poor aesthetics for the child.

References

[1] D. Ray, B. Bhattacharya, S. Sarkar, and G. Das, "Erupted maxillary conical mesiodens in deciduous dentition in a Bengali girl—a case report," *Journal of Indian Society of Pedodontics and Preventive Dentistry*, vol. 23, no. 3, pp. 153–155, 2005.

[2] A. Sharma, S. Gupta, and M. Madan, "Uncommon mesiodens—a report of two cases," *Journal of the Indian Society of Pedodontics and Preventive Dentistry*, vol. 17, no. 2, pp. 69–71, 1999.

[3] N. T. Prabhu, J. Rebecca, and A. K. Munshi, "Mesiodens in the primary dentition—a case report," *Journal of the Indian Society of Pedodontics and Preventive Dentistry*, vol. 16, no. 3, pp. 93–95, 1998.

[4] Y. Zilberman, M. Malron, and A. Shteyer, "Assessment of 100 children in Jerusalem with supernumerary teeth in the premaxillary region," *Journal of Dentistry for Children*, vol. 59, no. 1, pp. 44–47, 1992.

[5] G. van Buggenhout and I. Bailleul-Forestier, "Mesiodens," *European Journal of Medical Genetics*, vol. 51, no. 2, pp. 178–181, 2008.

[6] A. Shah, D. S. Gill, C. Tredwin, and F. B. Naini, "Diagnosis and management of supernumerary teeth," *Dental Update*, vol. 35, no. 8, pp. 510–520, 2008.

[7] J. R. Luten Jr., "The prevalence of supernumerary teeth in primary and mixed dentitions," *Journal of Dentistry for Children*, vol. 34, no. 5, pp. 346–353, 1967.

[8] R. D. Howard, "The unerupted incisor. A study of the postoperative eruptive history of incisors delayed in their eruption by supernumerary teeth," *The Dental Practitioner and Dental Record*, vol. 17, no. 9, pp. 332–341, 1967.

[9] M. Bhat, "Supplemental mandibular central incisor," *Journal of Indian Society of Pedodontics and Preventive Dentistry*, vol. 24, pp. S20–S23, 2006.

[10] A. Stellzig, E. K. Basdra, and G. Komposch, "Mesiodens: incidence, morphology, etiology," *Journal of Orofacial Orthopedics*, vol. 58, no. 3, pp. 144–153, 1997.

[11] H. O. Sedano and R. J. Gorlin, "Familial occurrence of mesiodens," *Oral Surgery, Oral Medicine, Oral Pathology*, vol. 27, no. 3, pp. 360–362, 1969.

[12] N. B. Nagaveni, K. V. Umashankara, Sreedevi, B. P. Reddy, N. B. Radhika, and T. S. Satisha, "Multi-lobed mesiodens with a palatal talon cusp—a rare case report," *Brazilian Dental Journal*, vol. 21, no. 4, pp. 375–378, 2010.

[13] A. Sharma, "Familial occurence of mesiodens—a case report," *Journal of the Indian Society of Pedodontics and Preventive Dentistry*, vol. 21, no. 2, pp. 84–85, 2003.

13

Cone Beam Computed Tomography Evaluation of the Periapical Status of Nonvital Tooth with Open Apex Obturated with Mineral Trioxide Aggregate: A Case Report

Vijay Shekhar and K. Shashikala

Department of Conservative Dentistry and Endodontics, D.A.P.M.R.V. Dental College and Hospital, Bangalore, Karnataka 560078, India

Correspondence should be addressed to Vijay Shekhar; ruchi_dolly_arora@yahoo.co.in

Academic Editors: D. W. Boston, L. Junquera, A. Kasaj, C. Ledesma-Montes, A. Markopoulos, and A. Milosevic

Management of a tooth with open apex is a challenge to the dental practitioners. Evaluation of the periapical healing is required in such cases by radiographic techniques. The objective of this paper was to assess the healing of a periapical lesion in a non-vital tooth with open apex treated with mineral trioxide aggregate (MTA) obturation using cone beam computed tomography (CBCT). The endodontic treatment of a fractured non-vital discolored maxillary left lateral incisor with an open apex was done with MTA obturation. The clinical and radiographic followup done regularly showed that the tooth was clinically asymptomatic and that the size of the periapical lesion observed by intraoral periapical (IOPA) radiographs and CBCT was decreased remarkably after two years. CBCT and IOPA radiographs were found to be useful radiographic tools to assess the healing of a large periapical lesion in a non-vital tooth with open apex managed by MTA obturation.

1. Introduction

Periapical lesion of endodontic origin is one of the most frequently occurring pathologic conditions found in the alveolar bone. It represents an inflammatory response to bacterial infection of the root canals. Periapical lesions may progress from the inflammation of the periodontal ligament around the root apex (apical periodontitis) into a variety of pathologic conditions, like apical abscess, periapical granuloma, and radicular cyst. Besides the possible clinical signs and symptoms associated with the periapical lesions, there are changes in the mineralization and structure of the periradicular bone which results in resorption. This can be visualized by various radiographic techniques as periapical radiolucencies. Their management is initially done with nonsurgical endodontic treatment. Surgical intervention is recommended when nonsurgical procedures have been unable to resolve the periapical lesions. Studies have reported high success rate (upto 94%) of healing of periapical lesions following nonsurgical endodontic therapy [1].

Complete asepsis and three-dimensional obturation of the root-canal system is essential for long-term endodontic success [2, 3]. Cessation of root development caused by trauma or pulpal disease presents both endodontic and restorative challenges. The thin fragile root-canal dentin walls may be too weak to withstand the normal forces of mastication, making them prone to fracture [3, 4]. The divergent apical architecture (blunderbuss canal) and absence of normal apical constriction of root canal make complete debridement, canal disinfection, and control of obturation material nearly impossible [3–7]. Occasionally, the filling is inadequate or the filling materials extrude beyond apex into periradicular tissues, which may have harmful effect on the prognosis of endodontic treatment. The use of biomaterials has been advocated to encourage periapical regeneration and prevent complications if overfilling occurs [8, 9].

Apexification with calcium hydroxide was the treatment of choice in necrotic teeth with open apex in the last decades [3, 4, 6–11]. The long-term use of calcium hydroxide had several disadvantages, including multiple appointments, possible recontamination of the root canal during the treatment period, and increased brittleness of the root dentin [2–4, 8, 9]. The new treatment concept involves eliminating the gutta-percha obturation step after apexification. MTA, placed in an apexification technique, could become the sole obturation material, preserving and restoring the open apex [4].

Mineral trioxide aggregate (MTA; ProRoot, Dentsply, Tulsa, OK, USA) has been proposed as obturation material as it can completely seal the root-canal system [1, 4, 5]. According to the manufacturer, MTA is a mixture of three powder ingredients: Portland cement, bismuth oxide, and gypsum. When mixed with sterile water, hydration reaction occurs and MTA sets, even in the presence of moisture. The pH of MTA increases from 10 to 12.5, three hours after mixing. It is assumed that in a high pH environment, calcium ions, that are released from MTA, react with phosphates in the tissue fluid to form hydroxyapatite. This would explain its favorable sealing ability and biocompatibility [1, 10, 11]. MTA has shown potential as a root-end filling material, root/furcal perforations sealing material, and a direct pulp capping agent after pulp exposure, pulpotomy agent, and root-canal filling material in teeth with complete and incomplete root development. Despite its outstanding tissue biocompatibility, MTA has few disadvantages, which include delayed setting time, poor handling characteristics, unpredictable antibacterial effects, and high cost [1].

It has long been debated whether bone healing after endodontic treatment is ongoing or whether the treatment effort has been futile. The endodontic treatment is considered successful when there is absence of periapical radiolucency at periapex of endodontically treated roots. The newer diagnostic method such as cone beam computed tomography (CBCT) is considered as a useful diagnostic tool for assessing periapical healing by measuring true size of the periapical lesion three-dimensionally, which is mostly underestimated by intraoral periapical (IOPA) radiographs [12–15].

CBCT is one of the latest and most advanced types of digital radiography. Here, an object is exposed to multiple cone-shaped beams that travel 360° around the patient with the motion center placed in the area of interest and the X-ray detector on the opposite side of the circle. Later, serial sagittal, coronal, and axial section images are obtained, allowing the clinician to visualize morphologic features and pathologies from different three-dimensional perspectives eliminating the superimposition of anatomical structures. For endodontic purposes, the limited volume or focused CBCT scanners are used which capture small volumes of data encompassing just 3-4 individual teeth. CBCT may also be useful in the evaluation of the root-canal anatomy, canal preparation, obturation, retreatment, coronal microleakage, and periapical lesions, including their relatively true size, extent, nature, and position.

The following case report describes evaluation of healing of a large periapical lesion in an asymptomatic non-vital left maxillary lateral incisor with an open apex treated with MTA obturation using CBCT and IOPA radiographs over a period of two years.

2. Case Report

A 24-year-old healthy female patient was reported with the chief complaint of broken left upper front teeth. Patient had history of fall 15 years back which resulted in fracture of the crowns and occasional mild pain in left upper front teeth since then, for which she took painkillers prescribed by a local doctor to provide symptomatic relief. There was no history of discharge or swelling. The patient came for definite treatment six months back.

On clinical examination, Ellis class 2 fracture was noted in teeth 21 and 22 (Figure 1(a)). Vitality (heat, cold and electric) tests revealed that both teeth were non-vital. Tooth 22 was discolored. There were no signs of maxillofacial fracture or swelling or mobility. The soft tissue examination was noncontributory. Radiographic examination with IOPA radiograph revealed a well-defined radiolucency with respect to the apex of both teeth and a wide open apex in tooth 22 (Figure 1(b)).

Based on the clinical and radiographic findings, a diagnosis of periapical granuloma involving teeth 21 and 22 was established. A treatment plan involving endodontic therapy was proposed, with MTA obturation in tooth 22, followed by ceramic crowns.

The endodontic treatment was done under rubber dam isolation. First, access opening was done, followed by working length determination (Figure 1(c)). Cleaning and shaping were done by circumferential filing in tooth 22. Obturation of tooth 21 was done with conventional lateral condensation of gutta-percha. In tooth 22, calcium hydroxide dressing was placed in the first appointment, which was removed one week later, with alternate sodium hypochlorite and saline irrigation. The canals were thoroughly dried with paper points. The ProRoot gray MTA was mixed to a paste consistency with sterile water and delivered to the canal using Messing gun. A plugger was used to condense MTA homogeneously into the canal (Figure 1(d)). A moist cotton pellet was sealed inside for setting of MTA. It was noteworthy that there was inadvertent extrusion of MTA into the periapical region during its compaction.

The composite core build-up and tooth preparation was done on both teeth for ceramic crowns in the next appointment (Figure 2(a)). Temporization was done with acrylic crowns (Figure 2(b)). The occlusion was carefully checked and adjusted. Permanent crowns were not placed immediately as they would have interfered with the planned postoperative followup of the healing of periapical lesion using CBCT. The patient was given instructions to avoid any activities that could lead to trauma to the teeth and was recalled for followup. The permanent crowns, that is, porcelain fused-to-metal (PFM) crowns, were cemented on both teeth six months after the endodontic treatment and followup with CBCT (Figure 2(c)).

The postoperative evaluation of the periapical lesion was done clinically as well as radiographically, with both IOPA radiographs and CBCT. The IOPA radiographic evaluation revealed a decreasing size of the periapical radiolucency at each visit after one month, three months, six months, one year, and two years (Figures 3(a)–3(e)). The follow-up

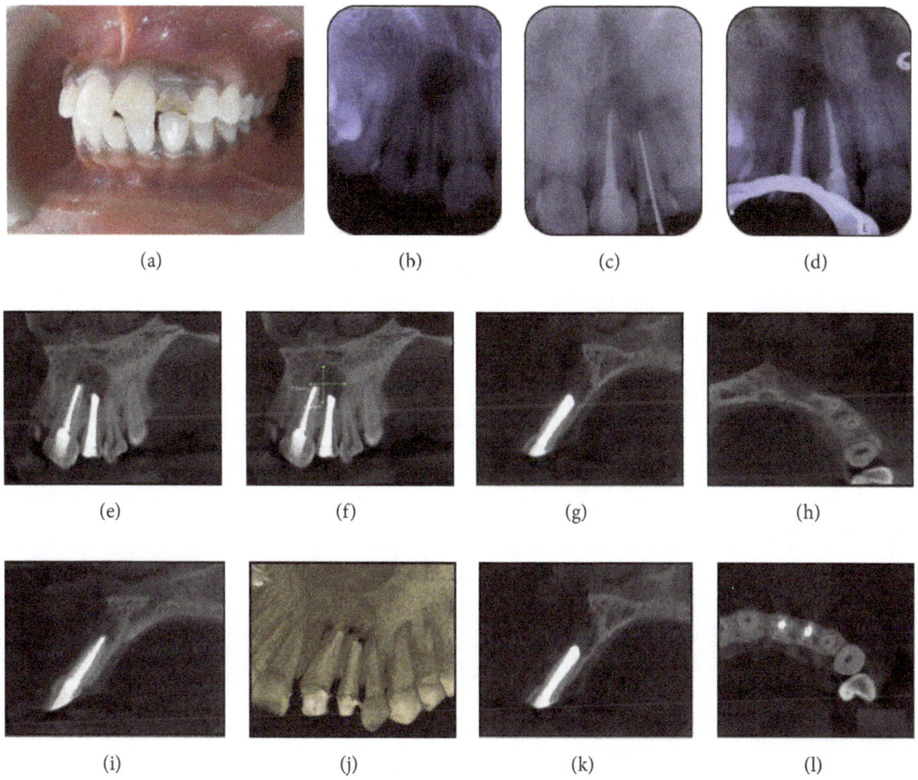

FIGURE 1: (a) Preoperative photo showing crown fracture and discoloration in left maxillary lateral incisor. (b) IOPA radiograph showing well-defined radiolucency and open apex. (c) Working length IOPA radiograph. (d) IOPA radiograph showing MTA obturation. (e) Coronal plane CBCT image showing size of periapical lesion immediately after MTA obturation. (f) Coronal plane CBCT image showing size of periapical lesion; dimensions 9.8 mm/7.5 mm. (g) Sagittal plane CBCT image showing size of periapical lesion immediately after MTA obturation. (h) Axial plane CBCT image showing size of periapical lesion immediately after MTA obturation. (i) Sagittal plane CBCT image showing size of periapical lesion immediately after endodontic treatment in tooth 21. (j) Three-dimensional CBCT image of periapical lesion immediately after MTA obturation. (k) Sagittal plane CBCT image showing status of MTA obturation. (l) Axial plane CBCT image showing status of MTA obturation.

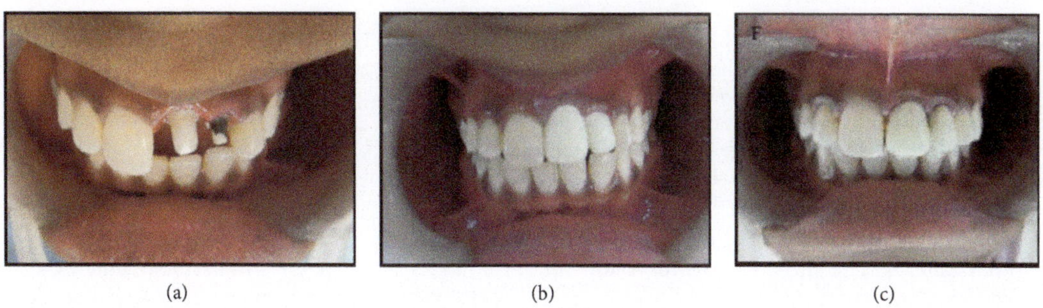

FIGURE 2: (a) Build-up with composite and tooth preparation. (b) Temporization with acrylic crowns. (c) Permanent cementation of PFM crowns.

radiograph taken two years after treatment revealed that the periapical radiolucency was almost unnoticeable, in relation to both teeth.

CBCT examination was done immediately after MTA obturation (Figures 1(e)–1(l)) using limited field of view CBCT unit (9000 3D, KODAK, USA). The second CBCT evaluation done after six months revealed a decrease in the size of periapical radiolucency in all the three planes—coronal, sagittal, and axial and in three-dimensional reconstruction images (Figures 3(f)–3(j)). The status of MTA obturation as evaluated with CBCT revealed a well compacted filling up to the apex with no voids, even after six months (Figures 3(k)-3(l)). The patient when observed clinically after two years was asymptomatic and had no complaint of

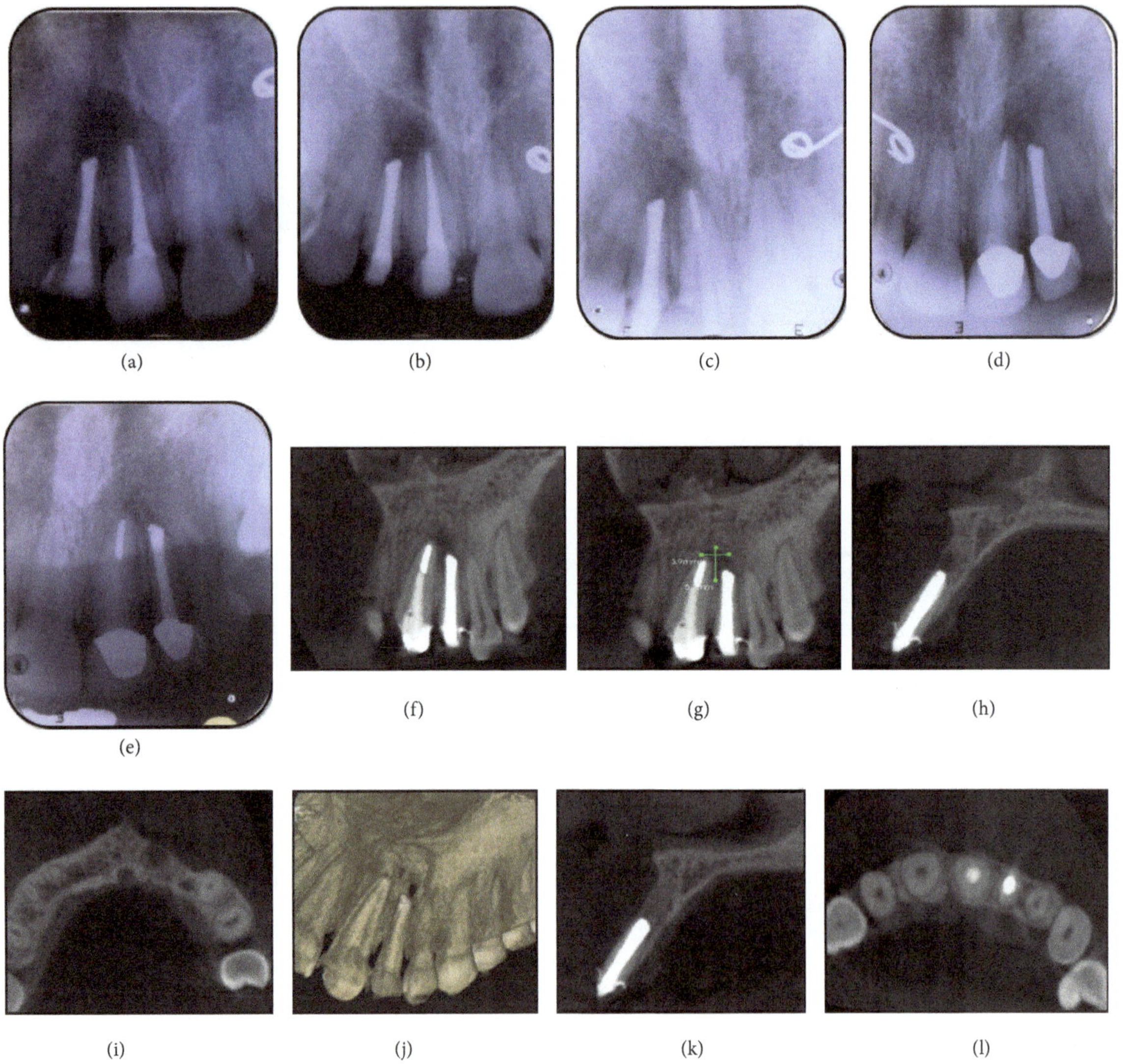

FIGURE 3: (a) IOPA radiograph at one month. (b) IOPA radiograph at three months. (c) IOPA radiograph at six months. (d) IOPA radiograph at one year. (e) IOPA radiograph at two-year followup. (f) Coronal plane CBCT image showing decreased size of periapical lesion at six months. (g) Coronal plane CBCT image showing measurement of periapical lesion; dimensions 5.7 mm/3.9 mm. (h) Sagittal plane CBCT image showing decrease in size of periapical lesion at six months. (i) Axial plane CBCT image showing decrease in size of periapical lesion at six months. (j) Three-dimensional CBCT image showing periapical lesion six months. (k) Sagittal plane CBCT image showing status of MTA obturation at six months. (l) Axial plane CBCT image showing status of root-canal filling at six months.

discomfort. The patient is scheduled to come for follow-up yearly in the department.

3. Discussion

Bacterial infection of the dental pulp may lead to periapical lesion. Its treatment involves eradicating or substantially reducing the number of root-canal pathogens and preventing reinfection by three-dimensional obturation. When endodontic treatment is done properly, healing of the periapical lesion occurs with hard tissue regeneration, which is characterized by gradual resolution of the periapical radiolucency [1].

In the present case, the radiographic evaluation of the periapical lesion after two years revealed an excellent treatment outcome which is comparable with similar previously reported cases of successful MTA apexification in necrotic open apex teeth with periradicular lesions. In such teeth, the outcome of conventional gutta-percha fillings would be doubtful, while MTA has the potential to provide an effective seal, even in the presence of moisture such as in a blunderbuss root canal [5]. Furthermore, several studies have confirmed the superior biocompatibility of MTA as a root-end filling material for the periodontal tissues and the regeneration of periradicular tissues to an almost normal condition [8].

When treating non-vital teeth, a main issue is eliminating bacteria from the root canal system. In this case, in order to limit bacterial infection before obturation with MTA, irrigation with sodium hypochlorite was done and short-term intracanal calcium hydroxide medication was placed within the canal for one week. The rationale was to enhance the difficult task of debriding the canal system with an open apex [6]. Researchers showed that the remains of calcium hydroxide on the dentinal walls had no significant effect on MTA microleakage. Others have suggested that the combination of MTA and calcium hydroxide in apexification procedures may favorably influence the regeneration of the periodontium.

In necrotic teeth with open apex, the absence of apical constriction complicates the adaptation of MTA to root canal. A hand condensation technique was used in this case to overcome this difficulty. This technique resulted in improved adaptation and fewer voids than the thermoplasticised gutta-percha techniques used traditionally. Due to the physical and handling properties of MTA, this material is more likely to extrude apically in an open apex. When the extruded root-canal filling material contacts periradicular tissues, reactions like mild to severe inflammation, allergic reactions, and neurotoxic effects may occur. Gutta-percha and calcium hydroxide are the most common materials associated with these complications. Conversely, the extrusion of MTA root-canal filling biomaterial into a periradicular lesion does not produce complications, which was confirmed with CBCT in this case. Recently, the biological basis for the favorable properties of MTA has been attributed to the production of hydroxyapatite. Furthermore, the deposition of cellular cementum adjacent to MTA as a root filling has been demonstrated. The case reported here demonstrated that when MTA is used as an obturation material in necrotic tooth with open apex, the canal can be effectively sealed. It has an added advantage of speed of completion of therapy and periapical healing that follows [7].

Followup is of utmost importance to observe success of the treatment. Various studies have recommended that followup should be performed for a minimum of one year. In this study, followup was done for two years and the patient is scheduled for further recall visits yearly. The clinical and radiographic examinations by CBCT and IOPA radiographs done at each visit revealed a remarkable decrease in the size of the periapical radiolucency.

CBCT has enabled the early and accurate detection of periapical lesion and the spatial relationship of these lesions to important anatomic landmarks. A major advantage of limited (small field of view) CBCT scanner, which was used in this case, is the relatively low-effective radiation dose the patient is exposed to. It yields radiation doses similar to that from two to three intraoral radiographs. However, the difference in information is considerably larger as compared to periapical radiography. The use of CBCT has also provided new capabilities for assessment of the periapical healing. In this case, an immediate postoperative radiograph was taken along with a CBCT scan, which showed the extent of MTA extrusion into periapical area as well as the extent and size of the periapical lesion. The latter has an advantage of evaluation using the same radiographic criteria at each appointment postoperatively. The IOPA radiographs and CBCT images show how distinctly different they are and how futile it is to compare one with the other. Our results also show how superior the CBCT images are, particularly in evaluation of status of MTA obturation and periapical healing in traumatized teeth with open apex.

4. Conclusion

This paper revealed that CBCT is a better and more accurate radiographic tool as compared to IOPA radiographs to assess the healing of a large periapical lesion associated with a nonvital tooth with open apex. Also, MTA obturation in such a case was found to result in favourable treatment outcome two years postoperatively.

Conflict of Interests

The authors deny any conflict of interests related to this study.

References

[1] M. Jyothi, "Conservative management of periapical lesions: case report," *Indian Journal of Stomatology*, vol. 3, pp. 190–193, 2012.

[2] G. C. Kubasad and S. B. Ghivari, "Apexification with apical plug of MTA—report of cases," *sOral Science Research*, vol. 1, pp. 104–107, 2011.

[3] S. A. Patil, A. A. Patil, and P. K. Dodwad, "Management of nonvital teeth with open apices using MTA as an apical plug: two case reports," *World Journal of Dentistry*, vol. 2, pp. 45–48, 2011.

[4] D. R. Hachmeister, W. G. Schindler, W. A. Walker 3rd. W.A., and D. D. Thomas, "The sealing ability and retention characteristics of mineral trioxide aggregate in a model of apexification," *Journal of Endodontics*, vol. 28, no. 5, pp. 386–390, 2002.

[5] J. B. Park and J. H. Lee, "Use of mineral trioxide aggregate in the open apex of a maxillary first premolar," *Journal of Oral Science*, vol. 50, no. 3, pp. 355–358, 2008.

[6] D. P. Raldi, I. Mello, S. M. Habitante, J. L. Lage-Marques, and J. Coil, "Treatment options for teeth with open apices and apical periodontitis," *Journal of Canadian Dental Association*, vol. 75, no. 8, pp. 591–596, 2009.

[7] V. Giuliani, T. Baccetti, R. Pace, and G. Pagavino, "The use of MTA in teeth with necrotic pulps and open apices," *Dental Traumatology*, vol. 18, no. 4, pp. 217–221, 2002.

[8] S. Asgary and S. Ehsani, "MTA resorption and periradicular healing in an open-apex incisor: a case report," *Saudi Dental Journal*, vol. 24, pp. 55–59, 2012.

[9] R. Sharma, A. Dhingra, and R. Nayar, "Delayed MTA apical plug in immature open apex- a case report," *Endodontology*, pp. 49–52, 2012.

[10] G. T. J. Huang, "Apexification: the beginning of its end," *International Endodontic Journal*, vol. 42, no. 10, pp. 855–866, 2009.

[11] S. Dogra, K. S. Mukunda, and S. M. Rao, "Apexification: review," *Journal of Dental Sciences Research*, vol. 3, pp. 1–4, 2012.

[12] S. Desai and N. Chandler, "The restoration of permanent immature anterior teeth, root filled using MTA: a review," *Journal of Dentistry*, vol. 37, no. 9, pp. 652–657, 2009.

[13] D. F. Brun, R. K. Scarparo, P. M. P. Kopper, and F. S. Grecca, "Apical internal inflammatory root resorption and open apex treated with MTA: a case report," *Revista Odonto Ciência*, vol. 25, pp. 213–215, 2010.

[14] H. W. Roberts, J. M. Toth, D. W. Berzins, and D. G. Charlton, "Mineral trioxide aggregate material use in endodontic treatment: a review of the literature," *Dental Materials*, vol. 24, no. 2, pp. 149–164, 2008.

[15] M. Parirokh and M. Torabinejad, "Mineral trioxide aggregate: a comprehensive literature review—part 3: clinical applications, drawbacks, and mechanism of action," *Journal of Endodontics*, vol. 36, no. 3, pp. 400–413, 2010.

14

Osteosarcoma of the Mandible Masquerading as a Dental Abscess: Report of a Case

Sukumaran Anil,[1] Anitha P. Krishnan,[2] and R. Rajendran[3]

[1] *Department of Periodontics and Community Dentistry, College of Dentistry, King Saud University, P.O. Box 60169, Riyadh 11545, Saudi Arabia*
[2] *Department of Oral and Maxillofacial Pathology, College of Dentistry, Salman Bin Abdulaziz University, P.O. Box 153, Al-Kharj 11942, Saudi Arabia*
[3] *College of Dentistry, King Saud bin Abdulaziz University for Health Sciences, P.O. Box 22490, Riyadh 11426, Saudi Arabia*

Correspondence should be addressed to Sukumaran Anil, drsanil@gmail.com

Academic Editors: M. Feichtinger, S. R. Watt-Smith, and E. F. Wright

An aggressive and fatal case of osteosarcoma of the mandible in a 19-year-old female is reported. Six weeks after the clinical appearance of the swelling, the patient died. This paper is unique in that the age of occurrence and the biologic behavior of the tumor were not consistent with the reported literature. The case report is followed by a brief review of osteosarcoma of the jaw with a note on its clinical presentation, diverse radiologic appearance, varied histopathologic picture, and prognosis.

1. Introduction

Osteosarcomas are rare malignant neoplasms with a high rate of mortality. They are malignant connective tissue tumors originating from undifferentiated mesenchymal cells that are able to form bone or osteoid tissue [1]. The most common location is the metaphyseal region of long bones, with the area directly above or below the knee accounting for almost half of all cases [2]. Approximately 7% of all osteosarcomas arise in the jawbones [3–5]. The occurrence of osteosarcoma of the jaws is about a decade later than in patients with long bone tumors. The peak age for jaw tumors is 30 to 39 years. Males slightly outnumber females in reported cases [1, 4, 6].

Maxilla and mandible are affected equally, with males showing a predilection for occurrence in the mandible and females in the maxilla [6, 7]. Mandibular lesions are located in the body, symphysis, angle, or ramus in descending order of frequency, while maxillary lesions most often involve the alveolar ridge, antrum, sinus floor, and palate [8, 9]. Clinical symptoms include pain, swelling, loose teeth, separation of teeth, and paresthesia [10].

Radiographically, osteosarcoma can appear with a variable bone density depending on the amount of bone formed by the neoplasm. In some cases, the typical "sunray" appearance is observed at the periphery of the tumor. The changes may be very subtle and difficult to recognize in the early course of the disease. Widened periodontal ligament space has been described as a classical sign of early osteosarcoma [11]. Computed tomography and magnetic resonance imaging are valuable adjuncts in evaluating the extent of the tumor and its relationship with neighboring tissues [12].

Histologically, osteosarcomas are composed of malignant spindle cells which produce foci of osteoid or immature bone. In the jaws, about half of the lesions demonstrate a cartilaginous differentiation [13]. In general, osteosarcomas of the jaws tend to be better differentiated than their long bone counterparts, with some tumors exhibiting a deceptively bland histological appearance [14, 15]. Therefore, correlation of the histological features with the clinical and radiographic findings is essential for the diagnosis.

2. Case Report

A 19-year-old, single, female was referred to the Dental College and Hospital, University of Kerala, India, by a general dental practitioner after treating her in vain with antibiotics

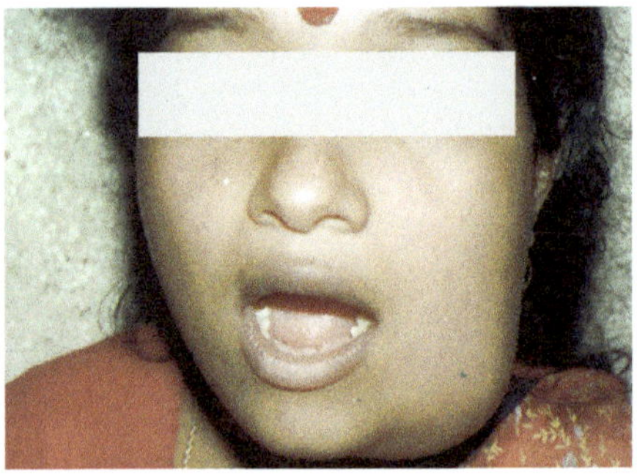

FIGURE 1: Clinical appearance of the swelling showing the diffuse borders.

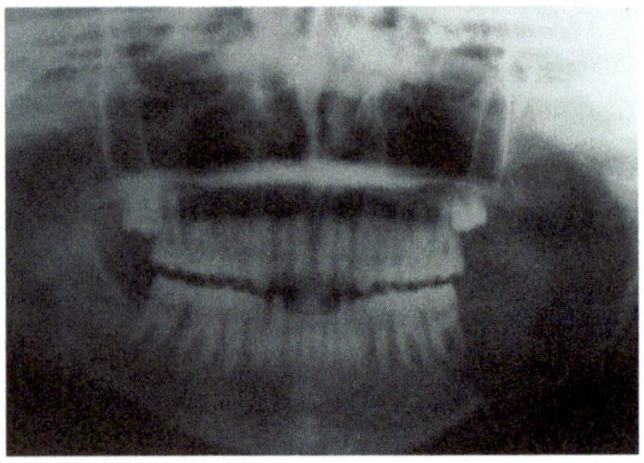

FIGURE 2: Panoramic radiograph showing the tumor at the left ramus of the mandible.

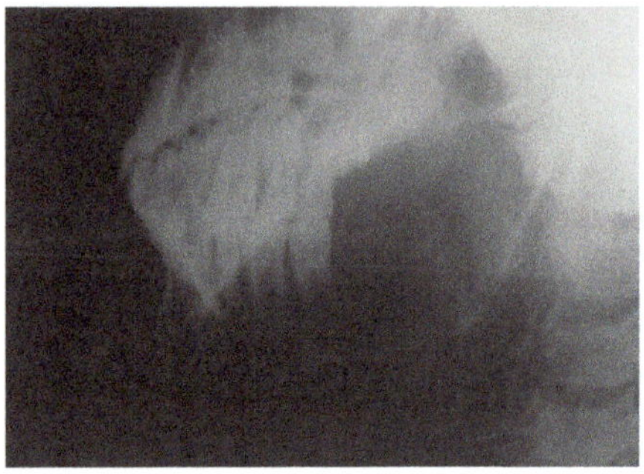

FIGURE 3: Lateral oblique view of the mandible showing the extent of the tumor.

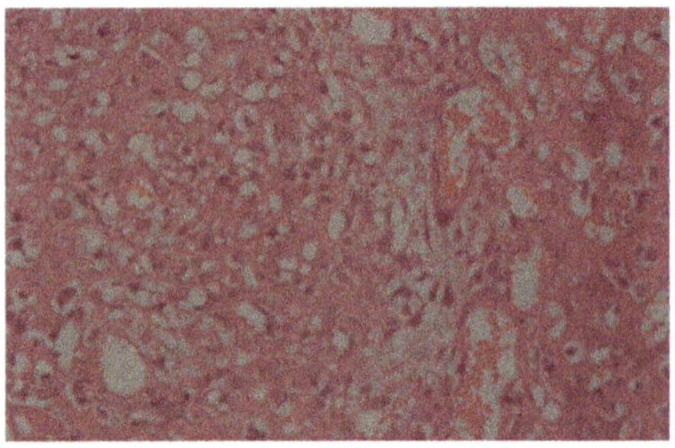

FIGURE 4: Showing proliferating spindle and oval-shaped mesenchymal cells with tumor osteoid and tumor bone formation HE ×96.

for dental abscess for a period of ten days. The patient presented with a complaint of a diffuse swelling on the left side of the mandible, large enough to cause her aesthetic anxiety. She had mild tenderness on palpation of the swelling and slight discomfort in the last molar region of the affected side while chewing. History revealed nothing of significance. At the time of clinical examination, the swelling was of two weeks duration. On examination, the swelling was circumscribed, bony hard, and roughly about 6 × 5 cm in size at the angle of the mandible. The swelling showed diffuse borders. The skin overlying the swelling was of normal color but had a glossy appearance, probably due to tautness of the skin over the swelling (Figure 1). Intraorally, the swelling was evident on the mandibular buccal vestibule adjacent to the second molar. There was apparent expansion of the buccal cortical plate. Lingual cortical plate also showed expansion but to a lesser extent. The mandibular third molar was missing, and the patient explained that both her mandibular wisdom teeth were extracted due to recurrent infection a couple of years ago.

Premolars and the first molar on the affected side were healthy with no carious or periodontal involvement. The second molar showed grade I mobility. Bidigital palpation did not reveal any lymph node enlargement anywhere in the cervicofacial chain.

Panoramic and lateral oblique views of the mandible were ordered. The orthopantogram showed a large radiolucency at the angle of the mandible on the left side, involving the second molar (Figure 2). The tooth appeared to float in space with bony attachment apparent only mesially. The circumscribed cortical plate expansion showed a centrifugal growth pattern involving the angle and major part of ramus of the mandible (Figure 3). The maxillary third molar of the affected side was present within the bone, but the mandibular third molar was absent corroborating the history and clinical finding. There was no widening of the periodontal ligament space and there was no sign of periodontal bone loss anywhere else. The inferior margin of the body of the mandible on the affected side had a moth eaten appearance in the lateral oblique view and a discontinuity in the inferior border suggestive of a pathologic fracture was apparent at the junction of the body and ramus.

An incision biopsy was performed. The histopathologic picture showed tissue lined with stratified squamous epithelium. Numerous proliferating spindle and oval-shaped mesenchymal cells with tumor osteoid and tumor bone formation were strewn subepithalially. Some areas showed highly pleomorphic cells with hyperchromatic nucleus and bizarre nuclear-cytoplasmic ratio with numerous vascular channels (Figure 4). Without much difficulty a diagnosis of osteosarcoma, osteoblastic variant, of the mandible was arrived.

Patient was recalled and interrogated for any paresthesia or numbness over the affected area. She admitted to a tingling sensation which had been present for a long time. Since it had not caused her any discomfort, she deemed it irrelevant to be mentioned. The serum alkaline phosphatase level was within normal limits. The patient was referred to the Regional Cancer Center for expert management. We followed up the patient's progress and learned that her CT scan did not show any metastatic lesion in the body and also her nuclear bone scan showed an increased isotope uptake at the lesional site. The patient was planned for a radical hemi-mandibulectomy, but before the scheduled date she died. Death was due to massive uncontrolled local disease. It had been a mere six weeks from the time she reported to a dental clinic with the complaint of swelling to her demise. At the time of her death, the swelling on her jaw had doubled in size and the skin over the swelling was stretched tighter and had a deep bluish hue to it.

3. Discussion

The clinical presentation of the case was classic with minimal symptoms for such a large swelling and involving posterior mandible. But the rapid rate of growth of the lesion from the time the patient was seen initially to the time of her death was not consistent with the general growth pattern of jaw osteosarcomas. Osteosarcomas of the jaws are usually biologically distinct from those of long bones in that they behave better than their long bone counterparts [16, 17].

The numbness due to compression or infiltration of the inferior alveolar nerve in the mandibular canal of the affected area has been well documented in osteosarcoma and could be an indication of poor prognosis. In this case, even though numbness was not a presenting complaint of the patient, she was having the tingling sensation much before the swelling become apparent. Numbness or paresthesia of the affected area as an early diagnostic feature of osteosarcoma is thus highlighted by our case [18]. The dark hue over the rapidly growing swelling that was noticed towards the end of her days is attributed probably to telangiectasia of superficial vessels due to tumor compression.

The radiographic picture of the case did not show any widening of the periodontal ligament space of either the affected or the adjacent teeth. The circumscribed bilateral centrifugal cortical plate expansion could mimic a central benign neoplasm, although ossifying fibroma is a slow growing benign lesion and does not cause numbness of the affected area or pathological fracture of the bone. There was loss of lamina dura of both the mesial and distal roots of the second molar associated with the bone swelling. This could also be found in periodontal infections, odontogenic cysts and tumors, metastatic tumors, and so forth. Even though the patient had numbness of the affected area, radiographic feature of mandibular canal involvement was not evident. Probably, the extensive periostitis reaction masked this finding [10]. The characteristic sunray appearance and Codman's triangle seen in osteosarcoma of the long bones is less commonly encountered in jaw lesions [2]. The difficulty in diagnosing osteosarcomas by radiological means is mainly because of its wider spectrum of variable.

Rise in serum alkaline phosphatase is reported in osteosarcoma but is not considered to be a consistent finding [19]. However, the present case did not show an elevation in serum alkaline phosphatase. The short clinical course of the tumor could be an explanation for this finding.

Differentiation of osteosarcoma from other bony lesions like Paget's disease, fibrous dysplasia, multiple myeloma, and metastatic tumors is based more on microscopical than radiological evidence [19]. Even then different levels of cell differentiation may create difficulty in distinguishing this tumor from reactive stromal proliferations such as fractured callus or from cellular forms of Paget's disease [20].

Besides the size of the lesion, the histologic type and grading of the tumor are important factors in determining the prognosis. Conventional osteosarcoma can be subdivided into osteoblastic, chondroblastic, and fibroblastic histologic variants depending on the extracellular matrix produced by the tumor cells [1].

Other histologic variants include the myxomatous type, telangiectatic type, small cell osteosarcoma, giant cell osteosarcoma, giant cell predominant osteosarcoma, large cell type, fibrous histiocytoma-like type, and epithelioid osteosarcoma [16]. Histologic picture of the present case showed areas of osteoblastic differentiation with some foci of highly pleomorphic cells and cellular anaplasia. This type has a poorer prognosis when compared with the chondroblastic variety. In fact, in our opinion, the histological grading is more important than all the other features combined in determining the prognosis.

The prognosis of osteosarcoma of the jaws is better than that of long bone, with a 5-year-survival rate of 25.8 percent for the maxilla and 34.8 percent for the mandible. The median survival time for the maxilla is 2.9 years and 6.5 years for the mandible [21]. The progress of the neoplastic growth in this case was so rapid that in contrast to the literature, the time span between diagnosis and death was barely six weeks. Probably the swelling had been present for a longer time but went unnoticed by the patient due to lack of any appreciable clinical symptoms. The patient is aware that its presence began only when it grew large enough to be of aesthetic concern. Usually, the prognosis of a jaw osteosarcoma gets better as the age at which it occurs increases [6]. Older patients are reported to have increased resistance to the tumor, thus increasing the chances of a better prognosis [10]. In our case, the patient was younger than the mean age of occurrence for jaw osteosarcomas. Also, the tumor ran a very aggressive biologic course, a feature uncommon for gnathic lesions [16].

Local recurrence and metastasis occur frequently in patients with osteosarcoma. Rate of metastasis in jaw osteosarcomas is lower than those of the long bones [6, 22]. But metastasis is relatively higher in case of postradiation osteosarcoma of the jaws [23]. Metastasis is usually via the bloodstream and in most cases occurs within 2-3 years. The absence of any metastatic spread seen in this case could be attributed to the very rapid rate of growth of the tumor and short clinical course.

Osteosarcomas of the jaws are cytologically unremarkable. Hence, it is important to separate them from benign or reactive lesions like fibrous dysplasia and osteoblastoma, [24]. It is crucial to completely investigate the lesion and arrive at accurate diagnosis in the initial biopsy. To assist in the identification of malignancy besides histopathological examination, special investigations have been carried out. Bone matrix protein is suggested to assist in recognizing malignant osteoid [25]. Osteocalcin is a bone specific protein that may be useful in differentiating osteosarcoma from malignant fibrous histiocytoma [26].

Early diagnosis and complete tumor resection are the most important factors in increasing prognosis of jaw osteosarcomas [27]. Treatment of osteosarcoma is radical surgery [28]. This usually is accompanied by radiotherapy or chemotherapy. Anatomic limitations in the orofacial region cause difficulties in achieving uninvolved margins and for this reason local recurrence of the lesions is high between 33% and 39%. Tumor-free margins in surgery, chemotherapy with multidrugs, and radiotherapy after surgery have effects in the prognosis of osteosarcoma [29].

4. Conclusion

The case reported here emphasizes the importance of histopathology in the diagnosis and predicting prognosis of osteosarcomas of the jaws. Eliciting simple but important clinical symptoms like numbness or paresthesia of the affected area is highlighted. X-ray, CT scan, and MRI imaging along with bone scan are valuable adjuncts to microscopy in the early diagnosis and staging of this malignancy.

References

[1] J. H. Bennett, G. Thomas, A. W. Evans, and P. M. Speight, "Osteosarcoma of the jaws: a 30-year retrospective review," *Oral Surgery, Oral Medicine, Oral Pathology, Oral Radiology, and Endodontics*, vol. 90, no. 3, pp. 323–333, 2000.

[2] J. L. Clark, K. K. Unni, D. C. Dahlin, and K. D. Devine, "Osteosarcoma of the jaw," *Cancer*, vol. 51, no. 12, pp. 2311–2316, 1983.

[3] O. Mardinger, N. Givol, Y. P. Talmi, and S. Taicher, "Osteosarcoma of the jaw: the Chaim Sheba Medical Center experience," *Oral Surgery, Oral Medicine, Oral Pathology, Oral Radiology, and Endodontics*, vol. 91, no. 4, pp. 445–451, 2001.

[4] M. O. Ogunlewe, O. F. Ajayi, W. L. Adeyemo, A. L. Ladeinde, and O. James, "Osteogenic sarcoma of the jaw bones: a single institution experience over a 21-year period," *Oral Surgery, Oral Medicine, Oral Pathology, Oral Radiology, and Endodontics*, vol. 101, no. 1, pp. 76–81, 2006.

[5] A. J. Ajura and S. H. Lau, "A retrospective clinicopathological study of 59 osteogenic sarcoma of jaw bone archived in a stomatology unit," *Malaysian Journal of Pathology*, vol. 32, no. 1, pp. 27–34, 2010.

[6] G. E. Garrington, H. H. Scofield, J. Cornyn, and S. P. Hooker, "Osteosarcoma of the jaws. Analysis of 56 cases," *Cancer*, vol. 20, no. 3, pp. 377–391, 1967.

[7] H. Dorfman and B. Czerniak, "Bone tumors," *The New England Journal of Medicine*, vol. 1998, pp. 1088–1089, 1998.

[8] F. Schajowicz, H. Sissons, and L. Sobin, "The World Health Organization's histologic classification of bone tumors," *Cancer*, vol. 75, pp. 1208–1214, 1995.

[9] D. C. Doval, R. V. Kumar, V. Kannan et al., "Osteosarcoma of the jaw bones," *British Journal of Oral and Maxillofacial Surgery*, vol. 35, no. 5, pp. 357–362, 1997.

[10] P. J. Slootweg and H. Muller, "Osteosarcoma of the jaw bones. Analysis of 18 cases," *Journal of Maxillofacial Surgery*, vol. 13, no. 4, pp. 158–166, 1985.

[11] D. G. Gardner and D. M. Mills, "The widened periodontal ligament of osteosarcoma of the jaws," *Oral Surgery Oral Medicine and Oral Pathology*, vol. 41, no. 5, pp. 652–656, 1976.

[12] D. Wilner, *Radiology of Bone Tumors and Allied Disorders*, 1982.

[13] D. S. Vege, A. M. Borges, K. Aggrawal, G. Balasubramaniam, D. M. Parikh, and B. Bhaser, "Osteosarcoma of the craniofacial bones. A clinico-pathological study," *Journal of Cranio-Maxillo-Facial Surgery*, vol. 19, no. 2, pp. 90–93, 1991.

[14] K. K. Unni, D. C. Dahlin, R. A. McLeod, and D. J. Pritchard, "Intraosseous well differentiated osteosarcoma," *Cancer*, vol. 40, no. 3, pp. 1337–1347, 1977.

[15] R. Fernandes, N. G. Nikitakis, A. Pazoki, and R. A. Ord, "Osteogenic Sarcoma of the Jaw: a 10-year experience," *Journal of Oral and Maxillofacial Surgery*, vol. 65, no. 7, pp. 1286–1291, 2007.

[16] M. J. Klein and G. P. Siegal, "Osteosarcoma: anatomic and histologic variants," *American Journal of Clinical Pathology*, vol. 125, no. 4, pp. 555–581, 2006.

[17] A. W. Woźniak, M. T. Nowaczyk, K. Osmola, and W. Golusinski, "Malignant transformation of an osteoblastoma of the mandible: case report and review of the literature," *European Archives of Oto-Rhino-Laryngology*, vol. 267, no. 6, pp. 845–849, 2010.

[18] S. Yamaguchi, H. Nagasawa, T. Suzuki et al., "Sarcomas of the oral and maxillofacial region: a review of 32 cases in 25 years," *Clinical Oral Investigations*, vol. 8, no. 2, pp. 52–55, 2004.

[19] A. N. Roca, J. L. Smith, and B. S. Jing, "Osteosarcoma and parosteal osteogenic sarcoma of the maxilla and mandible: study of 20 cases," *American Journal of Clinical Pathology*, vol. 54, no. 4, pp. 625–636, 1970.

[20] L. B. Kahn, F. W. Wood, and L. V. Ackerman, "Fracture callus associated with benign and malignant bone lesions and mimicking osteosarcoma," *American Journal of Clinical Pathology*, vol. 52, no. 1, pp. 14–24, 1969.

[21] S. G. Patel, P. Meyers, A. G. Huvos et al., "Improved outcomes in patients with osteogenic sarcoma of the head and neck," *Cancer*, vol. 95, no. 7, pp. 1495–1503, 2002.

[22] M. S. Weinfeld and H. R. Dudley Jr., "Osteogenic sarcoma. A follow-up study of the ninety-four cases observed at the Massachusetts General Hospital from 1920 to 1960," *Journal of Bone and Joint Surgery*, vol. 44, pp. 269–276, 1962.

[23] J. J. Kasthoori and M. L. Wastie, "Radiation-induced osteosarcoma of the maxilla," *Singapore Medical Journal*, vol. 47, no. 10, pp. 907–909, 2006.

[24] M. E. Koury, J. A. Regezi, D. H. Perrott, and L. B. Kaban, "'Atypical' fibro-osseous lesions: diagnostic challenges and treatment concepts," *International Journal of Oral and Maxillofacial Surgery*, vol. 24, no. 2, pp. 162–169, 1995.

[25] S. Ushigome, T. Shimoda, M. Fukunaga, T. Takakuwa, and H. Nakajima, "Immunocytochemical aspects of the differential diagnosis of osteosarcoma and malignant fibrous histiocytoma," *Surgical Pathology*, vol. 1, pp. 347–357, 1988.

[26] D. Lajeunesse, C. Frondoza, B. Schoffield, and B. Sacktor, "Osteocalcin secretion by the human osteosarcoma cell line MG-63," *Journal of Bone and Mineral Research*, vol. 5, no. 9, pp. 915–922, 1990.

[27] J. E. Russ and R. H. Jesse, "Management of osteosarcoma of the maxilla and mandible," *American Journal of Surgery*, vol. 140, no. 4, pp. 572–576, 1980.

[28] L. E. Smeele, J. E. Van Der Wal, P. J. Van Diest, I. Van Der Waal, and G. B. Snow, "Radical surgical treatment in craniofacial osteosarcoma gives excellent survival. A retrospective cohort

study of 14 patients," *European Journal of Cancer Part B: Oral Oncology*, vol. 30, no. 6, pp. 374–376, 1994.

[29] M. August, P. Magennis, and D. Dewitt, "Osteogenic sarcoma of the jaws: factors influencing prognosis," *International Journal of Oral and Maxillofacial Surgery*, vol. 26, no. 3, pp. 198–204, 1997.

15

Condylar Aplasia and Hypoplasia: A Rare Case

Peeyush Shivhare, Lata Shankarnarayan, Usha, Mahesh Kumar, and Malliger Basavaraju Sowbhagya

Department of Oral Medicine and Radiology, Raja Rajeswari Dental College, and Hospital, Rajiv Gandhi University, Ramohalli Cross, kumbalgodu, Bangalore, Karnataka 560074, India

Correspondence should be addressed to Peeyush Shivhare; drshivharepeeyush3@gmail.com

Academic Editors: M. O. Sayin and K. H. Zawawi

Aplasia of condyle is very rare, when this condition not seen as a part of a syndrome. We report a case of condylar aplasia on the right side and hypoplasia on the left side in a 21-year-old female. The patient reported to the department with a chief complaint of underdeveloped lower jaw. Clinical examination, conventional radiographs, and 3D CBCT images revealed complete absence of condyle on the right side and hypoplasia on the left side.

1. Introduction

The temporomandibular joint (TMJ) is one of the most complex joints of the human body. It is considered a ginglymus diarthrodial joint capable of both rotational and translatory movements. It consists of the mandibular condyle and the articular eminence of the temporal bone. The condyle is very special because the expression of mandibular growth is provided by mandibular condyle. In compared to other diarthrodial joints, during prenatal life the TMJ lags morphologically behind other synovial joints in both the timing of its appearance and its progress, so that at birth the joint is still largely underdeveloped. The TMJ first appears in the 8th week of gestation, when two separate areas of mesenchymal blastemas appear near the eventual location of the mandibular condyle and glenoid fossa [1, 2]. Bone and cartilage are first seen in the mandibular condyle at approximately the 10th gestational week. First condylar blastema developed from which the mandibular condyle cartilage, the aponeurosis of the lateral pterygoid muscle, and the disc and capsule component composing the lower portion of the joint are derived. Next is the temporal blastema, which eventually forms the articular surface of the temporal component and the structures of the upper portion of the joint. The mandibular condyle and temporal blastemas begin their growth at relatively distant sites; they then move towards each other as the joint develops by the 12th week. At birth, the articular surfaces of both the mandibular condyle and temporal bones are covered with fibrous connective tissue. Later, this tissue is slowly converted to fibrocartilage as the fossa deepens and the mandibular condyle develops under functional influences [3, 4].

Growth disturbances in the development of mandibular condyle may occur in utero late in the first trimester and may result in disorders such as aplasia or hypoplasia of the mandibular condyle. As compared to hypoplasia, hyperplasia of the mandibular condyle is not visible at birth and seems to be gradually acquired during growth [5].

2. Case Report

A 21-yr-old female was presented to the oral medicine and radiology department with a chief complaint of underdeveloped lower jaw, which was first noticed during childhood and gradually progressed. Due to unfavorable socioeconomic conditions, it was not possible to get the treatment done for the patient. At the anamnesis there was no history of any trauma or any systemic diseases. Patient's parents gave a history of consanguineous marriage. There was no family history of the present problem.

General Physical examination did not reveal any abnormalities. Her vital signs were within normal limits. Extraoral examination revealed facial asymmetry with severe retruded mandible giving a bird face appearance (Figures 1 and 2).

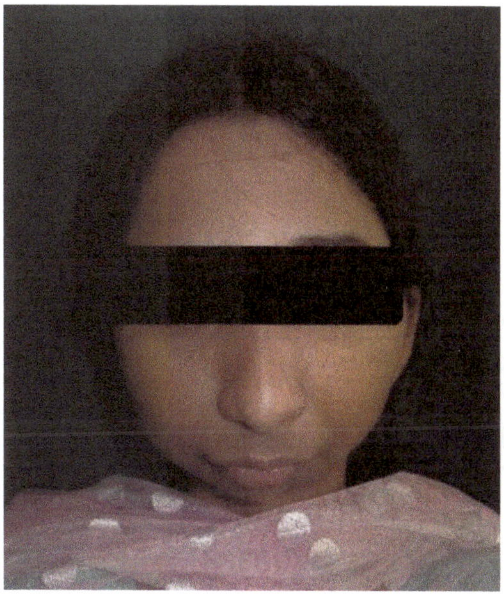

Figure 1: Frontal view of patient.

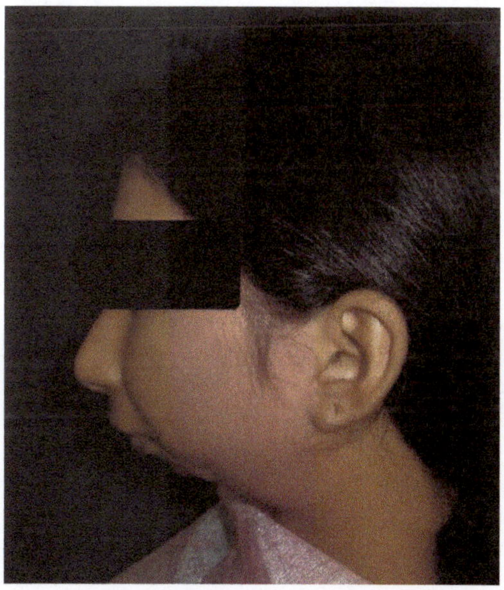

Figure 2: Lateral view of patient shows severe retruded mandible.

Mouth opening was restricted (10 mm) with no deviation or deflection (Figure 3). On palpation condyles were not detected on both sides. Intraorally there was crowding in upper and lower anterior teeth with increased overjet and overbite (Figure 4). Molar relation was Angle's Class II bilaterally. She had deep palate and generalized enamel hypoplasia (fluorosis). No other important clinical extraoral or intraoral findings were observed. Based on clinical findings, a provisional diagnosis of bilateral ankylosis and differential diagnosis of bilateral condylar hypoplasia or aplasia were given.

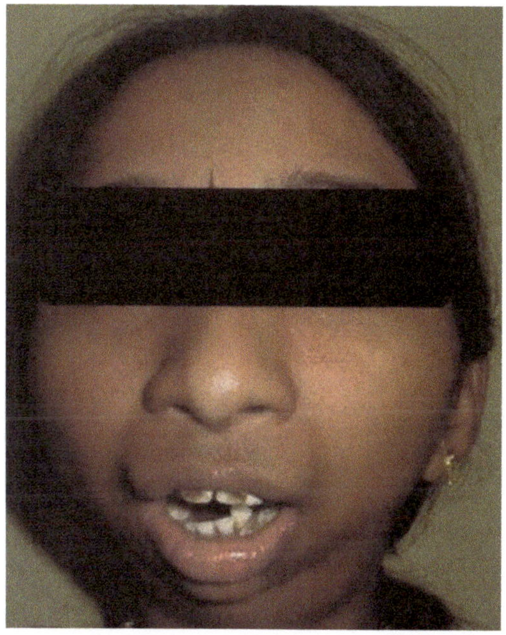

Figure 3: Restricted mouth opening.

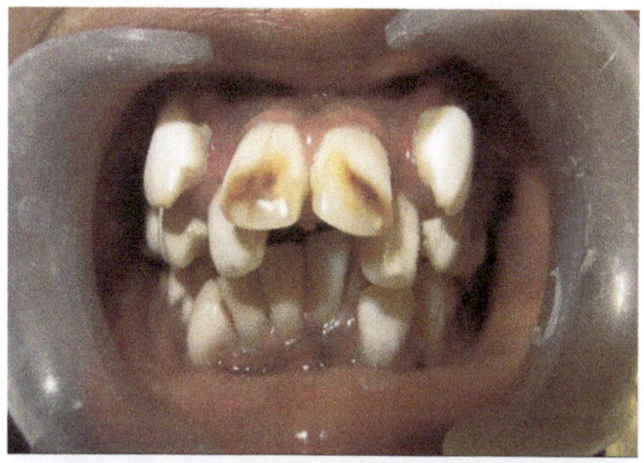

Figure 4: Severe crowding in upper and lower anteriors with fluorosis.

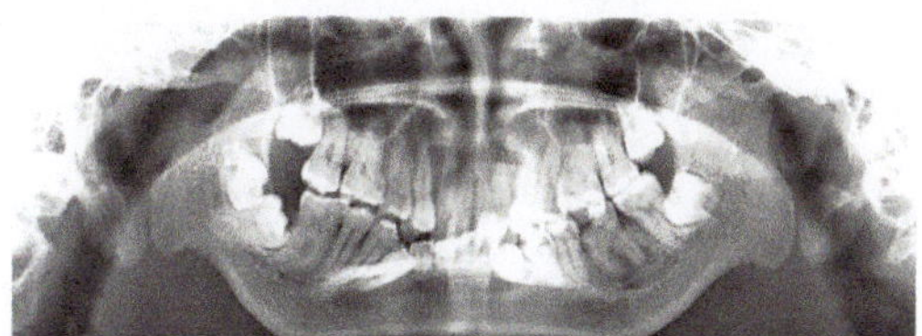

Figure 5: OPG shows condylar aplasia on the right side, condylar hypoplasia on the left side, prominent antigonial notch, and hypoplasia of mandible.

After clinical examination, radiographic examinations were performed. Panoramic radiograph showed complete absence of condyle on the right side and rudimentary condyle on the left side. Glenoid fossa was not developed on the right side and underdeveloped on the left side. Antegonial notch was prominent bilaterally (Figure 5). PA view findings were

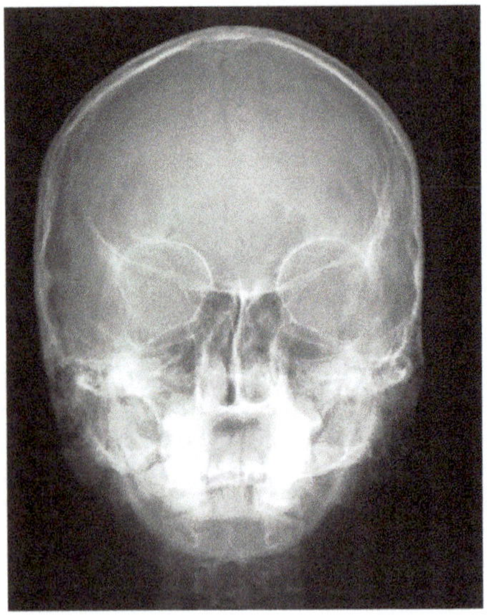

Figure 6: PA view reveals no significant asymmetry.

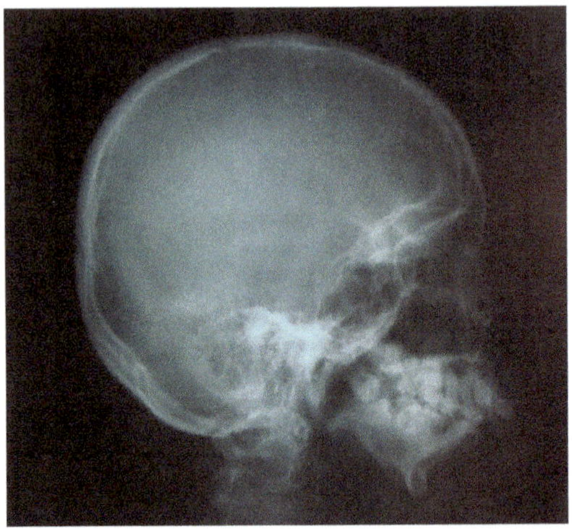

Figure 7: Lateral skull. Radiograph shows severe retruded mandible.

inconclusive (Figure 6). Lateral skull views showed severe retruded and micrognathic mandible (Figure 7). Findings of panoramic radiograph were confirmed by lateral skull radiographs. CBCT was advised for additional information. CBCT also confirmed the findings of OPG and lateral skull radiographs (Figures 8, 9, 10, and 11). After radiographic confirmation patient was advised complete systemic evaluation and referred to general medicine, cardiology, ophthalmology, ENT, and orthopedics to rule out any syndromes. Medical evaluation revealed no abnormalities. Based on the clinical and radiographic findings, a final diagnosis of nonsyndromic agenesis of the right condyle and hypoplasia of the left condyle was given. Patient was referred to oral surgeon and orthodontist for the best possible treatment.

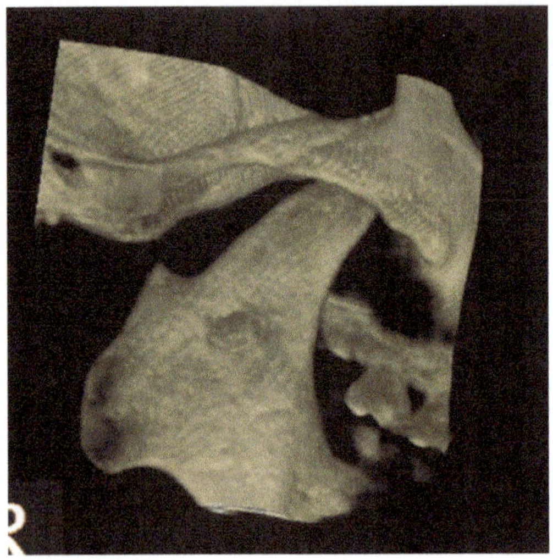

Figure 8: 3D CBCT right oblique lateral shows absence of glenoid fossa and complete absence of the condyle.

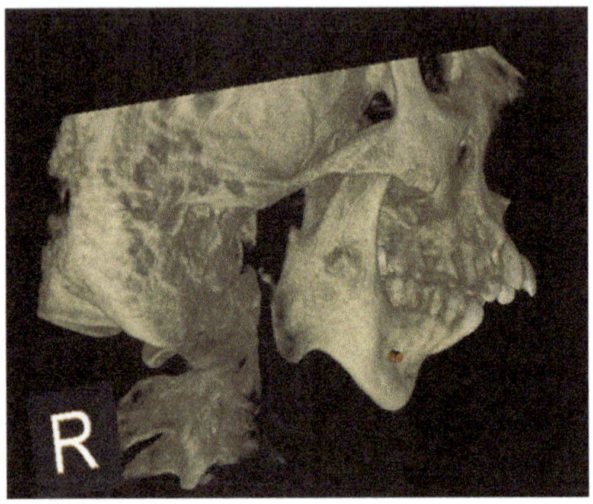

Figure 9: 3D CBCT right lateral shows absence of glenoid fossa and complete absence of the condyle.

3. Discussion

The congenital deformities and developmental abnormalities of the mandibular condyle can be classified as hypoplasia or aplasia, hyperplasia, and bifidity. Hypoplasia or aplasia of the mandibular condyle indicates underdevelopment or nondevelopment associated mainly with various craniofacial abnormalities. These may be either congenital or acquired [5].

Congenital (primary) condylar hypoplasia is characterized by unilateral or bilateral underdevelopment of the mandibular condyle and usually occurs as a part of some systemic condition originating in the first and second branchial arches, such as Mandibulofacial dysostosis (Treacher Collins syndrome), Hemifacial microsomia (first and second branchial arch syndrome), Oculoauriculovertebral syndrome (Goldenhar syndrome), Oculomandibulodyscephaly (Hallermann-Streiff syndrome), Hurler's syndrome, Proteus syndrome, Morquio syndrome and Auriculocondylar syndrome [5–8].

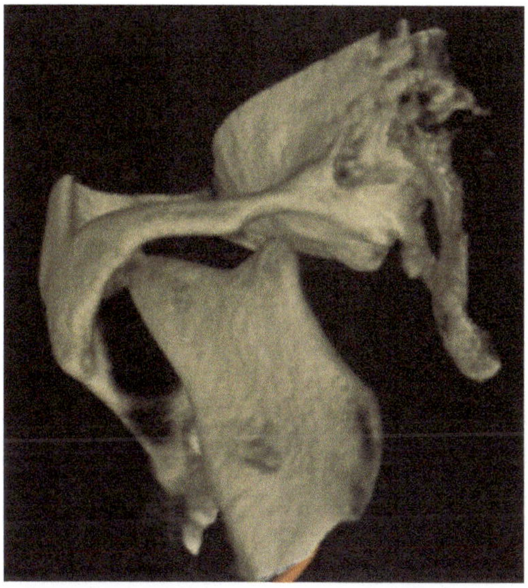

FIGURE 10: 3D CBCT left oblique lateral—shows hypoplasia of glenoid fossa and condyle.

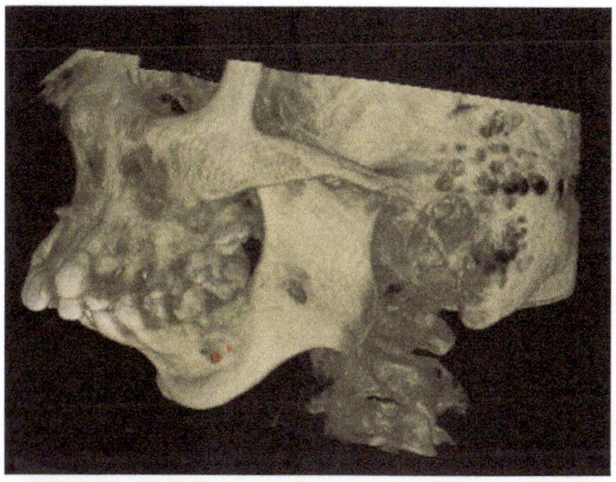

FIGURE 11: 3D CBCT left lateral—shows hypoplasia of glenoid fossa and condyle.

As a rule, in each of these conditions some soft tissue manifestations accompany the condylar agenesis and/or condylar malformations [9].

Acquired (secondary) condylar hypoplasia takes place if the condyle is injured during active growth, because of which development may be arrested. The most common causes are mechanical injury, such as trauma (before the age of 2), infection of the joint itself or the middle ear, childhood rheumatoid arthritis, radiotherapy, and parathyroid hormone-related protein deficiency which affect bone formation and chondrocyte differentiation [5, 9, 10].

Several authors confirmed that mandibular deficiency can occur without any defined etiology [11]. Aplasia of the mandibular condyle without any other facial malformations is an extremely rare condition [8].

The cases of nonsyndromic mandibular condyle aplasia have been previously reported by Krogstad [9], Prowler and Glossman [11], Akihiko et al. [12], Santos et al. [13], Bowden Jr. and Kohn [14], Canger and Celenk [15] and so forth. Our case also presented condylar aplasia and hypoplasia without any other features suggestive of any syndrome.

The TMJ develops from initially widely separated temporal and condylar blastemata which appear at about the 8th week of conception. Eventually they grow towards each other and ossify to form a functional joint by about the 20th week of intrauterine life [5]. In our case, total absence of the condyle and glenoid fossa on the right side and hypoplastic condyle and glenoid fossa on the left side constitute an evidence that the defect originated in the prenatal period.

Various treatment approaches have been proposed for treating condylar aplasia and possibilities for influencing mandibular growth. Most of the time it is treated by multimode with the help of oral surgeon, general surgeon, plastic surgeon, and orthodontist [9, 15, 16].

The treatment could then be a costochondral graft transplant, preferably before the growth spurt, orthognathic surgery at the end of the growth period, or both [16]. Krogstad reported that effective results were obtained through the application of a form of orthodontic activator which aimed to swing the mandible to the unaffected side and promote formation of a mandibular condyle, albeit irregular in shape [9]. Surgery is often required, but the timing and regimen of this choice is still an issue to be resolved [15].

4. Conclusion

In conclusion we report a rare case of total condylar aplasia on the right side and condylar hypoplasia on the left side, not related to any clear pathological disorder. This case of unknown etiology was thoroughly examined; based on clinical and radiographic findings, we suggest that this case is of congenital origin. Nonsyndromic condylar hypoplasia and aplasia are exceedingly rare conditions and very few case reports are published till date. In this context, our case is an important addition to the literature. Early detection and prompt treatment are imperative to restore esthetics and thus provide psychologic benefit to these patients.

References

[1] D. Buchbinder and A. S. Kaplan, "Biology," in *Temporomandibular Disorders Diagnosis and Treatment*, A. S. Kaplan and L. A. Assael, Eds., pp. 11–23, Saunders, Philadelphia, Pa, USA, 1991.

[2] J. W. Choi, J. T. Kim, J. H. Park et al., "gp130 is important for the normal morphogenesis of Meckel's cartilage and subsequent mandibular development," *Experimental & Molecular Medicine*, vol. 39, pp. 295–303, 2007.

[3] J. F. Cleall, "Postnatal craniofacial growth and development," in *Oral and Maxillofacial Surgery Volume One*, D. M. Laskin, Ed., pp. 70–107, Mosby, St Louis, Mo, USA, 1980.

[4] S. Pruzansky, "Postnatal development of craniofacial malformations," *Journal of Dental Research*, vol. 47, no. 6, p. 936, 1968.

[5] K. Kaneyama, N. Segami, and T. Hatta, "Congenital deformities and developmental abnormalities of the mandibular condyle in the temporomandibular joint," *Congenital Anomalies*, vol. 48, no. 3, pp. 118–125, 2008.

[6] D. R. Delone, W. D. Brown, and L. R. Gentry, "Proteus syndrome: craniofacial and cerebral MRI," *Neuroradiology*, vol. 41, no. 11, pp. 840–843, 1999.

[7] K. A. Morgan, M. A. Rehman, and R. E. Schwartz, "Morquio's syndrome and its anaesthetic considerations," *Pediatric Anesthesi*, vol. 12, pp. 641–644, 2002.

[8] S. Ozturk, M. Sengezer, S. Isik, D. Gul, and F. Zor, "The correction of auricular and mandibular deformities in auriculocondylar syndrome," *Journal of Craniofacial Surgery*, vol. 16, no. 3, pp. 489–492, 2005.

[9] O. Krogstad, "Aplasia of the mandibular condyle," *European Journal of Orthodontics*, vol. 19, no. 5, pp. 483–489, 1997.

[10] S. Shibata, N. Suda, K. Fukada, K. Ohyama, Y. Yamashita, and V. E. Hammond, "Mandibular coronoid process in parathyroid hormone-related protein-deficient mice shows ectopic cartilage formation accompanied by abnormal bone modeling," *Anatomy and Embryology*, vol. 207, no. 1, pp. 35–44, 2003.

[11] J. R. Prowler and S. Glassman, "Agenesis of the mandibular condyles. Diagnostic findings and treatment of deformity by polyethylene implant," *Oral Surgery, Oral Medicine, Oral Pathology*, vol. 7, no. 2, pp. 133–139, 1954.

[12] I. Akihiko, T. Ritsuo, F. Junichi, I. Nobuyuki, and T. Yutaka, "Agenesis of bilateral mandibular condyle- report of a case," *Journal of the Japanese Stomatological Society*, vol. 55, pp. 187–192, 2006.

[13] K. C. P. Santos, M. E. P. Dutra, C. Costa, C. A. Lascala, and J. X. de Oliviera, "Aplasia of mandibular condyle: case report," *Dentomaxillofacial Radiology*, vol. 36, pp. 420–422, 2007.

[14] C. M. Bowden Jr. and M. W. Kohn, "Mandibular deformity associated with unilateral absence of the condyle," *Journal of Oral Surgery*, vol. 31, no. 6, pp. 469–472, 1973.

[15] E. M. Canger and P. Celenk, "Aplasia of mandibular condyle associated with some orthopedic abnormalities: a case report," *Dentomaxillofacial Radiology*, pp. 1–5, 2011.

[16] K. Vargervik and L. B. Kaban, "Hemifacial microstomia diagnosis and management," in *Modern Practice in Orthognathic and Reconstructive Surgery*, W. H. Bell, Ed., vol. 2, pp. 1533–1560, W B Saunders Company, Philadelphia, Pa, USA, 1992.

16

Stafne Bone Defect: Report of Two Cases

A. P. Münevveroğlu[1] and K. C. Aydın[2]

[1] *Pedodonti Ana Bilim Dalı, Dişhekimliği Fakültesi, İstanbul Medipol Üniversitesi, 34083 Fatih, Turkey*
[2] *Diş ve Çene Radyolojisi Anabilim Dalı, Dişhekimliği Fakültesi Ağız, İstanbul Medipol Üniversitesi, 34083 Fatih, Turkey*

Correspondence should be addressed to A. P. Münevveroğlu, apatir@medipol.edu.tr

Academic Editors: A. C. B. Delbem, A. Markopoulos, and A. Milosevic

Stafne bone defects are asymptomatic lingual bone depressions of the lower jaw. In 1942, Stafne described for the first time 35 asymptomatic, radiolucent cavities, unilaterally located in the posterior region of the mandible, between the mandibular angle and the third molar, below the inferior dental canal and slightly above the basis mandibulae. In this study, the clinical and radiological characteristics of 2 cases of Stafne bone defects were described. Orthopantomograph and CBCT were used for diagnosing the defects. The bone defects of two patients in this study were asymptomatic and any other bone lesions, such as cysts and tumors, were excluded because no signs of inflammatory or tumoral changes were evident Therefore, surgery was not considered and the patients were followed for 1 year. Stafne bone defect was an incidental finding, presenting no evolutionary changes, and as such conservatory therapy based on periodic controls was indicated. Currently, complementary techniques such as CT are sufficient to establish a certain diagnosis.

1. Introduction

In 1942, Stafne [1] described for the first time 35 asymptomatic, radiolucent cavities, unilaterally located in the posterior region of the mandible, between the mandibular angle and the third molar, below the inferior dental canal and slightly above the basis mandibulae [1–6]. Radiographically, the cortical outline of the bone defect is denser and thicker than that of odontogenic cysts [2].

The exact pathogenesis is still obscure. Stafne suggested that the cavity could result from a failure of normal bone deposition in the region formerly occupied by cartilage [1, 5, 7]. However, the most widely accepted view is that the cavities develop as a result of a localized pressure atrophy of the lingual surface of the mandible from the adjacent salivary gland [5, 8]. Due to the multiple explanations offered as to its etiopathogenesis, this entity has been given numerous names, particularly, static bone cyst, lingual mandibular bone defect, Stafne bone cavity, idiopathic bone cavity, and lingual mandibular bone depression [8]. The shape of a lingual bone cavity can be round or oval, and it varies from 1 to 3 cm in diameter [2].

Bone defects of Stafne frequently affect men in their fifth or seventh decade of life and show a prevalence between 0.10% and 0.48% [3, 9]. They usually contain ectopic salivary gland tissue and do not require surgery [3, 4, 10].

In addition to occurring more commonly in the posterior region of the mandible (posterior variant), Stafne bone defect may also appear in the anterior region (anterior variant) and in the ascending ramus of the mandible (mandibular ramus variant) [11]. Posterior Stafne bone defects can be readily diagnosed because of their unique location in the radiographic examination; however, anterior bone defects may be misdiagnosed and confused with several pathologic entities, such as traumatic and cystic lesions or tumors of the jaw [3]. Normally, it is unilateral, with some reports of bilateral occurrence [3–6]. Double unilateral occurrence is rare, and bilocular occurrence is even rarer [3].

The objective of this study is to describe the clinical and radiological characteristics of 2 cases of Stafne bone defect.

Case 1. A 31-year-old asymptomatic male patient was referred to Istanbul Medipol University, Faculty of Dentistry, Department of Dentomaxillofacial Radiology in order to undergo routine panoramic radiography. The patient was misdiagnosed in behalf of a cystic lesion of his left mandible by a former dentist. Medical history and dental history were not contributory. Palpation of the defect was not painful,

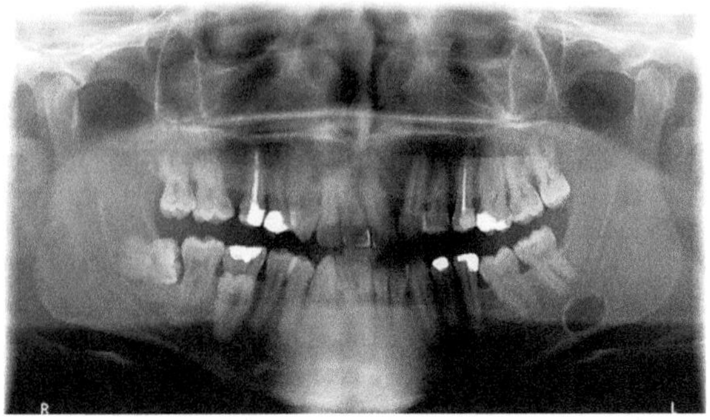

FIGURE 1: Panoramic radiography showing the radiolucent area.

and the cavity could be palpated by bidigital palpation. Cone beam computerized tomography (CBCT) was found appropriate for further evaluation (see Figures 2 and 4). Results showed an oval-shaped, radiolucent area of cystic aspect and regular, well-defined cortical outline with a little buccal cortical resorpton. Its longest axis was placed horizontally in the left hemimandible. This lithic area, located under the lower left second molar, was anterior to the mandibular angle. The lower wall of the mandibular canal which was visible within the radiolucent area showed that there could be a neighboring relationship, but not an involvement, of the inferior alveolar nerve (Figure 1). Patient displayed no pain or paresthesia. Lingual wall of the basal bone displayed involvement of the lesion and dimensions of the defect 14 × 10 × 6.4 mm depth (mesiodistal length, inferosuperior height, buccolingual depth).

A diagnosis of idiopathic bone defect was made and it was decided that the patient would undergo a 6-month follow-up period.

Case 2. A 57-year-old asymptomatic male patient was referred to Istanbul Medipol University, Faculty of Dentistry, Department of Dentomaxillofacial Radiology in order to undergo routine periodontal treatment. Medical history and dental history were not contributory. Defect of the right mandibular corpus was detected during routine panoramic imaging. Palpation of the defect was not painful with no discomfort. Cone beam computerized tomography (CBCT) was found appropriate for further evaluation. Results showed an oval-shaped, radiolucent area of cystic aspect. This lithic area, located under the lower right second and third molar. The lower wall of the mandibular canal was visible within the radiolucent area showed that there could be a neighboring relationship, but not an involvement, of the inferior alveolar nerve (Figure 3). Lingual wall of the basal bone displayed involvement of the lesion and dimensions of the defect were 22.5 × 10 × 5.5 mm depth (mesiodistal length, inferosuperior height, and buccolingual depth).

2. Discussion

The Stafne bone defect was first described by Stafne in 1942 [1]. Since then, numerous cases have been reported [1–4, 7, 11, 12]. The exact pathogenesis is still obscure. Stafne suggested that the cavity could result from a failure of normal bone deposition in the region formerly occupied by cartilage [1, 5]. However, the most widely accepted view is that the cavities develop as a result of a localized pressure atrophy of the lingual surface of the mandible from the adjacent salivary gland [13].

Stafne bone defect has anterior and posterior variants. The posterior variant is the most known variant of the defect and is located between the mandibular angle and first mandibular molar tooth below the inferior dental canal [1–11, 14–17]. The defect in our first case was located on the second molar region and soft tissue content was connected with the mouth floor through the lingual cortex. For the second case, the defect was located on the edentulous third molar region.

Stafne bone defects were asymptomatic, with a predilection for men between 50 and 70 years [2, 5, 7, 8]. Distinctively, ın the first case, Stafne bone defect was described for 31-year-old asymptomatic male patient. And the prevalence in published series ranges from 0.10% to 0.48% [1–4, 7–14]. In our clinic, 7922 patients were diagnosed in 1 year and it can be assumed that the prevalence of Stafne bone defect is nearly 0.025%.

The diagnosis of this defect is incidental, since patients do not usually present clinical symptoms [9]. In the orthopantomograph, the technique which usually first identifies this entity, a radiolucent image with a well-defined sclerotic border is generally observed, situated at a posterior location of the mandible, below the inferior dental canal [16, 17].

Surgery is not necessary for the treatment of anterior or posterior Stafne bone defect. Surgical exploration or biopsy should be performed in atypical cases or other suspected lesions. The bone defects of two patients in this study were asymptomatic and any other bone lesions, such as cysts and tumors, were excluded because no signs of inflammatory or tumoral changes were evident [3]. Therefore, surgery was not considered and the patients were followed for 1 year. No remarkable changes of the defects were seen during the follow-up period; thus, justifying the accuracy of the initial diagnosis of posterior Stafne bone defect.

The differential diagnosis of SBC includes benign and malign jaw lesions such as odontogenic cystic lesion, nonossifying fibroma, fibrous displasia, vascular malformation,

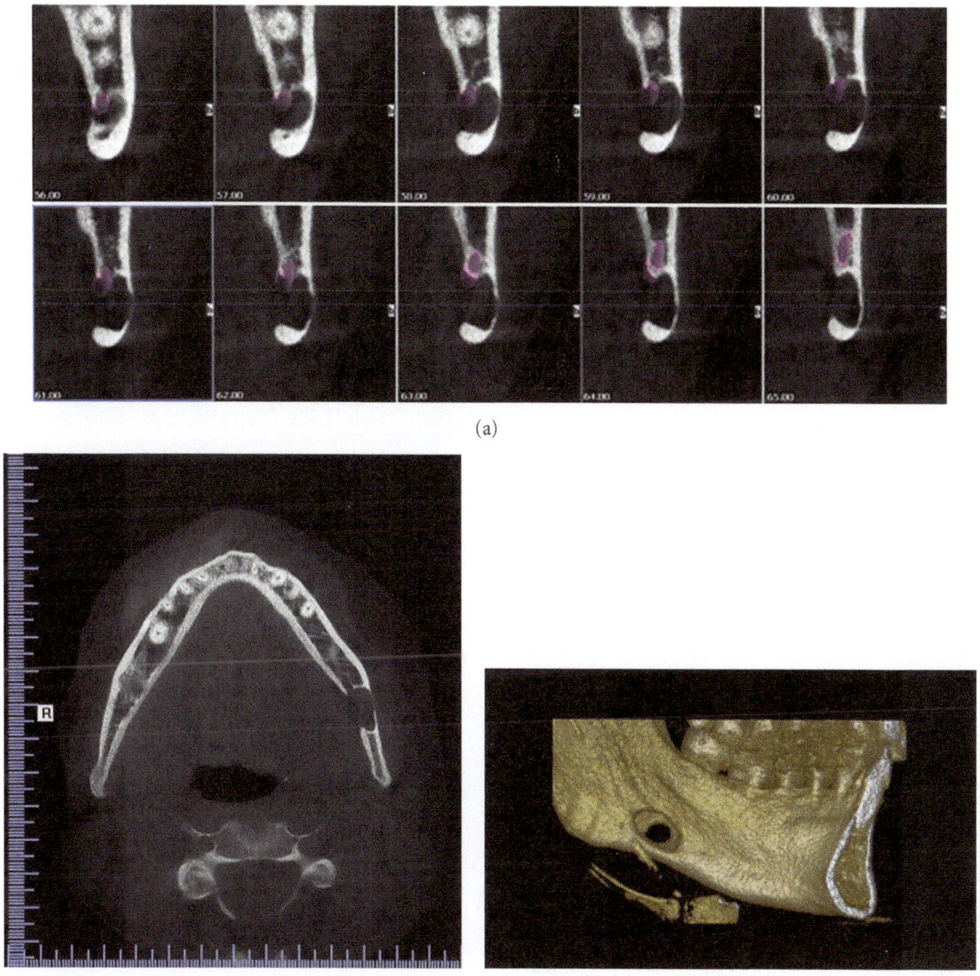

(a)

(b) (c)

FIGURE 2: CBCT images: (a) sagital view displaying continuous 1 mm width sections, (b) horizontal view displaying the cavity outline with diminished buccal cortical bone, and (c) 3D reconstruction of the left mandible displaying buccal cortical bone reduction.

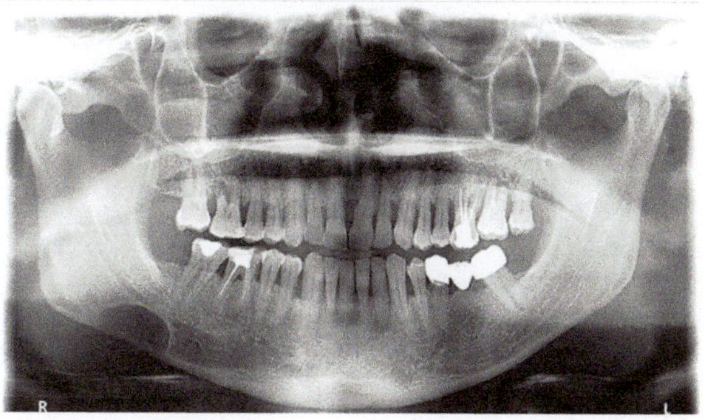

FIGURE 3: Panoramic radiography showing the radiolucent area.

focal osteoporotic bone marrow defect, brown tumor of hyperparathyroidism, ameloblastoma, basal cell nevus syndrome, giant cell tumor, or a metastasis from a primary malignant tumor. Therefore, in some cases more confirmatory diagnostic tools are mandatory [2–5, 12, 18]. Sialography is able to depict salivary tissue in the bony cavity and has been used to confirm the diagnosis [19]. However, there were case reports of surgically proved Stafne bone cavity with negative results in sialography [20]. CT, currently considered as the complementary test of choice, has the great

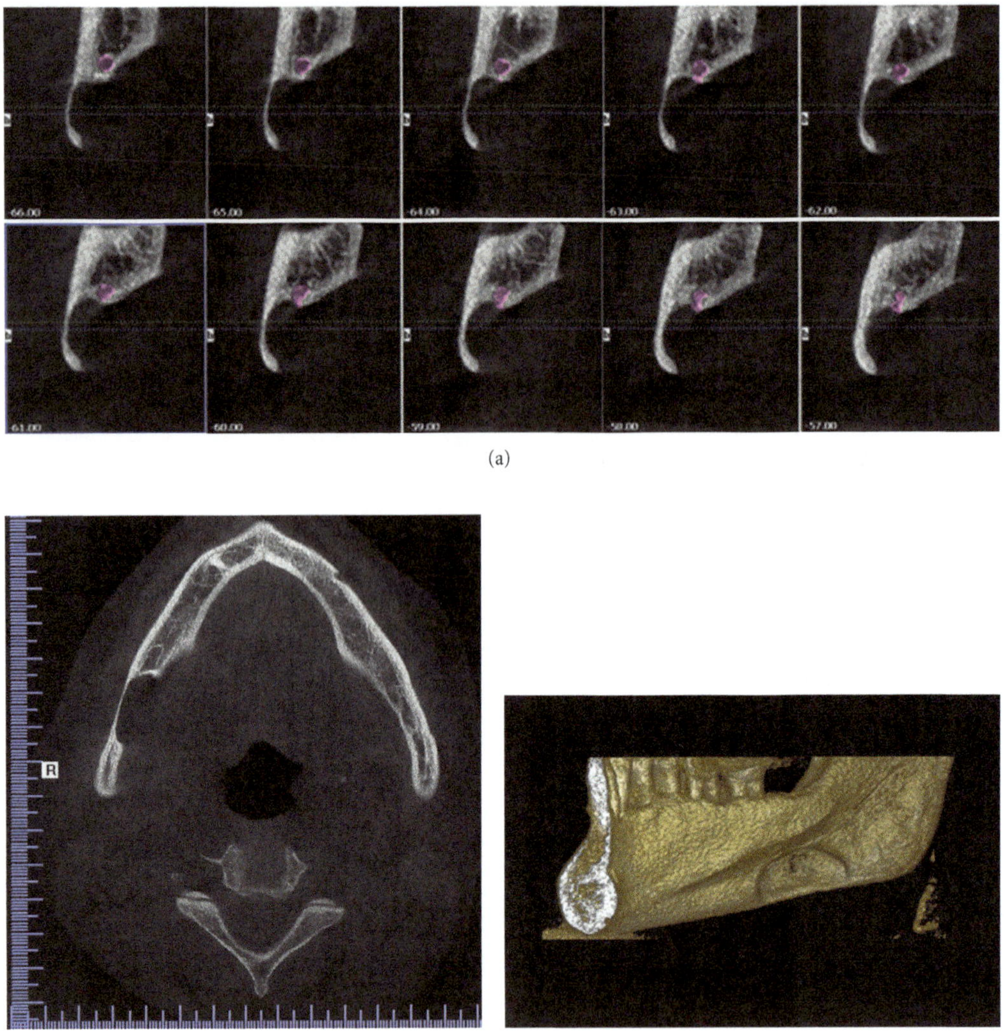

(a)

(b) (c)

Figure 4: CBCT images: (a) sagital view displaying continuous 1 mm width sections, (b) horizontal view displaying the cavity outline, and (c) 3D reconstruction of the right mandible displaying buccal cortical bone reduction.

advantage of verifying the peripheral origin of the lesion and the conservation of the lingual cortical, which are essential characteristics for discounting other pathologies such as apical or residual cysts, fibrous dysplasia, and traumatic osseous cyst, among others [8, 17]. The fact that CT is more specific to bone lesions of the jaws and much less so to soft tissue have led some authors to advocate MR imaging as the primary diagnostic technique [6, 8]. Branstetter et al. [6] were the first to establish a diagnosis of SBC merely on MR imaging with no further treatment. The main advantage of MR imaging is its superior soft tissue characterization and discrimination. The superior soft tissue contrast of MR imaging should be adequate to make the diagnosis of SBC, even without any intravenous contrast material. Its major disadvantage is the high cost and the distortion artifacts produced by dental material [5]. In this paper, orthopantomograph and CBCT are used for diagnosing the defect.

3. Conclusion

Stafne bone defect was an incidental finding, presenting no evolutionary changes, and as such conservatory therapy based on periodic controls was indicated. Currently, complementary techniques such as CT are sufficient to establish a certain diagnosis.

References

[1] E. C. Stafne, “Bone cavities situated near the angle of the mandible,” *Journal of the American Dental Association*, vol. 29, pp. 1969–1972, 1942.

[2] P. S. Campos, J. A. C. Oliveira, J. A. Dantas et al., “Stafne's defect with Buccal cortical expansion: a case report,” *International Journal of Dentistry*, vol. 2010, Article ID 515931, 3 pages, 2010.

[3] O. Dereci and S. Duran, “Intraorally exposed anterior Stafne bone defect: a case report,” *Oral Surgery, Oral Medicine, Oral*

Pathology, Oral Radiology, and Endodontology, vol. 113, no. 5, pp. e1–e3, 2012.

[4] K. Turkoglu and K. Orhan, "Stafne bone cavity in the anterior mandible," *Journal of Craniofacial Surgery*, vol. 21, no. 6, pp. 1769–1775, 2010.

[5] Y. Segev, M. Puterman, and L. Bodner, "Stafne bone cavity-magnetic resonance imaging.," *Medicina Oral, Patología Oral y Cirugía Bucal*, vol. 11, no. 4, pp. E345–347, 2006.

[6] B. F. Branstetter, J. L. Weissman, and S. B. Kaplan, "Imaging of a Stafne bone cavity: what MR adds and why a new name is needed," *American Journal of Neuroradiology*, vol. 20, no. 4, pp. 587–589, 1999.

[7] L. B. V. Aguiar, F. S. Neves, L. C. Bastos, I. Crusoé-Rebello, G. M. B. Ambrosano, and P. S. F. Campos, "Multiple Stafne bone defects: a rare entity," *ISRN Dentistry*, vol. 2011, Article ID 792145, 3 pages, 2011.

[8] T. J. Grellner, D. E. Frost, and R. B. Brannon, "Lingual mandibular bone defect: report of three cases," *Journal of Oral and Maxillofacial Surgery*, vol. 48, no. 3, pp. 288–296, 1990.

[9] C. Quesada-Gómez, E. Valmaseda-Castellón, L. Berini-Aytés, and C. Gay-Escoda, "Stafne bone cavity: a retrospective study of 11 cases.," *Medicina Oral, Patología Oral y Cirugía Bucal*, vol. 11, no. 3, pp. E277–280, 2006.

[10] E. L. Layne, A. F. Morgan, and T. H. Morton Jr, "Anterior lingual mandibular bone concavity: report of case," *Journal of Oral Surgery*, vol. 39, no. 8, pp. 599–600, 1981.

[11] M. Şahin, S. Görgün, and O. Güven, "Stafne kemik kavitesi," *Türkiye Klinikleri Journal of Dental Sciences*, vol. 11, pp. 39–42, 2005.

[12] H. P. Philipsen, T. Takata, P. A. Reichart, S. Sato, and Y. Suei, "Lingual and buccal mandibular bone depressions: a review based on 583 cases from a world-wide literature survey, including 69 new cases from Japan," *Dentomaxillofacial Radiology*, vol. 31, no. 5, pp. 281–290, 2002.

[13] C. A. Boyle, K. Horner, P. Coulthard, and G. J. Fleming, "Multiple Stafne bone cavities: a diagnostic dilemma.," *Dental Update*, vol. 27, no. 10, pp. 494–497, 2000.

[14] M. Dorman and D. Pierse, "Ectopic salivary gland tissue in the anterior mandible: a case report," *British Dental Journal*, vol. 193, no. 10, pp. 571–572, 2002.

[15] A. de Courten, R. Küffer, J. Samson, and T. Lombardi, "Anterior lingual mandibular salivary gland defect (Stafne defect) presenting as a residual cyst," *Oral Surgery, Oral Medicine, Oral Pathology, Oral Radiology, and Endodontics*, vol. 94, no. 4, pp. 460–464, 2002.

[16] G. R. Barker, "Xeroradiography in relation to a stafne bone cavity," *British Journal of Oral and Maxillofacial Surgery*, vol. 26, no. 1, pp. 32–35, 1988.

[17] I. Reuter, "An unusual case of Stafne bone cavity with extra-osseous course of the mandibular neurovascular bundle," *Dentomaxillofacial Radiology*, vol. 27, no. 3, pp. 189–191, 1998.

[18] S. Prapanpoch and R. P. Langlais, "Lingual cortical defect of the mandible: an unusual presentation and tomographic diagnosis," *Dentomaxillofacial Radiology*, vol. 23, no. 4, pp. 234–237, 1994.

[19] K. Tonigana, Y. Kuga, K. Kubota, and T. Ohba, "Stafne's bone cavity in the anterior mandible," *Dentomaxillofacial Radiology*, vol. 19, pp. 28–30, 1990.

[20] V. J. Oikarinen, J. Wolf, and M. Julku, "A sterosialographic study of developmental mandibular bone defects (Stafne's idiopathic bone cavities)," *International Journal of Oral Surgery*, vol. 4, pp. 51–54, 1975.

Aberrant Anatomical Variation of Maxillary Sinus Mimicking Periapical Cyst: A Report of Two Cases and Role of CBCT in Diagnosis

Ahmet Ercan Sekerci, Yildiray Sisman, Meryem Etoz, and Duygu Goller Bulut

Department of Oral and Maxillofacial Radiology, Faculty of Dentistry, Erciyes University, 38039 Kayseri, Turkey

Correspondence should be addressed to Ahmet Ercan Sekerci; aercansekerci@hotmail.com

Academic Editors: J. Asaumi, R. S. Brown, G. Schierano, and K. H. Zawawi

Most periapical lesions are associated with microorganisms from infected root canal systems. Maxillary sinus can pose a diagnostic dilemma radiographically because of its anatomical variation which can mimic a periapical pathosis. The aim of this study was to describe two cases of aberrant anatomical variation of the maxillary sinus that presented radiographic similarities to a periapical cyst in order to call the attention of clinicians to the fact that several different diseases are able to mimic endodontic periapical lesions. An accurate assessment of this morphology was made with the help of cone-beam computed tomography (CBCT).

1. Introduction

Several cases of benign and malignant lesions mimicking radiographically periapical inflammatory lesions, such as carcinoma [1], odontogenic cyst [2], periapical cemental dysplasia [3], benign tumors, and locally aggressive or malignant neoplasias [4], have been described in the literature. Film-processing errors have also been reported to mimic the appearance of periapical infection and cause diagnostic confusion [5]. Plain radiographs play an important role in the management of dentomaxillofacial lesions especially for detection, treatment, and followup of bone lesion. However, routine radiographic procedures do not demonstrate reliably the presence of every lesion. Furthermore, advanced imaging techniques can influence the diagnosis [6].

In the present report, two unique cases of anatomical variation of the maxillary sinus manifesting as a well-defined periapical radiolucency in relation to the roots of the upper left first molar and right second premolar, which were initially misdiagnosed as a periapical cyst, are described. This variation may have been interpreted as a periapical inflammatory lesion. The value of cone-beam computed tomography (CBCT) as a prognostic determinant was highlighted.

2. Case Report

2.1. Patient I. A 25-year-old man was referred by his general dental practitioner to the Department of Oral and Maxillofacial Radiology regarding a periapical lesion related to the apex of the upper right molar teeth and prosthetic management. Intraoral examination revealed that there were a few teeth with caries in different regions. Panoramic radiography revealed a well-defined radiolucency involving the root apices of the upper right maxillary first molar (Figure 1(a)). The borders exhibited dense radiopaque features. Provisional diagnosis of the radicular cyst was established, and root canal treatment was carried out. Endodontic retreatment was initiated by his dentist, but after a followup of several months, no changes were observed in the ovoid radiolucency, and the patient was referred for consultation to our department. The patient's medical history was unremarkable, included no trauma of the jaws, and he had not undergone any jaw surgery. He was not aware of the radiolucent area before his routine dental examination and had no sensory or motor deficiency. The tooth was asymptomatic and it also presented with a poor root canal filling. The overlying mucosa of the lesion was quite normal, and there was no sign of infection

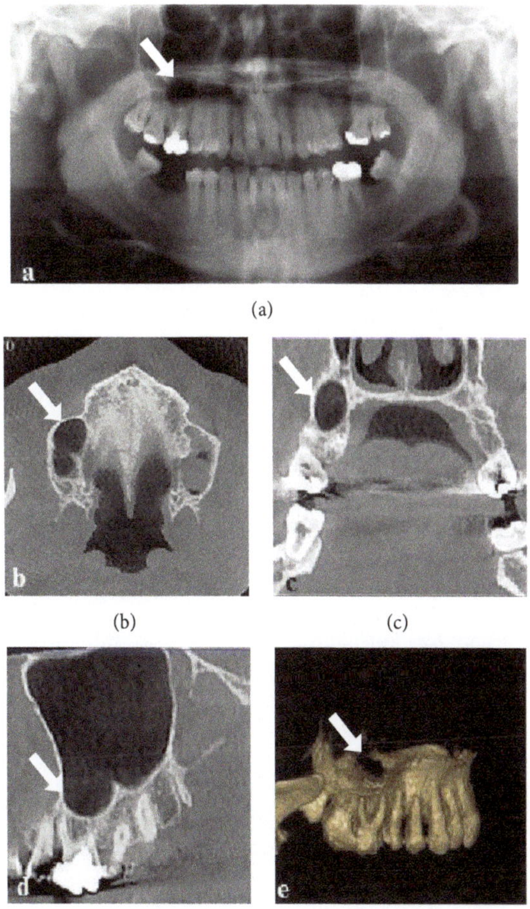

(a)

(b) (c)

(d) (e)

FIGURE 1: Panoramic radiograph showing well-defined periapical radiolucency in relation to maxillary first molar, extending to involve the root of canine and suggestive of a periapical cyst (a). Axial (b), coronal (c), sagittal, and three dimensional view of the aberrant anatomical variation of maxillary sinus.

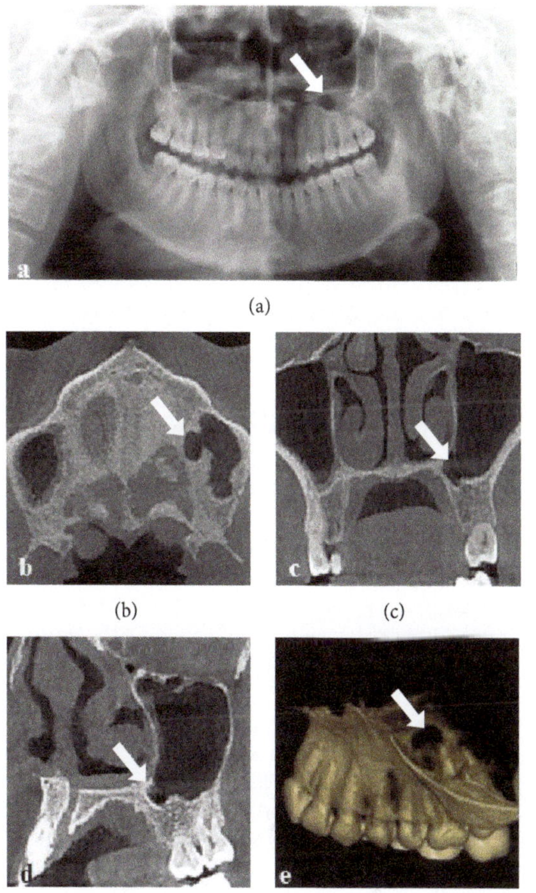

(a)

(b) (c)

(d) (e)

FIGURE 2: Panoramic radiograph showing well-defined periapical radiolucency in relation to apices of the maxillary left second premolar and first molar (a). Axial (b), coronal (c), sagittal, and three dimensional view of the anatomical variation of maxillary sinus.

or fistula. The overall appearance of the lesion seemed to be that of a radicular cyst of the right maxillary first molar. On performance of vitality tests, all the teeth except the first molar- in the mentioned area appeared to be vital.

To reveal the exact location definition of the pathologic features, he was referred for a CBCT (NewTom 5G, QR, Verona, Italy) scan. After this, a CBCT was taken which revealed the maxillary sinus with its border extending but not involving the roots of the mentioned teeth, which is one of the anatomical variations of maxillary sinus (Figure 1(b)–1(e)). The dimensions of the defect were 13.2 × 14.2 × 9.3 mm depth (mesiodistal length, inferosuperior height, and buccolingual depth).

2.2. Patient II. A 29-year-old otherwise healthy woman was referred to our clinic for routine dental examination and periodontal management. Panoramic radiography showed a unilocular, oval, and radiolucent lesion with well-defined sclerotic borders situated at the apices of the second left premolar and first molar teeth in the maxilla (Figure 2(a)). The radiolucency was located superior to, but not continuous with, the periodontal area of the tooth. The patient's history included no trauma of the jaws, and she had not undergone any jaw surgery. The patient was not aware of the radiolucent area before her routine dental examination and had no sensory or motor deficiency, and there was no pain. The overlying mucosa of the lesion was quite normal, and there was no sign of infection or fistula. The overall appearance of the lesion seemed to be that of a radicular cyst of the right maxillary first molar, On performance of vitality tests, all the teeth in the mentioned area appeared to be vital.

To reveal the exact location definition of the pathologic features, she was referred for cone-beam computed tomography (CBCT: Newtom 5G, QR, Verona, Italy) scan. The dimensions of the defect were 7.3 × 6.7 × 4.7 mm depth (mesiodistal length, inferosuperior height, and buccolingual depth).

Then by combining the results of the patients from clinical examination, radiographic examinations, results from vitality tests, and CBCT examination of the patients, the final diagnosis was made as one of the anatomical variations of the maxillary sinus (Figures 1 and 2).

3. Discussion

The present report deals with one such diagnostic problem, where a maxillary sinus was interpreted in a panoramic radiograph as a periapical lesion. The maxillary sinus is a pyramid-shaped cavity with thin walls corresponding to the orbital, alveolar, facial, and infratemporal aspects of the maxilla. The size, shape, and wall thickness of the sinus vary from one to another even on the two sides of an individual skull [7]. It develops by the invagination of mucous membrane from the nasal cavity. The borders of the maxillary sinus appear on periapical radiographs as a thin, delicate, and tenuous radiopaque line (actually a thin layer of cortical bone). In the absence of disease, it appears continuous, but on close examination, it can be seen to have small interruptions in its smoothness or density. These discontinuities are probably illusions caused by the superimposition of small marrow spaces [8]. Superiorly, the roof is formed by the orbital plate and inferiorly it is bordered by the alveolar process of maxilla [5].

The degree of extension of the maxillary sinus into the alveolar process is extremely variable. The floor of the maxillary sinus is seen on dental radiographs at approximately the same level around the age of puberty. In some projections the floor of the sinus will be well above the apices of the posterior teeth. The roots of the molars usually lie in close apposition to the maxillary sinus. Root apices may project anatomically into the floor of the sinus, causing small elevations or prominences. The thin layer of bone covering the root is seen as a fusion of the lamina dura and the floor of the sinus. When the rounded sinus floor dips between the buccal and palatal molar roots and is medial to the premolar roots, the projection of the apices is superior to the floor. This appearance conveys the impression that the roots project into the sinus cavity, which is an illusion [8]. There has been one case reported in which the maxillary sinus extended from the lateral incisors to the third molars [9]. The sinus floor usually has its most inferior point near the first molar region. Several conical elevations projecting into the sinus floor and corresponding to the roots of the first and second molar teeth sometimes perforate [10].

Frequently one or a number of radiopaque lines which are called septa traverse the image of the maxillary sinus. They are thin folds of cortical bone that project a few millimeters away from the floor and wall of the antrum, or they may extend across the sinus. They appear on many periapical intraoral radiographs and commonly on CBCT images. While septa appear to separate the sinuses into distinct compartments, this is rarely the case. Rather, the septa naturally extend only a few millimeters into the central volume of the sinus. Septa deserve attention because they sometimes mimic periapical disease, and the chambers they create in the alveolar recess may complicate the search for a root fragment displaced into the sinus [8].

Maxillary cysts are pathologic cavities with a liquid or semiliquid content delimited wholly or partially by epithelium; the origin of the latter allows one to distinguish cysts as odontogenic or nonodontogenic [11]. Radicular cysts are considered to be lesions of an odontogenic nature which originate from the epithelial residues present in the parodontium space, and their proliferation is activated by an inflammatory- type mechanism [12]. The radicular cyst is the most common cystic lesion, with a frequency of about 50% amongst all cystic lesions of odontogenic nature. This lesion is often diagnosed accidentally while taking normal radiographic tests. A rather convenient indication to address the diagnoses is the vitality test, as a radicular cyst is always associated with a necrotic dental element [13]. From a radiographic point of view, this neoformation appears as a unilocular radio transparency with very clear margins with a roundish shape still in relation with the radicular apex [14].

Basnet et al. [5] suggested that, when periapical radiolucency is seen in theradiograph, it may be a distinct pathologic lesion or it could just be an anatomical variation. The gathering of data by clinical and radiographic examinations helps clinicians to form an operational opinion. They also stated that only endodontic therapy should be initiated if these data support the diagnosis of radiolucent lesion associated with a nonvital tooth. If it does not, then further diagnostic data should be collected from various clinical tests, advance imaging techniques, biopsy, consultation with appropriate specialists, and so forth. In the present study, on performance of vitality tests, all the teeth appeared to be vital. Therefore, CBCT scan was performed for the diagnosis.

Therefore, thorough knowledge about the anatomy of the maxillary sinus and its variations, proper diagnostic aids and good interpretation skills are essential to form an accurate diagnosis.

4. Conclusion

The present report highlights the need for careful consideration of the causes of periapical radiolucency before making an actual diagnosis using CBCT and identifies a poorly recognized anatomical variation which may cause diagnostic confusion. In addition, it is necessary for dentists to be reasonably well informed on the radiographic appearances of the normal anatomy, as well as the abnormalities and diseases that occur in the maxilla.

Conflict of Interests

The authors declare no conflict of interests.

References

[1] R. Cutler, "Neoplasia masquerading as periapical infection," *British Dental Journal*, vol. 168, no. 9, pp. 348–349, 1990.

[2] M. A. F. Hancock Jr., C. E. Brown, and K. S. Hartman, "Orthokeratinized odontogenic cyst presenting as a periapical lesion," *Journal of Endodontics*, vol. 12, no. 11, pp. 539–541, 1986.

[3] S. Smith, K. Patel, and A. E. Hoskinson, "Periapical cemental dysplasia: a case of misdiasnosis," *British Dental Journal*, vol. 185, no. 3, pp. 122–123, 1998.

[4] C. C. García, F. V. Sempere, M. P. Diago, and E. M. Bowen, "The post-endodontic periapical lesion: histologic and etiopathogenic aspects," *Medicina Oral, Patología Oral y Cirugía Bucal*, vol. 12, no. 8, pp. 585–590, 2007.

[5] P. Basnet, M. P. Kamath, M. Kundabala, and A. Menda, "Anatomical variation of maxillary sinus mimicking a periapical cyst: a case report," *Kathmandu University Medical Journal*, vol. 3, no. 4, pp. 415–417, 2005.

[6] M. B. Saunders, K. Gulabivala, R. Holt, and R. S. Kahan, "Reliability of radiographic observation recordedon a performa using inter and intra observer variation: a preliminary study," *International Endodontic Journal*, vol. 33, no. 3, pp. 173–185, 2000.

[7] C. Arman, I. Ergür, A. Atabey et al., "The thickness and the lengths of the anterior wall of adult maxilla of the West Anatolian Turkish people," *Surgical and Radiologic Anatomy*, vol. 28, no. 6, pp. 553–558, 2006.

[8] S. C. White and M. J. Pharoah, *Oral Radiology Principles and Interpretation*, pp. 161–164, Mosby, St. Louis, Mo, USA, 6th edition, 2009.

[9] B. Srinivasan, *Textbook of Oral and Maxillofacial Surgery*, pp. 274–276, Elsevier, New Delhi, India, 2nd edition, 2004.

[10] J. P. A. van den Bergh, C. M. ten Bruggenkate, F. J. M. Disch, and D. B. Tuinzing, "Anatomical aspects of sinus floor elevations," *Clinical Oral Implants Research*, vol. 11, no. 3, pp. 256–265, 2000.

[11] E. Ciulli, M. Rocci, R. Bollero et al., "Maxillary cyst: description of a clinical case," *Oral Implantology*, vol. 2, no. 2, pp. 28–33, 2009.

[12] D. Ricucci, E. A. Pascon, T. R. Pitt Ford, and K. Langeland, "Epithelium and bacteria in periapical lesions," *Oral Surgery, Oral Medicine, Oral Pathology, Oral Radiology and Endodontology*, vol. 101, no. 2, pp. 239–249, 2006.

[13] G. Murmura, T. Traini, D. di Iorio, G. Varvara, G. Orsini, and S. Caputi, "Residual and inflammatory radicular cysts. Clinical and pathological aspects of 2 cases," *Minerva Stomatologica*, vol. 53, no. 11-12, pp. 693–701, 2004.

[14] J. Düker, "Radiographic diagnostics. Radicular cyst," *Quintessence International*, vol. 36, no. 4, article 317, 2005.

18

Hereditary Nonsyndromic Gingival Fibromatosis: Report of Family Case Series

Syed Wali Peeran,[1] Karthikeyan Ramalingam,[2] Syed Ali Peeran,[3] Marei Hamed Mugrabi,[4] and Khaled Awidat Abdulla[5]

[1] *Department of Periodontology and Oral Implantology, Faculty of Dentistry, Sebha University, Sebha, Libya*
[2] *Department of Oral Pathology & Microbiology, Faculty of Dentistry, Sebha University, Sebha, Libya*
[3] *Department of Oral and Maxillofacial Prosthodontics, Faculty of Dentistry, Jazan University, Jazan 45 142, Saudi Arabia*
[4] *Department of Periodontics, Faculty of Dentistry, Arab Medical University, Benghazi, Libya*
[5] *Department of Oral Biology and Orthodontics, Faculty of Dentistry, Sebha University, Sebha, Libya*

Correspondence should be addressed to Karthikeyan Ramalingam; drrkn79@gmail.com

Academic Editors: R. Crespi and A. Epivatianos

Hereditary gingival fibromatosis (HGF) is a rare, benign disorder with slowly progressive enlargement of maxillary and mandibular gingiva. Herewith, we report the first case series of HGF presenting among mother and all of her 3 children. Their complaints included unaesthetic appearance due to gingival growth, malocclusion, and difficulty in mastication. Conventional gingivectomy with oral hygiene measures and regular followup is the treatment of choice for such presentation.

1. Introduction

Hereditary gingival fibromatosis (HGF) is a rare type of gingival enlargement. HGF can present in two forms, a nodular form affecting the dental papillae or a symmetric uniform gingival enlargement. HGF is seen as pale-pink enlargements, firm and leathery in consistency [1].

The literature search in PubMed revealed only two case series on HGF [2, 3]. Herewith, we report the first case series to the best of our knowledge, comprising 4 patients with HGF involving the mother and all of her three children including 2 daughters and 1 son.

2. Case Presentation

A 14-year-old female was reported with her father to the Outpatient Department, Faculty of Dentistry, Sebha University, Sebha, Libya. Her chief complaint was gingival swellings in the posterior region of upper and lower jaws since her childhood. Previous medical and surgical histories were noncontributory. Family history revealed that similar presentations were seen in her elder sister, elder brother, and her mother. Her father was unaffected.

Clinical examination revealed diffuse, firm gingival enlargements symmetrically involving the maxillary and mandibular gingiva bilaterally (Figure 1). The enlargements were more severe in the molar region (Figure 2) and crowns were covered by soft tissue (Figure 3). Her family members were requested to report for clinical examination. Her elder sister was 25 years of age. She also had bilateral, symmetrical, and gingival enlargements in the posterior region of maxillary and mandibular gingiva (Figure 4). The teeth were displaced from their normal position. She also had retained deciduous teeth and multiple grossly decayed teeth (Figure 5). Her elder brother was 35 years of age. He also had bilateral, symmetrical enlargements, more prominent in the molar region (Figure 6). He also had severe malocclusion with arch collapse (Figures 7 and 8). Her mother was 62 years of age. She gave a history of similar enlargements in her gingiva and underwent multiple gingival surgeries for the same reason. Clinical examination revealed multiple

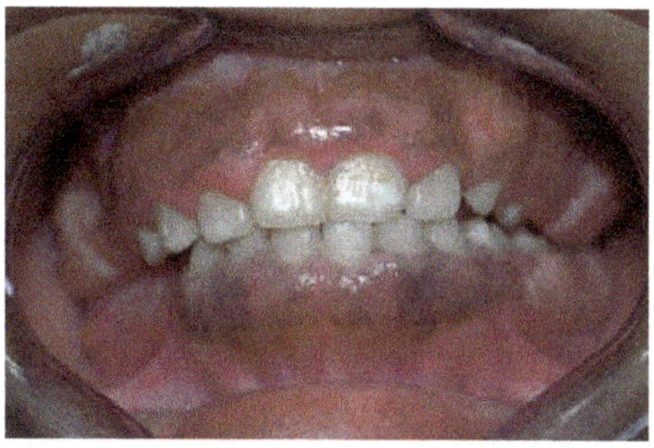

FIGURE 1: Clinical picture of 14-year-old female with gingival enlargement.

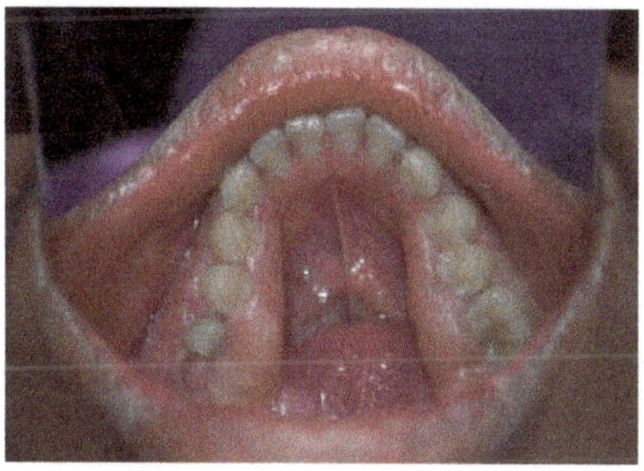

FIGURE 2: Clinical picture showing prominent enlargement in the posterior region.

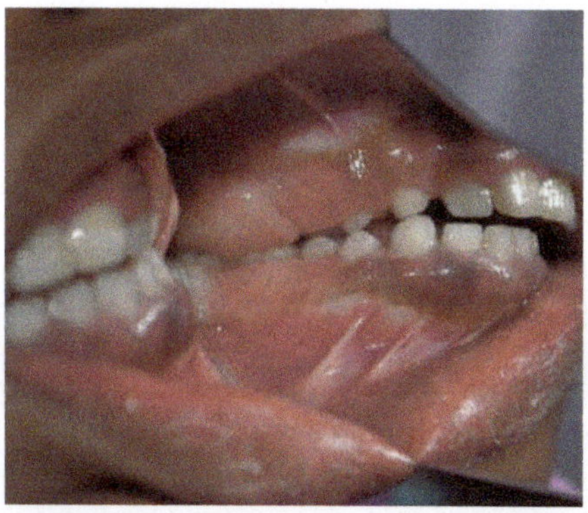

FIGURE 3: Clinical picture showing enlargement covering the crowns of molars.

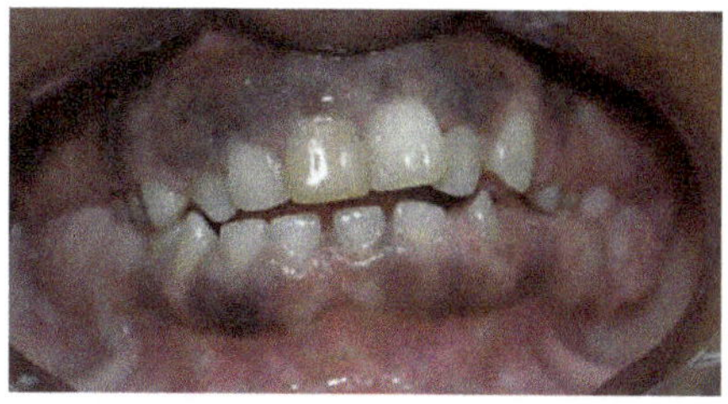

FIGURE 4: Clinical picture of 25-year-old sister with gingival enlargement.

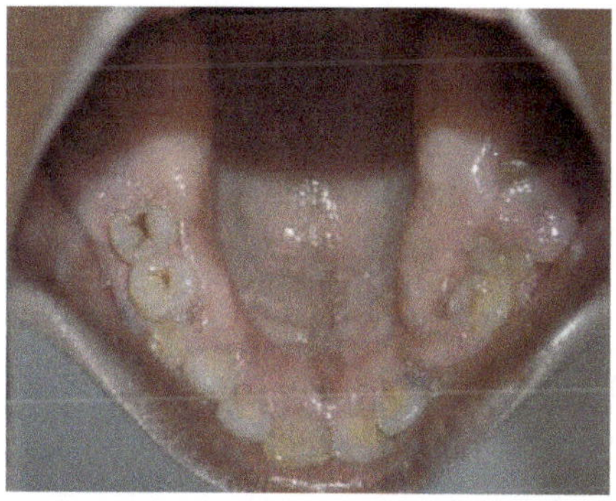

FIGURE 5: Clinical picture showing prominent gingival enlargement in posterior region.

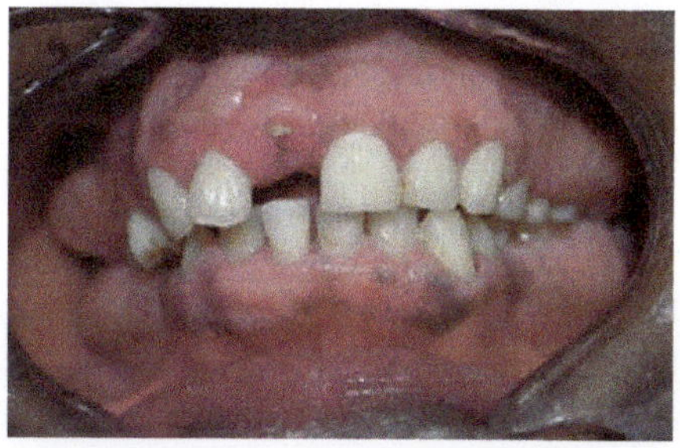

FIGURE 6: Clinical picture of 35-year-old brother with gingival enlargement.

missing teeth and remaining roots (Figure 9), and gingival enlargement was still evident in the molar region of mandible (Figure 10).

Correlating the family history and clinical presentations, it was diagnosed as hereditary nonsyndromic gingival fibromatosis.

The patients were advised for gingivectomy and regular oral hygiene maintenance with followup as treatment plan.

3. Discussion

HGF occurs due to congenital or hereditary causes. Studies reveal an autosomal dominant inheritance with chromosomal abnormality in 2p21-p22 and 5q13-q22 [1, 4]. It could arise due to nutritional and hormonal factors [5]. A mutation in the *Son of Sevenless-1* (*SOS-1*) gene has been suggested as a possible cause. Our case series also suggests autosomal dominant inheritance with HGF affecting the mother and all her children, whereas the father is unaffected.

HGF can present as a nonsyndromic isolated variant, occasionally with epilepsy, mental retardation, or hypertrichosis. HGF can also be associated with syndromes like Cowden's syndrome (multiple hamartomas), Zimmerman-Laband syndrome (defects of bone, nail, ear, nose, and splenomegaly), Murray-Purelie Drescher syndrome (multiple dental hyaline tumors), Rutherford syndrome (corneal dystrophy), Jones syndrome (sensori-neural deafness), and Cross syndrome (hypopigmentation with athetosis) [1, 6]. As our patients did not have any other manifestations, it can be diagnosed as the non-syndromic, idiopathic variant of HGF.

The gingival enlargement does not occur until the eruption of the primary or permanent dentition [5]. It affects

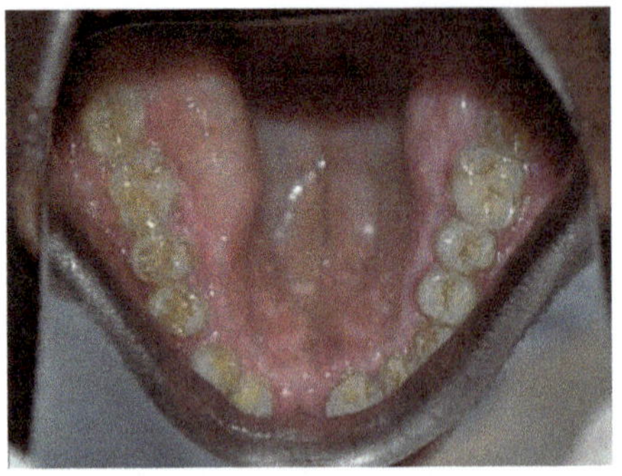

FIGURE 7: Clinical picture showing prominent enlargement in posterior region.

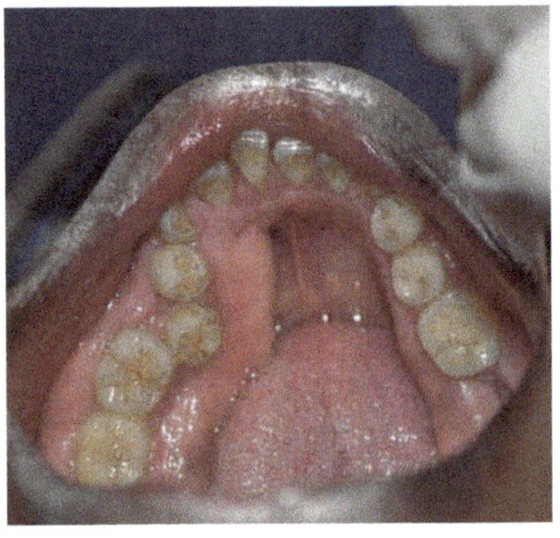

FIGURE 8: Clinical picture showing gingival enlargement and malocclusion.

interdental papillae and marginal and attached gingiva unlike drug induced enlargement in which attached gingiva is uninvolved. The severity may vary from mild involvement of one quadrant to severe involvement of all four quadrants [4]. The enlarged tissues can partially or totally cover the crowns, cause diastemas and pseudopockets, delay tooth eruption, and cause malocclusion. It can also present with abnormal swallowing pattern, difficulty in speech, and mastication. Our case series correlated with the literature in the clinical features of HGF.

The precise mechanism of HGF is unknown but could be confined to the fibroblasts in the gingivae. The continuing recurrence of the enlargement after repeated surgery and a permanent remolding of tissues after extraction of teeth suggest the importance of the presence of teeth and the gingival crevice environment in the pathogenesis of such enlargements [7]. Some authors report an increase in the proliferation of gingival fibroblasts, whereas others report slowerthan normal growth. Increased collagen synthesis rather than decreased levels of collagenase activity may be involved [8]. In our case series, gingival overgrowth has subsided in areas of prior extraction.

Histopathology of affected tissue reveals dense connective tissue rich in coarse connective tissue fibres, with young fibroblasts and scarce blood vessels. Small calcified particles,

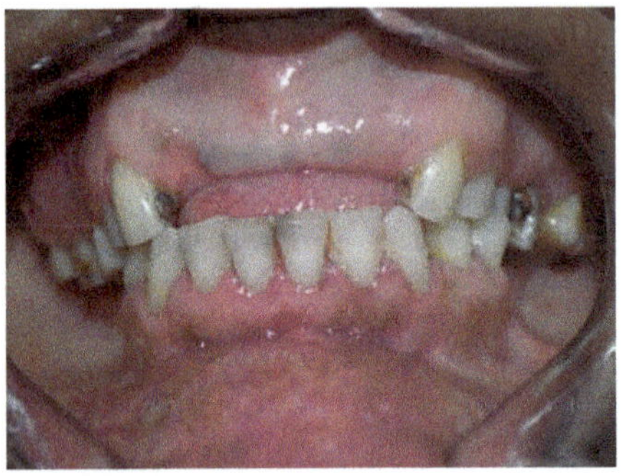

FIGURE 9: Clinical picture of 62-year-old mother with missing teeth.

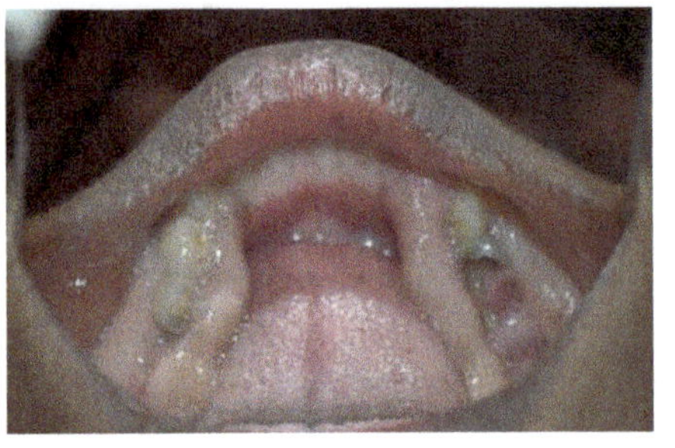

FIGURE 10: Clinical picture showing gingival enlargement in posterior region.

amyloid deposits, osseous metaplasia, and islands of odontogenic epithelium may be seen unusually. The overlying epithelium is of variable thickness and can show hyperkeratosis with elongated rete ridges [9].

The finest and suggested treatment modality for HGF is gingivectomy. The literature reports high recurrence rate after surgery and required a close followup. There is debate regarding the time of surgery. Eruption of complete set of permanent teeth is the recommended time for surgery [10]. The mother has previously undergone multiple gingivectomies and remained without recurrence. The treatment plan advised for the other affected patients is gingivectomy with regular oral hygiene measures and frequent followup.

To conclude, herewith we report the first case series to the best of our knowledge of HGF affecting the mother and all her children. A multidisciplinary management is advised to completely rehabilitate the patient.

References

[1] A. K. Tavergeri, S. S. Kulkarni, P. Sudha, and Basavprabhu, "Idiopathic gingival fibromatosis—a case report," *Journal of Indian Society of Pedodontics, Preventive Dentistry*, vol. 22, no. 4, pp. 180–182, 2004.

[2] E. G. Wagaiyu, R. N. Ng'ang'a, and A. M. Kemoli, "Hereditary gingival fibromatosis: report of family case series," *East African Medical Journal*, vol. 86, no. 10, pp. 491–493, 2009.

[3] J. Shi, W. Lin, X. Li, F. Zhang, and X. Hong, "Hereditary gingival fibromatosis: a three-generation case and pathogenic mechanism research on progress of the disease," *Journal of Periodontology*, vol. 82, no. 7, pp. 1089–1095, 2011.

[4] A. N. Prathibha, A. N. Ullal, K. Vishal, and N. Nupur, "Idiopathic gingival fibromatosis," *International Journal of Clinical Pediatric Dentistry*, vol. 4, no. 1, pp. 77–81, 2011.

[5] K. R. Indushekar, "Idiopathic gingival fibromatosis—case report," *Saudi Dental Journal*, vol. 14, pp. 143–145, 2003.

[6] R. J. Gorlin, J. J. Pindborg, and M. M. Cohen Jr., *Syndromes of Head and Neck*, pp. 329–336, McGraw Hill, New York, NY, USA, 2nd edition, 1976.

[7] P. S. Tiwana, I. J. De Kok, D. S. Stoker, and L. F. Cooper, "Facial distortion secondary to idiopathic gingival hyperplasia: surgical management and oral reconstruction with endosseous implants," *Oral Surgery, Oral Medicine, Oral Pathology, Oral Radiology and Endodontology*, vol. 100, no. 2, pp. 153–157, 2005.

[8] M. Jayachandran, S. Kapoor, and R. Mahesh, "Idiopathic gingival fibromatosis rehabilitation: a case report with two-year followup," *Case Reports in Dentistry*, vol. 2013, Article ID 513153, 5 pages, 2013.

[9] O. Günhan, D. G. Gardner, H. Bostanci, and M. Günhan, "Familial gingival fibromatosis with unusual histologic findings," *Journal of Periodontology*, vol. 66, no. 11, pp. 1008–1011, 1995.

[10] P. P. Jaju, A. Desai, R. Desai, and S. P. Jaju, "Idiopathic gingival fibromatosis: case report and its management," *International Journal of Dentistry*, vol. 2009, Article ID 153603, 6 pages, 2009.

19

Solitary Angiokeratoma of Oral Mucosa: A Rare Presentation

Shilpa Kandalgaonkar, Suyog Tupsakhare, Ashok Patil, Gaurav Agrawal, Mahesh Gabhane, and Shrikant Sonune

Department Oral Pathology & Microbiology, SMBT Dental College & Hospital, Sangamner, Maharashtra 422608, India

Correspondence should be addressed to Gaurav Agrawal; agrawalgaurav28@rediffmail.com

Academic Editors: R. S. Brown and A. C. B. Delbem

Solitary angiokeratoma of oral mucosa is rare entity. The term Angiokeratoma is used to refer to several lesions, whose common denominator is the presence of dilated blood vessels in association with epidermal hyperplasia. Mucosal involvement, including oral cavity is occasionally found either as a component of the systemic variety, cutaneous involvement or isolated oral involvement. Clinically, the lesion is irregular, whitish to dark brown in color, with female predominance. The etiological factors include injury, trauma, or chronic irritation to the wall of a papillary dermis. Histologically, it is characterized by hyperkeratosis, acanthosis, and dilated vascular spaces with or without organizing thrombi in papillary dermis. The vascular spaces are partly or completely enclosed by elongated ret-ridges. Along with this reporting a case of solitary angiokeratoma affecting tongue in a 38-year-old male patient, along with the literature review is presented.

1. Introduction

Angiokeratoma is an acquired vascular lesion which is characterized histologically as one or more dilated blood vessels lying directly subepidermally and showing an epidermal proliferative reaction especially acanthosis and hyperkeratosis with dilated capillaries in the papillary dermis [1].

Several clinical types have been described depending on the multiplicity and location of the lesions. They can be divided into localized and systemic types [2]. Mucosal involvement, including the oral cavity, has been described both as localized and systemic types, as a component of Fabry's disease, or as a component of fucosidosis [2–5]. To classify isolated oral mucosal angiokeratomas, other classification systems have been proposed by Ranjan and Mahajan [6].

However, solitary angiokeratomas of the oral mucosa seem to be a rather infrequent occurrence, and very few cases have been reported in the literature. According to the best of our knowledge, since 1997 till date, only 16 cases involving oral cavity have been reported.

2. Case Report

A 38-year-old male patient reported to the Department of Oral Pathology with chief complaint of growth on tip of tongue since last 10 years. The patient was apparently all right 10 years ago when he noticed small painless growth, and then the growth steadily increased in size up to present size involving right side of the tip of the tongue. Sometimes the Patient also experienced bleeding in that area which was associated with trauma during mastication. Bleeding subside, on its own, the patient had never taken any treatment for that growth and not even for bleeding episodes. No abnormality was reveled in his medical, personal histories and general examination. The patient had a habit of tobacco chewing for about 10–15 years.

On clinical examination, it was observed that well-circumscribed sessile growth is present on the dorsal surface of tip of the tongue, and the growth is of approximately 1 × 1 cm in dimension, ovoid in shape. Growth was dark brownish in color with a granular surface texture (Figure 1). On palpation, growth was non tender and rough. No other intra- or extraoral lesions are present.

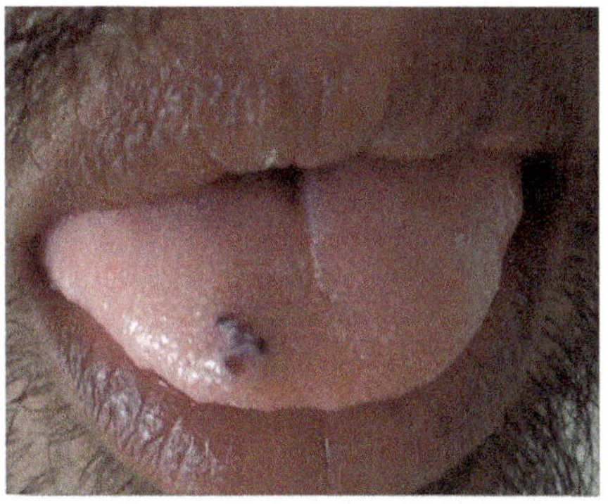

FIGURE 1: Brownish growth present on tip of tongue.

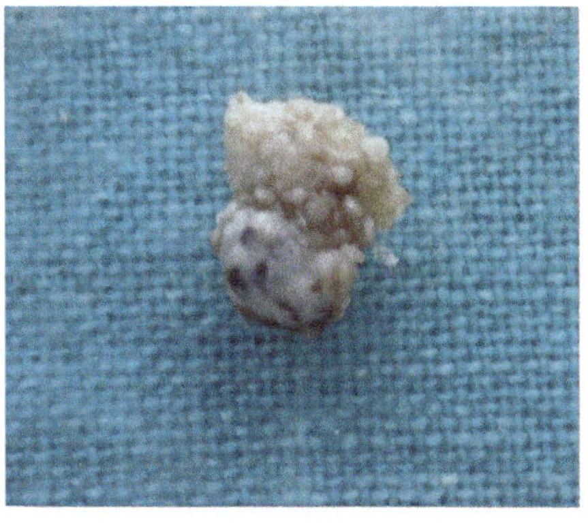

FIGURE 2: Excised specimen.

After routine hematological investigations, under local anesthesia, the lesion was completely excised and taken for histopathological investigation. The gross specimen is irregular in shape approximately 1 × 1 × 0.5 cm in size, brownish in color, and soft in consistency with rough surface (Figure 2).

Histopathologically, parakeratotic stratified squamous epithelium of varying thickness with long slender rete ridges and in some areas large bulbous rete ridges is evident. Papillary connective tissue shows numerous large dilated blood-filled spaces and lined by endothelial cells. Areas of extravasations of blood are also present. Chronic inflammatory cell infiltration around blood vessels and rete ridges is also present. All these features were suggestive of a diagnosis of angiokeratoma (Figures 3 and 4).

For the confirmation of proliferation of blood vessels, CD34 marker was used. The lesion was positive for CD34 (Figure 5).

After diagnosis, the patient underwent further examinations, and no lesions were found elsewhere in his skin or mucous membranes. The case was considered a solitary angiokeratoma affecting the tongue. In the last followup after six months, the patient was disease-free and asymptomatic.

3. Discussion

Solitary angiokeratoma was first described in 1967 by Imperial and Helwig [7]. These lesions are commonly found on the hips, thighs, buttocks, umbilicus, lower abdomen, scrotum, glans penis, and rarely oral mucosa [8]. Solitary angiokeratomas have been described in the oral cavity, mainly the tongue. Also, one case was also reported on the tonsillar pillar [9]. This lesion seems rather infrequent, and with thorough search, we found only 16 case reports of solitary angiokeratomas affecting oral cavity.

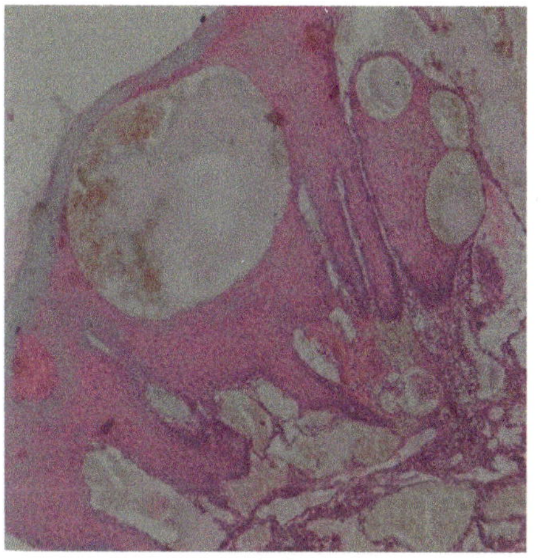

FIGURE 3: 100x magnification.

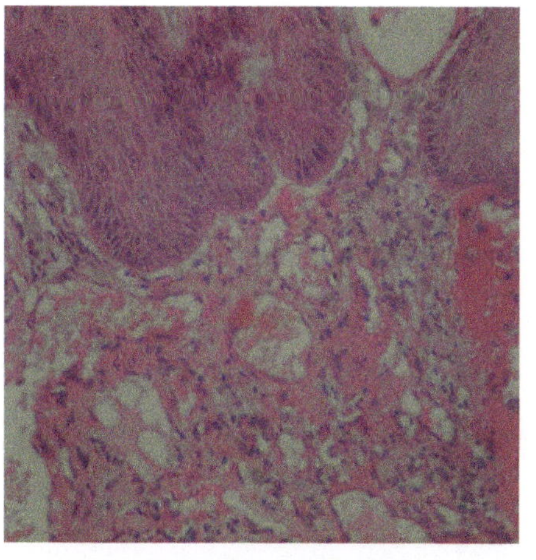

FIGURE 4: 400x magnification.

Pathogenesis of the lesion includes relation to trauma, high venous pressure, or vascular malformation [3]. It is thought that the primary event is vascular ectasia within the papillary dermis just beneath the basement membrane. The epidermal pathological changes seem to be a secondary reaction. It has been reported that the increased proliferative capacity on the surface of vascular malformation related to angiokeratoma [10]. The increase in proliferation of the epithelium is because of the close proximity of the vascular spaces. In case of angiokeratoma, the blood vessels are in close proximity to epithelium, and hence their close proximity to epithelium suggests the secondary proliferation of epithelium [10, 11]. In the present case, histopathology and immunohistochemistry confirm the proposed pathogenesis.

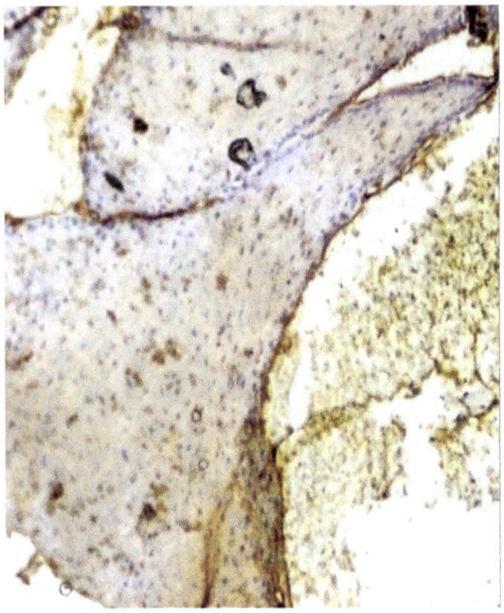

FIGURE 5: Immunohistochemical profile of the lesion with expression CD34 positive.

Review of all the past cases suggests that it is more common in female, but the present case patient was male. The most common site of involvement in the oral cavity is the tongue, the anterior dorsal surface. In present case the site of involvement was also the tongue.

The only clinical problems these lesions can cause are bleeding, discomfort or cosmetic changes [11]. However, most cases were asymptomatic. Therapy has usually been surgical excision in most of the published cases, mainly to discard alternative diagnosis. A recent report has employed diode laser in a 16-year-old woman [12]. Usually, no recurrences have been described [3]. However, few recent cases suggest the recurrence [5]. In the present case, after surgical excision, no recurrence is found after 6-month followup.

Oral mucosal involvement is a component of angiokeratoma corporis diffusum [8]. If further lesions elsewhere are present, then the possible association with systemic diseases could be expected in widespread cases [3]. Fabry's disease and fucosidosis can be suspected on histopathological grounds by the presence of swollen endothelial cells with a vacuolated cytoplasm in addition to the histology of angiokeratoma [1, 3]. The present case did not show swollen endothelial cells. Also, no other associated lesions were identified. Hence, the present case can be categorized as an isolated solitary angiokeratoma of oral cavity affecting tongue, a recent review by Ranjan and Mahajan. Solitary angiokeratoma of the tongue in adults has proposed a clinical classification for oral angiokeratomas [6].

Type 1: primary (purely mucocutaneous and not associated with systemic disorders)

Type 1A, isolated angiokeratomas of the oral cavity

Type 1As solitary
Type 1Am multiple

Type 1B, mucocutaneous angiokeratomas, that is, oral angiokeratomas associated with cutaneous angiokeratomas (e.g., angiokeratomas of vulva/scrotum)

Type 1Bs solitary
Type 1Bm multiple

Type 1C, angiokeratomas occurring simultaneously in oral cavity, skin (e.g., vulva/scrotum), and gastrointestinal mucosa

Type 1Cs solitary
Type 1Cm multiple

Type 2: secondary (as a component of a generalized systemic disorder)

Type 2A, As a component of Fabry's disease

Type 2As solitary
Type 2Am multiple

Type 2B, as a component of fucosidosis

Type 2Bs solitary
Type 2Bm multiple

Considering the same classification, the present case can be categorized as *Type 1As*, that is, *isolated solitary angiokeratoma*.

The main differential diagnosis on histopathological grounds was lymphangioma, to exclude the diagnosis and to confirm the proliferating blood vessels. Immunohistochemical staining is implied. In the previous literature, antigens used were CD31, CD34, and LYVE-1 (lymphatic vessel endothelial hyaluronan), and CD31 and CD34 were found positive and LYVE-1 (lymphatic vessel endothelial hyaluronan) was negative [3]. In the present case, antigen used was CD34. CD34 antigen that was used is considered as a reliable marker for the proliferating blood vessels. CD34 was positive in the present case which confirms the proliferating blood vessels.

The differential diagnosis of angiokeratoma is important because of its similarity to some other lesions [5, 12]. Other vascular lesions like hemangioma, and lymphangioma can be ruled out with the help of histopathological investigation. In case of hemangioma, small capillary lined by single layer of endothelial cells supported by connective tissue stroma is seen [13]. Also, endothelial cell proliferation is also noted. These blood vessels are completely lain within the connective tissue, while in case of angiokeratoma, blood vessels are supported by epithelium and lie very close to the epithelium [12].

In case of lymphangiomas, multiple intertwining lymph vessels lie very close to the epithelium and are seen also in papillary connective tissue. Presence of blood-filled spaces and endothelial lining also helped to differentiate angiokeratoma from lymphangiomas [12].

Angiokeratoma can be clinically confused with the aggressive lesions like malignant melanoma, especially in case of angiokeratoma when the vessels are thrombosed [14]. Histopathological examination can only differentiate angiokeratoma from malignant melanoma [1]. In malignant melanoma presence of atypical melanocytes, in clusters or groups, also singly placed. These cells show prominent nuclei often with prominent nucleoli [13]. Such appearances are not seen in case of angiokeratoma.

4. Conclusions

Oral angiokeratomas of the oral cavity are rare tumors. Although they can appear as isolated lesions, their presence should prompt further investigations to rule out systemic disease.

References

[1] O. Sangüeza and L. Requena, *Angiokeratoma in Pathology of Vascular Skin Lesions, Clinicopathologic Correlations*, Humana Press, New Jersey, NJ, USA, 2003.

[2] M. Siponen, T. Penna, M. Apaja-Sarkkinen, R. Palatsi, and T. Salo, "Solitary angiokeratoma of the tongue," *Journal of Oral Pathology and Medicine*, vol. 35, no. 4, pp. 252–253, 2006.

[3] M. J. Fernández-Aceñero, J. R. Biel, and G. Renedo, "Solitary angiokeratoma of the tongue in adults," *Romanian Journal of Morphology and Embryology*, vol. 51, no. 4, pp. 771–773, 2010.

[4] K. Karthikeyan, G. Sethuraman, and D. M. Thappa, "Angiokeratoma of the oral cavity and scrotum," *Journal of Dermatology*, vol. 27, no. 2, pp. 131–132, 2000.

[5] M. Nain, S. Agarwal, G. Singh, and R. Devenga, "Congenital solitary angiokeratoma of tongue: a rare case report," *International Journal of Oral and Maxillofacial Pathology*, vol. 3, no. 2, pp. 72–75, 2012.

[6] N. Ranjan and V. K. Mahajan, "Oral angiokeratomas: proposed clinical classification," *International Journal of Dermatology*, vol. 48, no. 7, pp. 778–781, 2009.

[7] R. Imperial and E. B. Helwig, "Angiokeratoma. A clinicopathological study," *Archives of Dermatology*, vol. 95, no. 2, pp. 166–175, 1967.

[8] U. Farooq, M. Mirzabeigi, and V. Vincek, "Solitary angiokeratoma of the tongue," *European Journal of Pediatric Dermatology*, vol. 15, no. 4, pp. 233–236, 2005.

[9] A. Fernandez-Flores and J. Sanroman, "Solitary angiokeratoma of the tonsillar pillar of the oral cavity," *Romanian Journal of Morphology and Embryology*, vol. 50, no. 1, pp. 115–117, 2008.

[10] H. K. Kar and L. Gupta, "A case report of angiokeratoma circumcriptum of the tongue, response with carbon dioxide and pulsed dye laser," *Journal of Cutaneous and Aesthetic Surgery*, vol. 4, pp. 205–207, 2011.

[11] P. I. Schiller and P. H. Itin, "Angiokeratomas: an update," *Dermatology*, vol. 193, no. 4, pp. 275–282, 1996.

[12] N. Sion-Vardy, E. Manor, M. Puterman, and L. Bodner, "Solitary angiokeratoma of the tongue," *Medicina Oral, Patologia Oral y Cirugia Bucal*, vol. 13, no. 1, pp. E12–E14, 2008.

[13] R. Rajendra and B. Shivprasadsundharam, *Shafers Textbook of Oral Pathology*, 6th edition, 2009.

[14] K. Aggarwal, V. K. Jain, S. Jangra, and R. Wadhera, "Angiokeratoma circumscriptum of the tongue," *Indian Pediatrics*, vol. 49, pp. 316–318, 2012.

20

Multilocular Unicystic Ameloblastoma of Mandible

Manas Bajpai,[1] Deshant Agarwal,[1] Anindya Bhalla,[2] Malay Kumar,[3] Rakesh Garg,[4] and Manish Kumar[5]

[1] *Department of Oral and Maxillofacial Pathology, NIMS Dental College, Jaipur, India*
[2] *Department of Public Health Dentistry, NIMS Dental College, Jaipur, India*
[3] *Department of Oral and Maxillofacial Pathology, Ahmedabad Dental College, Ahmedabad, India*
[4] *Department of Periodontics, NIMS Dental College, Jaipur, India*
[5] *Department of Prosthodontics Crown and Bridges, NIMS Dental College, Jaipur, India*

Correspondence should be addressed to Manas Bajpai; dr.manasbajpai@gmail.com

Academic Editors: M. Ashkenazi and A. Markopoulos

Introduction. We report a rare case of unicystic ameloblastoma (UA) of mandible which showed multilocular radiolucency on the left side of mandible on radiographic examination which is very unusual, and the majority of the cases of UAs till date has been reported of unilocular radiolucency. On histopathological examination, an odontogenic cystic lining that proliferates that intraluminally resembling ameloblastomatous epithelium was observed, leading to a definitive diagnosis of unicystic ameloblastoma. *Case Presentation*. A 42-year-old male patient presented with a swelling on the left side of the mandible extending from 33 to 36. Radiographically, it showed a multilocular radiolucent lesion resembling odontogenic cyst; however, the final diagnosis was made on histopathological ground with the inclusion of radiological and clinical features. *Conclusion*. It can be concluded that at present, histopathologic examination is the most sensitive tool for differentiating between odontogenic cysts and UAs. However, both clinical and radiologic findings share equal contribution to the final diagnosis.

1. Introduction

Ameloblastomas are benign tumors whose importance lies in its potential to grow into enormous size with resulting bone deformity. They are typically classified as unicystic, multicystic, peripheral, and malignant subtypes [1]. A solid or multicystic ameloblastoma is a benign epithelial tumor of odontogenic origin showing a strong tendency to recurrence and local aggression. Solid/multicystic, peripheral, desmoplastic, or unicystic ameloblastomas are other subtypes of ameloblastoma [2, 3].

Unicystic ameloblastoma (UA) represents an ameloblastoma variant, presenting as a cyst [3].

In 1977, Robinson and Martinez first used the term "unicystic ameloblastoma" (UA) for such lesions [4], but it was adopted in the second edition of the international histologic classification of odontogenic tumors by the WHO in 1992 [5]. The other name as recognised by WHO is "cystogenic ameloblastoma" [3].

Five to 15% of all ameloblastomas are of the unicystic type. Cases associated with an unerupted tooth show a mean age of 16 years as opposed to 35 years in the absence of an unerupted tooth. The mean age is significantly lower than that for solid/multicystic ameloblastoma. There is no gender predilection [3]. Unicystic ameloblastoma (UA) is a prognostically distinct entity. It has a recurrence rate of 6.7–35.7%, and the average interval for recurrence is approximately 7 years.

Six radiographic patterns have been identified for UA, ranging from well-defined unilocular to multilocular ones. When the radiographic appearance is divided into the two main patterns, unilocular and multilocular, there is a clear predominance of a unilocular configuration in all studies of UA where this feature has been evaluated, especially in cases associated with impacted teeth [6].

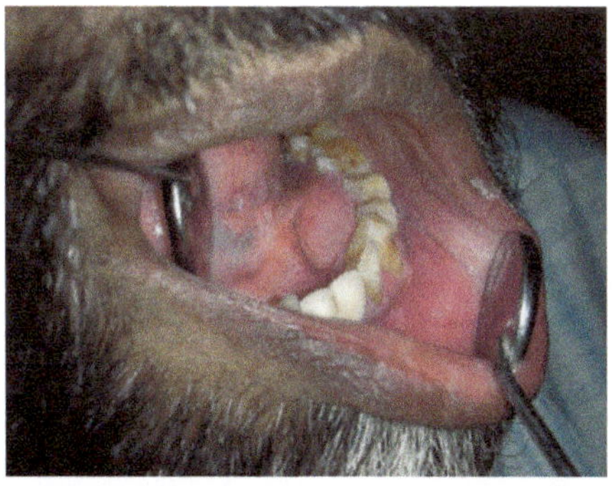

FIGURE 1: Swelling on lingual surface on the left side of the mandible extending from 33 to 36.

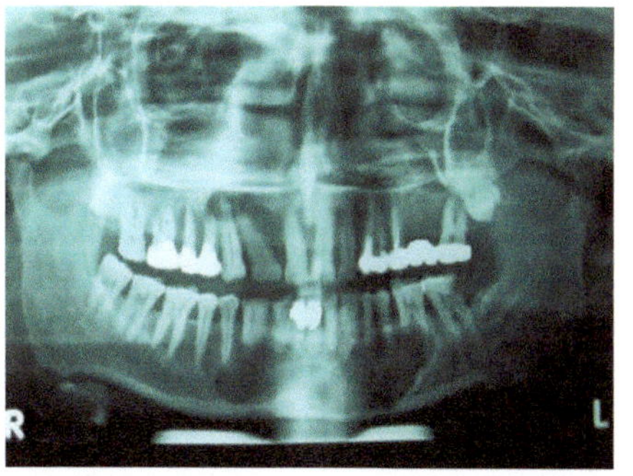

FIGURE 2: OPG of the patient reveals a large multilocular radiolucency.

2. Case Presentation

A 42-year-old male patient presented with the chief complains of swelling on the left side of the mandible since 1 month. On intraoral examination, solitary, oval swelling measuring 4 × 2 cm in size seen on the left side of the mandible extending from 33 to 36 was noticed (Figure 1). The swelling was hard in consistency with smooth surface, diffuse margins and was nontender on palpation. The buccal and lingual cortices were thinned out. Pain associated with the swelling was insidious in origin and dull, nonradiating, and intermittent in nature. A provisional diagnosis of odontogenic keratocyst was given. Panoramic radiograph revealed a huge osteodestructive lesion with well-defined multilocular radiolucency with thin corticated borders in the left side of the mandible extending from 36 to 45 (Figure 2). On fine needle aspiration, a serosanguinous aspirate was obtained which revealed acute inflammatory cells (consisting mainly of polymorphonuclear neutrophils) and cystic macrophages in an eosinophilic background on cytopathologic examination (Figure 3). Incisional biopsy was carried out to obtain a definitive diagnosis.

Histopathological examination demonstrated cystic lumen lined by nonkeratinized stratified squamous epithelium showing prominent basal cells with hyperchromatic nuclei which is polarized (Figure 4). The suprabasal layer resembles stellate reticulm like cells which are proliferating intraluminally with few vacuolated cells (Figure 5). The cystic lining shows squamous metaplasia of varying thickness at many places. The underlying connective tissue capsule shows inductive hyalinized eosinophilic band just beneath the epithelium (Figure 6). Thus, the histopathological findings confirmed the diagnosis of unicystic ameloblastoma (Table 1).

3. Discussion

The term unicystic ameloblastoma has been described as an ameloblastoma developing within the lining, lumen, or wall of a cyst as well as an invasive ameloblastoma that has a single cystic space rather than multicystic spaces [8]. Unicystic ameloblastoma, a variant of ameloblastoma, was first described by Robinson and Martinez [4]. This

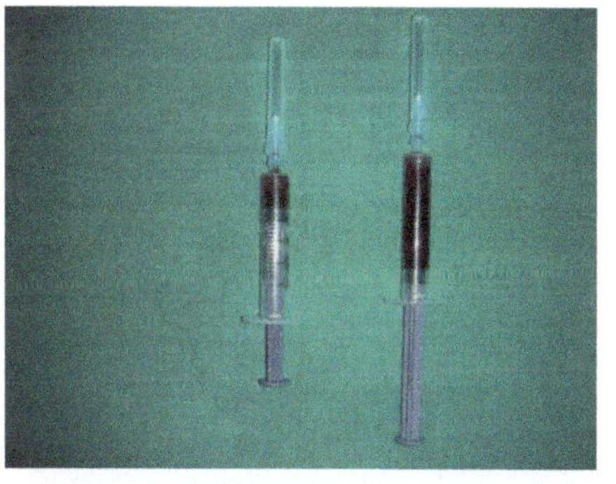

FIGURE 3: Serosanguinous aspirate with blood.

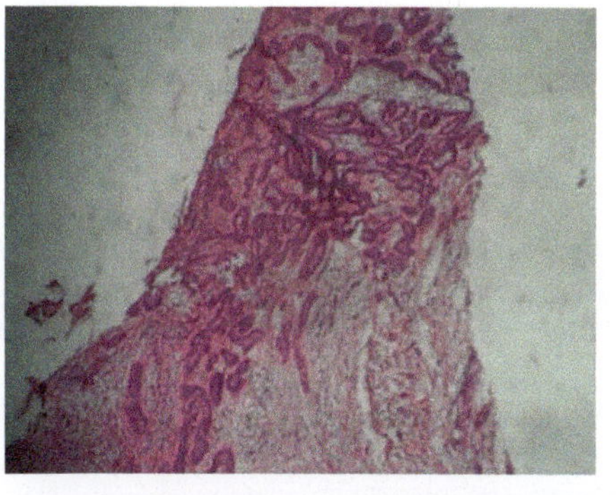

FIGURE 4: Cystic lumen lined by nonkeratinized stratified squamous epithelium showing prominent basal cells (H and E) 10x.

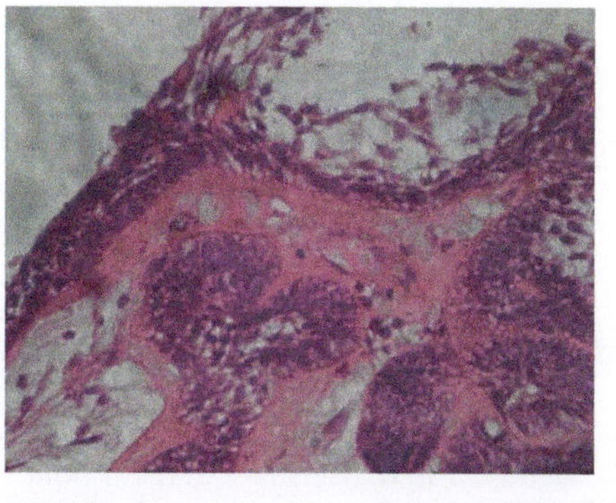

FIGURE 5: Suprabasal layer resembles stellate reticulum proliferating intraluminally with few vacuolated cells. (H and E) 40x.

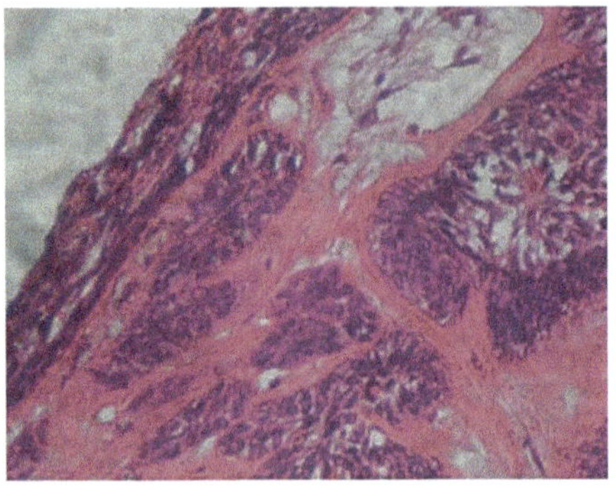

Figure 6: Squamous metaplasia of cystic lining and hyalinization of underlying connective tissue (H and E) 40x.

Table 1: Histopathological classification of unicystic ameloblastomas (UAs) [7].

Group	Interpretation
1	Luminal UA
1.2	Luminal and intraluminal UAs
1.2.3	Luminal, intraluminal, and intramural UAs
1.3	Luminal and intramural UAs

terminology may also represent an odontogenic cyst in which there has been ameloblastic transformation of the epithelial lining [5].

Various contradictory theories about the development of UAs have been proposed (Table 1). While some authors suggest that UAs develop by cystic degeneration of solid ameloblastomas, there are certain indications that UAs may develop by mural and/or luminal ameloblastomatous change in a preexisting cyst [2]. Robert and Diane have proposed three pathogenic mechanisms for the evolution of unicystic ameloblastoma: reduced enamel epithelium, from dentigerous cyst and due to cystic degeneration of solid ameloblastoma [9].

Some cases are asymptomatic, sometimes presenting as a swelling of the posterior mandible. More than 90% of cases involve the mandible, usually the posterior region. Up to 80% are associated with an unerupted mandibular third molar. The lesion presents radiographically as a well-corticated unilocular pattern, often pericoronal radiolucency [3].

The unilocular pattern is more common in the unicystic variant than the multilocular one, especially so in cases associated with tooth impaction [7].

Unicystic ameloblastoma may mimic other odontogenic cysts clinically and radiographically. Moreover, the histologic distinction between UAs and certain nonneoplastic odontogenic cysts can be difficult [10]. It appears to be more difficult to differentiate UAs in cases of dentigerous UAs (associated with an impacted tooth) than in cases of nondentigerous UAs (not associated with an impacted tooth). UAs that are not associated with an impacted tooth may mimic a residual cyst or a keratocystic odontogenic tumor (KCOT) [2]. Much confusion stems from the fact that a UA may appear not only as a unilocular but indeed also as a multilocular bone defect [7].

Since 1925, many had reported the development of ameloblastoma within the walls of odontogenic cysts, and the most commonly cited was the dentigerous cyst [4]. There have been many reports of ameloblastomas apparently arising from the epithelium of what initially was considered as an odontogenic cyst [7]. Hyperplastic epithelium may also resemble ameloblastomatous lining epithelium in radicular cyst and dentigerous cyst. However, since this type of feature was also associated with a dense inflammatory cell infiltrate where the stellate-reticulum like epithelium was a result of intercellular oedema arising from the presence of chronic inflammation in the area, it should be considered as not diagnostic of unicystic ameloblastoma [4]. In the present case, a lining epithelium resembling dentigerous cyst lining was evident in one specimen. However, a characteristic ameloblastomatous lining was evident on taking deeper sections of the other specimen that confirmed the diagnosis of unicystic ameloblastoma. This case, thus, highlights the role careful microscopic examination of all the sections in the biopsy specimen and of deeper and step sections in the diagnosis of unicystic ameloblastoma as also has been shown by Dunsche et al. [2]. In the past, other authors had suggested that in cases of small islands of ameloblastomatous epithelium within the cystic epithelium of a lesion, it might be necessary to examine the entire specimen to be sure of finding these islands [7, 11, 12].

In present case, the lesion presented as a localised swelling in the mandible and multilocular radiolucency on radiographic examination, which resembled a solid multicystic ameloblastoma or keratocystic odontogenic tumor (KCOT), and was difficult to diagnose clinically and radiographically. The final diagnosis was made on the basis of histopathological examination and also by the correlation of clinical and radiological features.

4. Conclusion

It can be concluded that at present, histologic examination is the most sensitive tool for differentiating between odontogenic cysts and UAs. However, both clinical and radiologic findings share equal contribution to the final diagnosis. This case also highlights the importance of careful examination of the entire specimen and the usefulness of deeper sections in diagnosis of unicystic ameloblastoma. Thus, it is of utmost importance to correlate the histopathologic findings with clinical and radiographic features to achieve at a correct definitive diagnosis as all such lesions may have prognostically different biologic behaviours and the final diagnosis may alter the therapeutic decision significantly.

References

[1] N. Gupta, S. Saxena, V. C. Rathod, and P. Aggarwal, "Unicystic ameloblastoma of the mandible," *Journal of Oral and Maxillofacial Pathology*, vol. 15, no. 2, pp. 228–231, 2011.

[2] A. Dunsche, O. Babendererde, J. Lüttges, and I. N. G. Springer, "Dentigerous cyst versus unicystic ameloblastoma: differential

diagnosis in routine histology," *Journal of Oral Pathology and Medicine*, vol. 32, no. 8, pp. 486–491, 2003.

[3] "WHO classification of tumours," in *Pathology and Genetics of Head and Neck Tumous*, L. Barnes, J. W. Everson, P. Reichart, and D. Sindransky, Eds., pp. 296–300, IARC Press, Lyon, France, 2005.

[4] L. Robinson and M. G. Martinez, "Unicystic ameloblastoma: a prognostically distinct entity," *Cancer*, vol. 40, no. 5, pp. 2278–2285, 1977.

[5] I. R. H. Kramer, J. J. Pindborg, and M. Shear, *Histological Typing of Odontogenic Tumors*, Springer, Berlin, Germany, 1992.

[6] L. R. Eversole, A. S. Leider, and D. Strub, "Radiographic characteristics of cystogenic ameloblastoma," *Oral Surgery Oral Medicine and Oral Pathology*, vol. 57, no. 5, pp. 572–577, 1984.

[7] H. P. Philipsen and P. A. Reichart, "Unicystic ameloblastoma: a review of 193 cases from the literature," *Oral Oncology*, vol. 34, no. 5, pp. 317–325, 1998.

[8] P. A. Reichart and H. P. Phillipsen, *Odontogenic Tumors and Allied Lesions*, Quintessence, Chicago, Ill, USA, 2004.

[9] E. M. Robert and S. Diane, *Oral and Maxillofacial Pathology: A Rationale for Diagnosis and Treatment*, Quintessence, Chicago, Ill, USA, 2003.

[10] A. S. Leider, L. R. Eversole, and M. E. Barkin, "Cystic ameloblastoma: a clinicopathologic analysis," *Oral Surgery Oral Medicine and Oral Pathology*, vol. 60, no. 6, pp. 624–630, 1985.

[11] H. Coleman, M. Altini, H. Ali, C. Doglioni, G. Favia, and E. Maiorano, "Use of calretinin in the differential diagnosis of unicystic ameloblastomas," *Histopathology*, vol. 38, no. 4, pp. 312–317, 2001.

[12] G. L. Ackermann, M. Altini, and M. Shear, "The unicystic ameloblastoma: a clinicopathological study of 57 cases," *Journal of Oral Pathology*, vol. 17, no. 9-10, pp. 541–546, 1988.

21

Breaking the Thumb Sucking Habit: When Compliance Is Essential

Orlando Tanaka, Wagner Oliveira, Melissa Galarza, Vanessa Aoki, and Bruno Bertaiolli

Graduate Dentistry Program in Orthodontics, School of Health and Biosciences, Pontifícia Universidade Católica do Paraná, Curitiba, PR, Brazil

Correspondence should be addressed to Orlando Tanaka; tanakaom@gmail.com

Academic Editor: Hüsamettin Oktay

The anterior open bite (AOB) and posterior cross bite are the most frequent malocclusions associated with prolonged sucking habits. This clinical case illustrates and discusses the use of a Haas-type palatal expander for stopping a thumb sucking habit. The improvement in closing the open bite with discontinuation of the habit was observed. But with the return of the habit and lack of cooperation, the relapse of anterior open bite occurred. Therefore, different approaches are necessary. The need of a multidisciplinary approach, consent, and cooperation are keys to a good prognosis.

1. Introduction

The oral habits can interfere with the growth and normal development of the jaws, favoring the onset of malocclusion and changes in normal swallowing and speech patterns depending on factors such as duration, frequency, intensity, and facial pattern [1].

The open bite is most frequently seen in the anterior region, having deleterious habits as one of its main etiological factors. The opposition of the teeth deformation and the alveolar processes exhibit a configuration that is more or less a negative impression of the thumb or fingers, when they are placed in the mouth during sucking [1].

The AOB has several etiologic factors besides the finger sucking habit, such as incomplete eruption of the anterior teeth, predominantly mouth breathing habits, poor tongue posture, speech and tongue thrusting, pacifier habit, and a continuous abnormal swallowing pattern of the child.

Regardless of the finger used during suction, the duration, intensity, and frequency, combined with the patient's facial pattern, and the will and compliance to eliminate the habit should be evaluated [2]. Besides that, the early mixed dentition phase is appropriate for treating skeletal open bites [3]. The act of sucking his or her thumb seems to be very enjoyable and it can arise for various reasons, from a psychological problem to a discovery of a way to achieve pleasure. However, if the act remains for a long time, it becomes a damaging habit. Some malocclusions are corrected when the sucking habit stops, since the pattern is normal and the skeletal deformity is mild. But in many cases, this does not happen and orthodontic correction is needed [4], and even an orthognathic surgery [5].

In order to eliminate the finger sucking habit, there is no ready-made recipe. The use of provided adhesive plasters on the child's fingers, removable or fixed appliances, and even suggestion can be advocated [2, 6]. The preference is for braces, once it does not require collaboration, and the lack of compliance is part of the problem [1, 6, 7].

This case report aims to describe the normalization of the overbite when the thumb sucking habit is interrupted and the relapse if the habit returns and also to focus on the importance of the patient's cooperation to remove the habit and attention to a multidisciplinary approach.

2. Case Report

A 6-year-old and 8-month-old female patient, in mixed dentition, presented a Class II division 1 malocclusion, overjet of 9.0 mm, and AOB of 4.0 mm. Constricted maxillary arch, slight diastema between the maxillary incisors and between the lower central incisors, and a slight midline deviation to the left were also present (Figure 1).

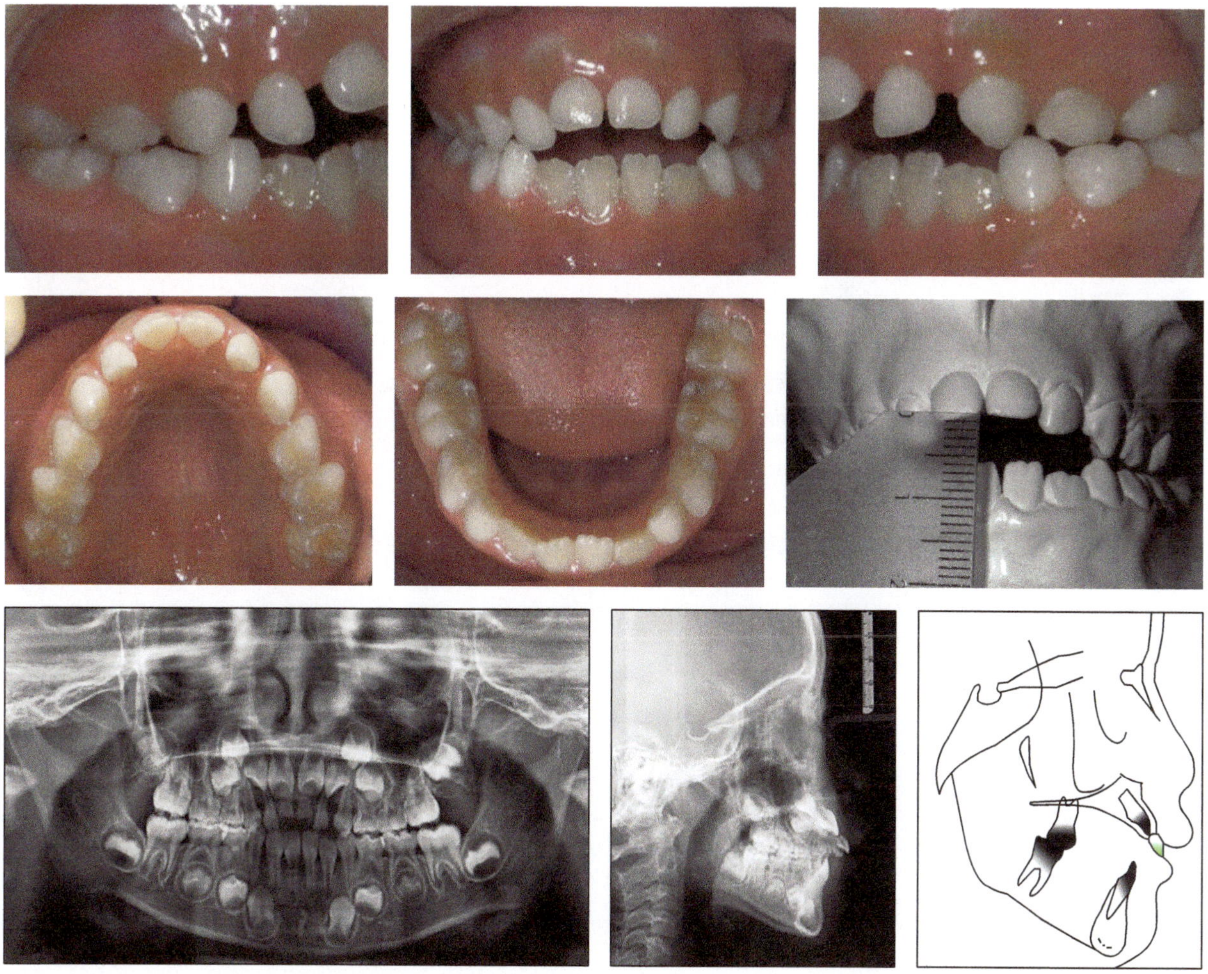

FIGURE 1: Pretreatment intraoral photographs, radiographs, and cephalometric tracing.

The absence of second maxillary premolars was detected in the panoramic radiograph (Figure 1). The cephalometric measurements showed a good relationship between the maxillary and mandibular bases (ANB = 2°), proclined maxillary incisors (1NA = 32°), and uprighted mandibular incisors (1NB = 21°), a vertical growth trend greater than an anteroposterior (Y-axis = 61°) and a convex lower third of the face (Z-angle = 67°) (Table 1).

And the most important anamnestic information was regarding the presence of the thumb sucking habit of her right hand, and she reported that she was eager to stop sucking her thumb (Figure 2).

2.1. Treatment Objectives. Remove the thumb sucking habit, close the AOB, and allow the physiological eruption of the maxillary incisors by using a Haas-type palatal expander (Figure 2).

2.2. Treatment Alternatives. Among the interception alternatives for stopping the thumb sucking habit, the following were explained: RME with palatal crib, Palatal Nance button, helicoidal fixed palatal arch, maxillary removable appliance with crib, and motivational psychology and suggestion.

2.3. Treatment Progress. In the interception phase, it was explained to the patient and his parents the importance of their cooperation in the elimination of the finger sucking habit. It was also explained to them how the device and the trader could help stop the habit.

A fixed Haas-type appliance for RPE was planned and fixed in order to achieve palatal expansion and serve as a "reminder" to curb the habit and indirectly promote the closure of the anterior open bite (Figure 3). Orthodontic treatment was started with the fixation of the palatal device to the first molars and bonding on the palatal surfaces of the molars and deciduous canines (Figure 4).

2.4. Treatment Results. During the first weeks of use of a palatal expander and in the subsequent months in the retention phase, the patient stopped her habit and the spontaneous correction of AOB was observed (Figure 5). The proposed objective of the RPE and stopping the thumb sucking habit

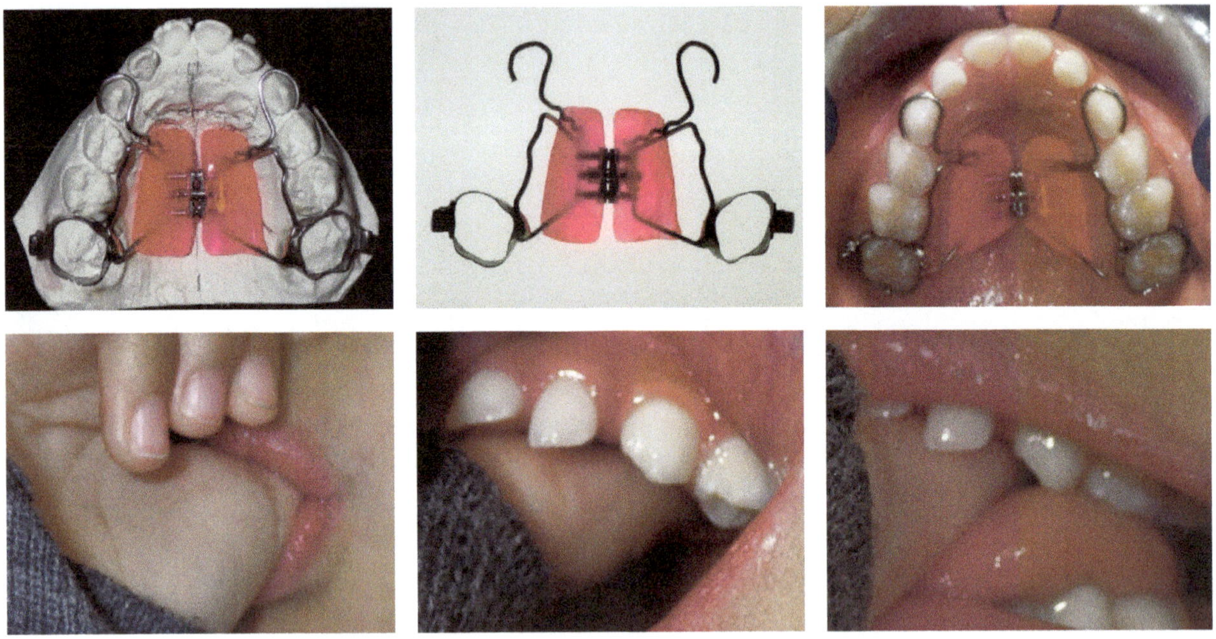

FIGURE 2: The expander before and after fixation. Thumb sucking position.

TABLE 1

JF	Mean	Author	6,9	7,3
SNA	82	Steiner	**78**	**83**
SNB	80	Steiner	**76**	**77**
ANB	2	Steiner	**2**	**6**
Convex	0	Downs	**7**	**12**
Y-axis	60	Downs	**61**	**63**
Facial	88	Downs	**85**	**85**
SN-GoGn	32	Steiner	**39**	**38**
FMA	25	Tweed	**29**	**29**
IMPA	90	Tweed	**86**	**86**
1.NA	22	Steiner	**32**	**17**
1_NA	4	Steiner	**9**	**1**
1.NB	25	Steiner	**21**	**20**
1¯NB	4	Steiner	**3**	**3**
Pog-NB		Holdaway	**0**	**1**
1 - 1	130	Downs	**125**	**138**
1¯A-Po	1	Ricketts	**1**	**−2**
LS - S	0	Steiner	**5**	**3**
LI - S	0	Steiner	**1**	**1**
Z-angle	75	Merrifield	**67**	**69**

were achieved with the functional reestablishment of occlusion. However, some months after the removal of the Haas-type palatal expander, the relapse of the habit was observed (Figure 6).

3. Discussion

Oral habits and AOB malocclusion have a high frequency in children. They hinder the normal development of dental and skeletal structures. As oral habits are risk factors for anterior open bite, the damaging habits most frequently associated are pacifier sucking, thumb sucking, and tongue thrust. Due to the correlation between the prevalence of anterior open bite and oral habits, prevention strategies incorporating psychological data related to children should be integrated into a national public health programme [8].

The AOB associated with deleterious habits can be successfully treated by means of interception at an early stage. However, the most important point in this therapeutic approach is the usual removal of the sucking habit [6, 9, 10]; otherwise, there will be a recurrence of malocclusion [11, 12].

The RPE is a common procedure in orthodontic mechanics and it is dedicated to expanding the maxillary arch; however, the preference for the Hyrax appliance has increased annually [13].

The etiologic factors most often associated with the development of an AOB are respiratory patterns [3], but age and growth factors also play an important role in AOB that is multifactorial, and there is an almost infinite variety to the dentoskeletal configuration and the magnitude of dysplasia associated with it [14].

Comforting behaviors, such as the use of finger or thumb sucking, are common in babies and young children but they tend to stop as children get older, under their own impetus or with support from parents and caretakers. However, if the habit continues whilst the permanent dentition is becoming established, it can contribute to, or cause, the development of a malocclusion. A diverse variety of approaches include advice, removal of the comforting object, fitting an orthodontic appliance to interfere with the habit, or behavior modification techniques. Some of these interventions are easier to apply than

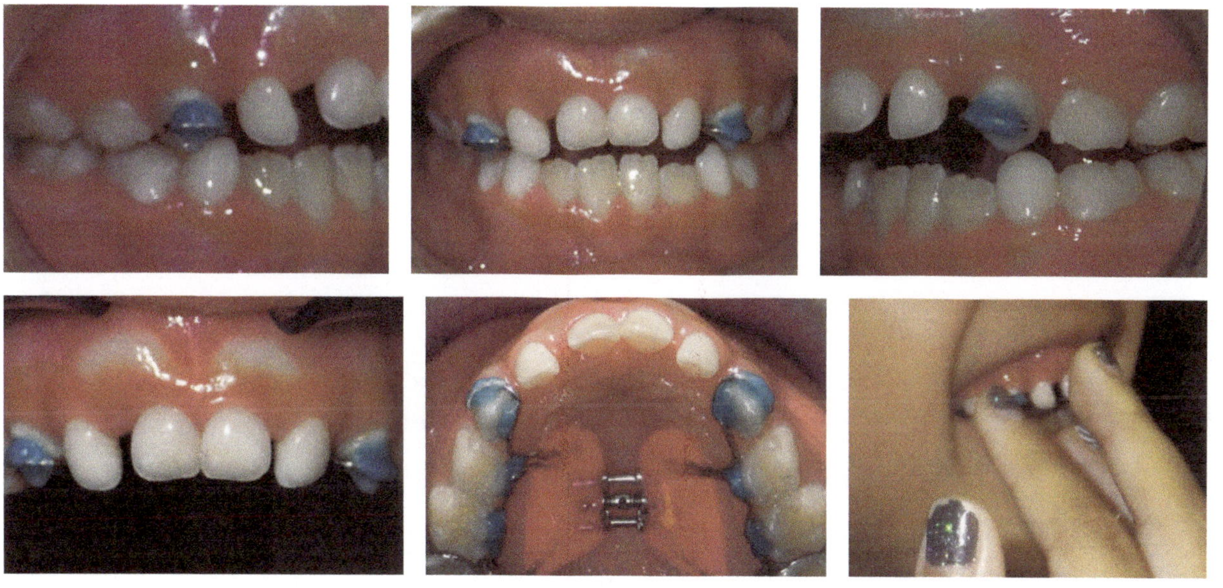

FIGURE 3: Progress after 3 weeks of palatal expansion. The appliance work as "reminder" and serve to curb the habit.

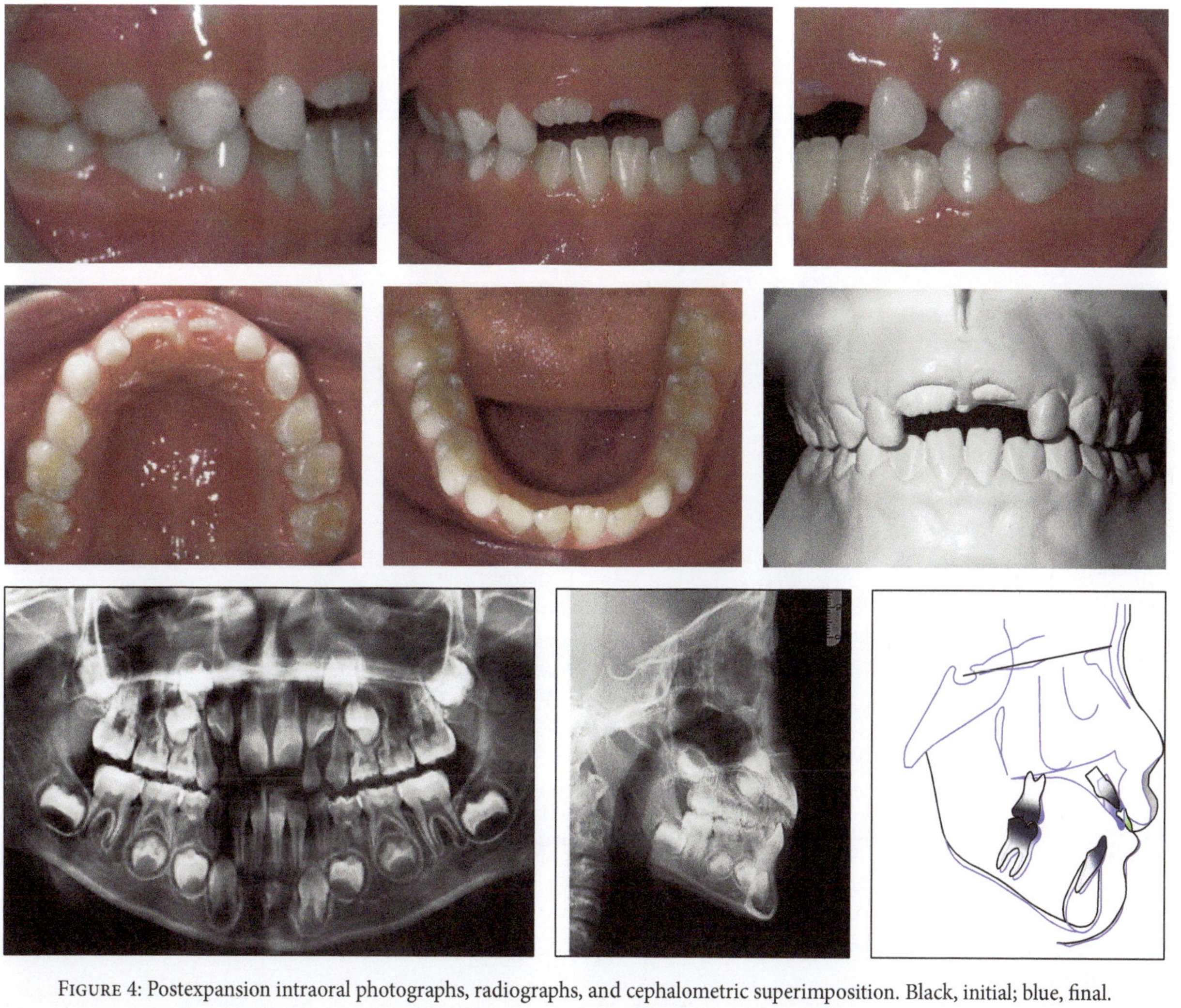

FIGURE 4: Postexpansion intraoral photographs, radiographs, and cephalometric superimposition. Black, initial; blue, final.

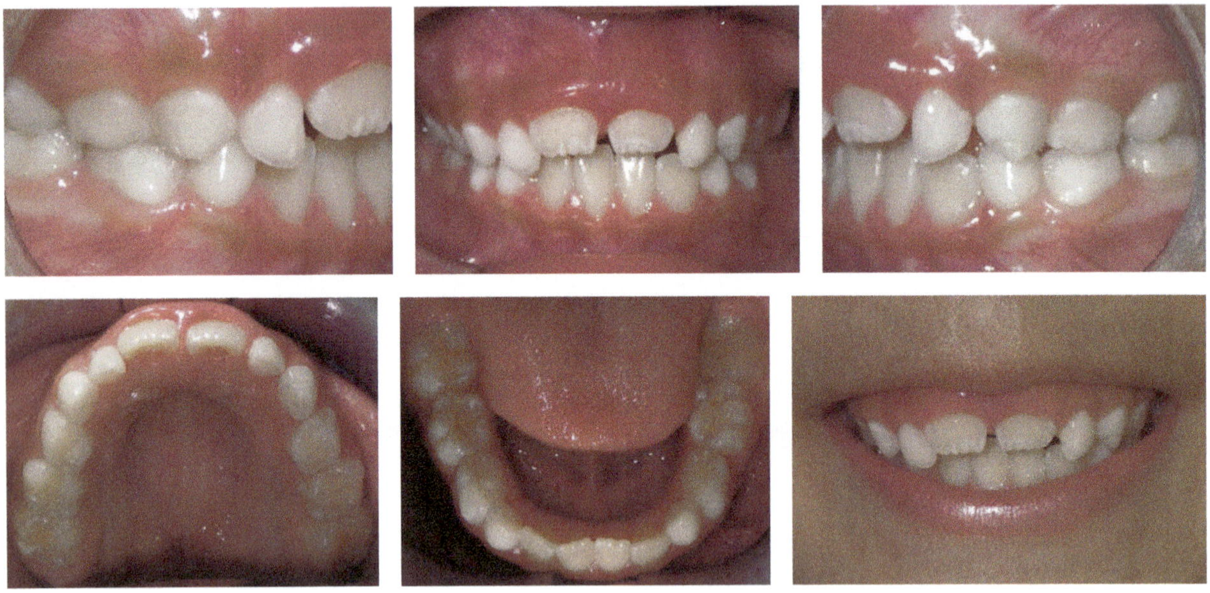

FIGURE 5: Nine months after removal of the palatal expander and no thumb sucking habit.

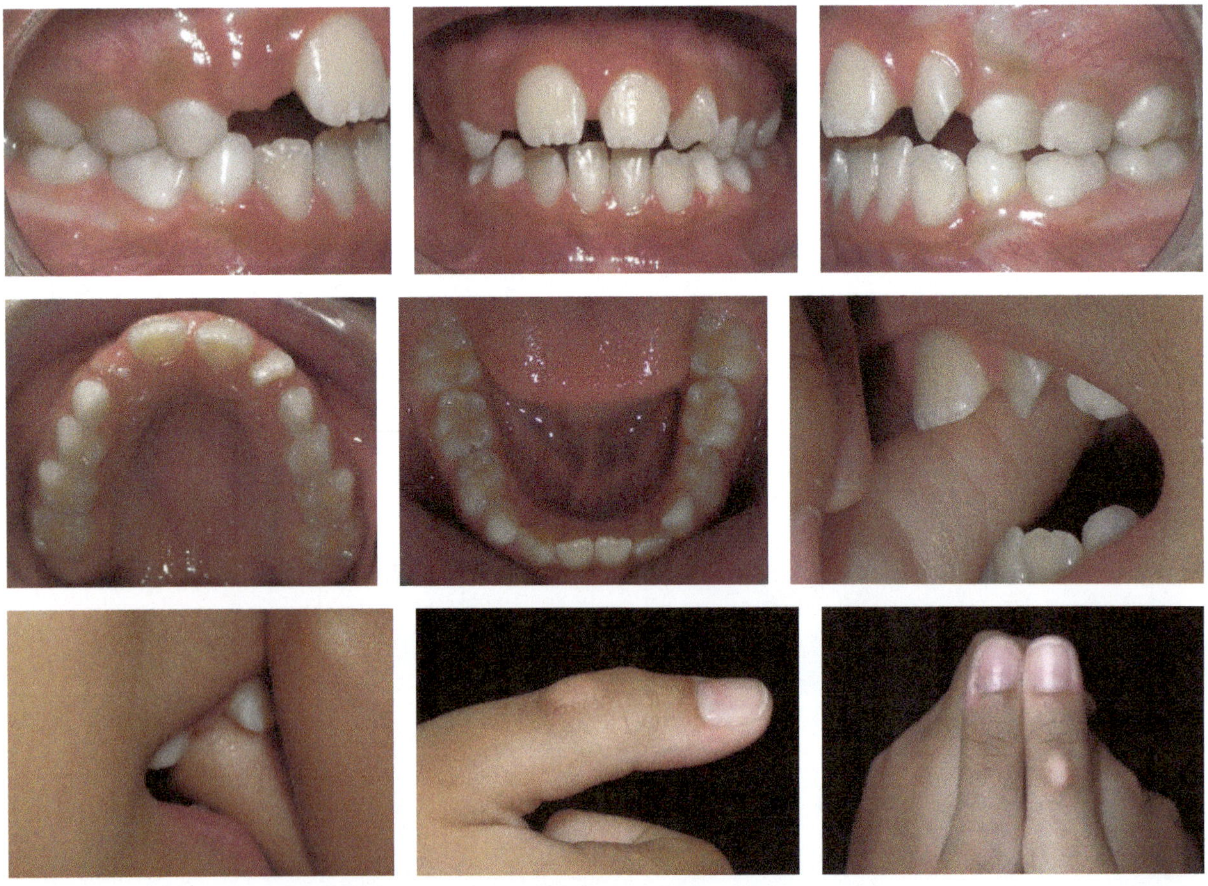

FIGURE 6: 18 months after removal of palatal expander appliance. Relapse of the anterior open bite due to relapse of the thumb sucking habit. Callus on the right thumb observed.

others and less disturbing for the child and their parents [15].

The maxillary removable or fixed appliance with crib is another alternative that not only prevents the suction of the finger or pacifier but also keeps the tongue in a more retruded position, preventing its interposition between the incisors during swallowing and speech. With the removal of the habit, there is a verticalization of the lower incisors and extrusion of the maxillary incisors closing the AOB [12] and similar results were observed in the present clinical case. The ideal age for the maxillary expansion is in mixed dentition, reducing the risk of damage and optimizing the procedure. As the patient progresses in skeletal age, the risk of damage to the supporting tissues increases particularly in growing patients.

The proposed results of maxillary expansion and stopping thumb sucking habit were fully achieved with the functional reestablishment of the occlusion. However, after the removal of the Haas-type appliance, it was observed the relapse of the thumb sucking habit with all its potential to harm the desired stability. Therefore, it is suggested that the desire to give up the habit must precede the presence of any type of appliance and that if after correction of the AOB the triggering factors of the usual reflexes are not completely eliminated.

There is low quality evidence that orthodontic appliances (palatal arch and palatal crib) and psychological interventions (including positive and negative reinforcement) are effective at improving sucking cessation in children [15]. When the habit is abandoned early, the malocclusion will usually revert without treatment. However, the absence of the habit is not a guarantee of having the malocclusion corrected [6] and the need for fixed appliances and complex biomechanics in the permanent dentition [16].

The fixed helicoid arch acts as a reminder and mechanical impediment of the habit and it causes discomfort for breaking the pleasure from the suction due to the volume of helicoids in the region where the pulp of the thumb should be [7]. During treatment, it should be clear to the patient, parents, or guardian that, for the successful removal of the finger sucking habit, it is not enough to use biomechanical orthodontic resources; the patient must be willing to stop the habit [6, 10].

A multidisciplinary approach should focus on efforts to build up the child's self-confidence and self-esteem.

4. Conclusion

The interception of the malocclusion at an early stage with the Haas-type fixed appliance was effective in RME and worked as an effective tool for stopping the thumb sucking habit and normalization of overjet and overbite. However, there was the recurrence of the habit with the relapse of the AOB, emphasizing the need of a multidisciplinary approach, consent, and cooperation as the keys to a good prognosis.

Conflict of Interests

The authors declare that there is no conflict of interests regarding the publication of this paper.

References

[1] W. R. Proffit, H. W. Fields, and D. Sarver, *Contemporary Orthodontics*, Elsevier Mosby, St. Louis, Mo, USA, 2007.

[2] O. Tanaka, T. B. Kreia, J. B. G. Bezerra, and H. Maruo, "Malocclusion and thumb-sucking habit," *Jornal Brasileiro de Ortodontia & Ortopedia Facial*, vol. 9, p. 276, 2004.

[3] A. Klocke, "Ask us," *American Journal of Orthodontics & Dentofacial Orthopedics*, vol. 123, no. 3, p. 13A, 2003.

[4] R. E. Moyers, *Ortodontia*, Guanabara Koogan, Rio de Janeiro, Brazil, 4th edition, 1991.

[5] O. M. Tanaka, O. Guariza-Filho, J. L. Carlini, D. D. Oliveira, M. M. Pithon, and E. S. Camargo, "Glossectomy as an adjunct to correct an open-bite malocclusion with shortened maxillary central incisor roots," *American Journal of Orthodontics and Dentofacial Orthopedics*, vol. 144, no. 1, pp. 130–140, 2013.

[6] O. M. Tanaka, R. W. F. Vitral, G. Y. Tanaka, A. P. Guerrero, and E. S. Camargo, "Nailbiting, or onychophagia: a special habit," *American Journal of Orthodontics and Dentofacial Orthopedics*, vol. 134, no. 2, pp. 305–308, 2008.

[7] D. F. Ferrari, J. C. B. Leão Filho, G. P. M. Silva, L. Z. Largura, and O. Tanaka, "Double helicoidal palatal arch. The undesirable arch for thumb sucking habit," *Orthodontic Science and Practice*, vol. 5, no. 17, pp. 86–93, 2011.

[8] V. Urzal, A. C. Braga, and A. P. Ferreira, "Oral habits as risk factors for anterior open bite in the deciduous and mixed dentition—cross-sectional study," *European Journal of Paediatric Dentistry*, vol. 14, no. 4, pp. 299–302, 2013.

[9] A. Locks, M. L. Sória, C. D. Derech, and G. L. U. Ribeiro, "Psychological aspects of non-nutritive sucking habit," *Jornal Brasileiro de Ortodontia e Ortopedia Facial*, vol. 6, no. 36, pp. 464–471, 2002.

[10] J. S. Ribeiro, T. B. Kreia, M. B. Moschetti, R. M. S. Mei, and O. Tanaka, "An usual forefinger sucking habit: case report," *Revista Clínica de Ortodontia Dental Press*, vol. 7, article 64, 2008.

[11] J. A. Bosio and R. Justus, "Treatment and retreatment of a patient with a severe anterior open bite," *American Journal of Orthodontics and Dentofacial Orthopedics*, vol. 144, no. 4, pp. 594–606, 2013.

[12] R. R. Almeida, R. R. Almeida-Pedrin, M. R. Almeida, F. P. C. Ferreira, A. Pinzan, and C. M. B. Insabralde, "Vertical dysplasias: anterior open bite treatment and stability," *Revista Dental Press de Ortodontia e Ortopedia Facial*, vol. 8, article 91, 2003.

[13] R. G. Keim, E. L. Gottlieb, D. S. Vogels III, and P. B. Vogels, "2014 JCO study of orthodontic diagnosis and treatment procedures, Part 1: results and trends," *Journal of Clinical Orthodontics*, vol. 48, no. 10, pp. 607–630, 2014.

[14] T. J. Cangialosi, "Skeletal morphologic features of anterior open bite," *American Journal of Orthodontics*, vol. 85, no. 1, pp. 28–36, 1984.

[15] F. R. Borrie, D. R. Bearn, N. P. Innes, and Z. Iheozor-Ejiofor, "Interventions for the cessation of non-nutritive sucking habits in children," *The Cochrane Database of Systematic Reviews*, vol. 3, Article ID CD008694, 2015.

[16] G. L. U. Ribeiro, S. Regis Jr., T. D. M. A. da Cunha, M. A. Sabatoski, O. Guariza-Filho, and O. M. Tanaka, "Multiloop edgewise archwire in the treatment of a patient with an anterior open bite and a long face," *American Journal of Orthodontics and Dentofacial Orthopedics*, vol. 138, no. 1, pp. 89–95, 2010.

22

Amalgam Tattoo Mimicking Mucosal Melanoma: A Diagnostic Dilemma Revisited

K. Lundin, G. Schmidt, and C. Bonde

Department of Plastic Surgery, Breast Surgery and Burns Treatment, Rigshospitalet-Copenhagen University Hospital, 2100 Copenhagen OE, Denmark

Correspondence should be addressed to K. Lundin; kira.lundin@dadlnet.dk

Academic Editors: N. Shah and E. F. Wright

Mucosal melanoma of the oral cavity is a rare but highly aggressive neoplasm. However, the clinicians need to be aware of the other and more frequent etiologies of intraoral pigmentation, such as amalgam tattoos. As amalgam has been extensively used for dental restorations and can cause pigmentations in the oral mucosa, this is a differential diagnosis not to be forgotten. We describe the characteristics of these two phenomena and present a case vignette illustrating the differential diagnostic issues. Other causes of intraoral pigmentation are summarized.

1. Introduction

Mucosal melanoma of the oral cavity is a highly aggressive neoplasm. The incidence and clinical course have been described in several studies despite its rarity [1–4]. However, the other etiologies of intraoral pigmentation need to be considered by the clinician. We here describe the characteristics of melanoma of the oral mucosa and the so-called amalgam tattoos. A case vignette of amalgam tattoo mimicking the more dire diagnosis of mucosal melanoma is presented, and other causes of intraoral pigmentation are summarized.

2. Case Vignette

A 51-year-old woman was referred to the Department of Plastic Surgery on suspicion of mucosal melanoma. She was a heavy smoker but otherwise healthy, with no prior family or personal history of melanoma.

The patient's dentist had noticed two dark discolorations in the gingiva from which the patient had no symptoms, though she suffered greatly from pain localised in the right side of the maxilla and mandible. The pain was thought to originate from extensive prosthetic dental treatment during the last six months.

The bluish-grey discolorations of the mucosa were localized in the buccal mucosa opposite the third upper molar on the right side and the first upper molar on the left side as seen in clinical photographs (Figures 1 and 2). No other suspect lesions or any enlarged lymph nodes were found, and the patient was treated with narrow excision of the elements under local anaesthesia.

Histopathological examination of the specimens showed brownish-black pigment along the collagenous fibres and in the vascular sheaths. No melanocytes or naevus cells were found, and there was no positive reaction in melanin stains. Both lesions were found to be consistent with amalgam tattoos. No other macules were identified in the oral mucosa, and the patient needed no further treatment or follow-up.

3. Discussion

Mucosal melanoma is very rare and reports are scarce, but it is considered one of the most aggressive malignancies known [1–7]. The recorded incidence is up to 1 or 2% of all melanomas [1–4, 7]; it is seen typically in the 4–7 decade and with no certain difference between sexes [1, 2, 4–6]. It is more frequent in African and Asian populations compared to Caucasians [1, 3, 5, 7, 8].

Clinical signs of mucosal melanoma of the oral cavity are usually dark brown, black, or bluish-greyish plaques with irregular pigmentation and an asymmetrical, irregular border

TABLE 1: Causes of intraoral pigmentation.

Endogenous	Exogenous
Hereditary or congenital	*Medicationand toxicity related*
Physiologic pigmentation (skin type 5-6)	Antimicrobial agents
Peutz-Jeghers syndrome	Antiarrhytchmic agents
Laugier-Hunziker syndrome	Oral contraceptives
	Cytostatics
Systemic or infectious	Smokers melanosis
Addison's disease	
Petechiae, varices, or thrombus	*Traumatic*
	Haematoma
Neoplastic or melanin related	Postinflammatory pigmentation
Naevi	Oral melanoacanthosis
Pigmented maculae	
Mucosal melanoma	*Other exogenous pigmentations*
Kaposi's sarcoma	Amalgam tattoos
Haemangioma	Accidental graphite tattoos
	Tribal tattoos

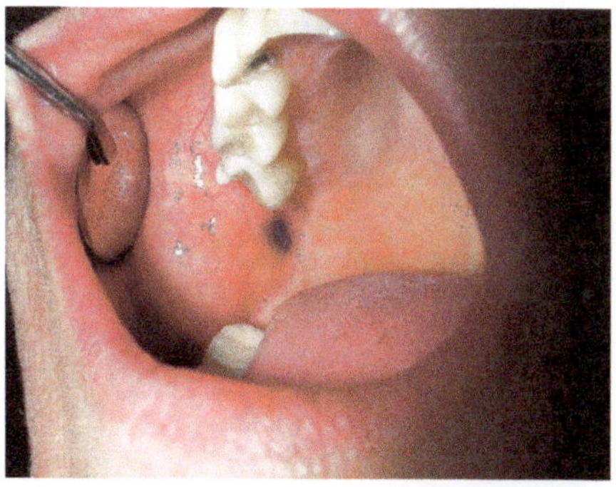

FIGURE 1: Clinical photograph of the 3 × 5 mm pigmented lesion of the left buccal mucosa mimicking mucosal melanoma.

[5, 6]. Swelling, ulceration, bleeding, pain/discomfort, and ill-fitting dentures are also common [2, 3, 5, 6]. Oral mucosal melanomas are typically of lentiginous or superficial type but may also be nodular [3, 9]. Most are localized to the maxillary mucosa and palate [2–6, 8]. Five to fifteen percent are reported to be amelanotic, though one study described up to two-thirds [2, 3, 5, 6, 8]. Mucosal melanomas are often preceded by a pigmented premalignant lesion, but due to the location, they tend to be diagnosed late and metastatic disease is not uncommon at the time of diagnosis [3, 5, 8]. Prognosis is uniformly described as poor and has been cited as below 15% five-year survival for oral mucosal melanoma [1].

However, studies are small and cannot provide certain stage-specific survival rates due to the rarity of the disease. Treatment is to a certain degree extrapolated from the regimens used for cutaneous melanoma [2, 9]. First choice treatment is wide radical excision. Though sentinel lymph node biopsy is state of the art for cutaneous melanoma, its role in mucosal melanomas remains uncertain and is not part of the recent guidelines from the National Comprehensive Cancer Network [1, 9–12]. Treatment of the clinically node-negative neck also remains controversial. Radiation has been used as adjuvant postoperative therapy and is also used for palliation [1, 12]. For metastatic disease, systemic therapy is suggested [1, 3, 4, 12].

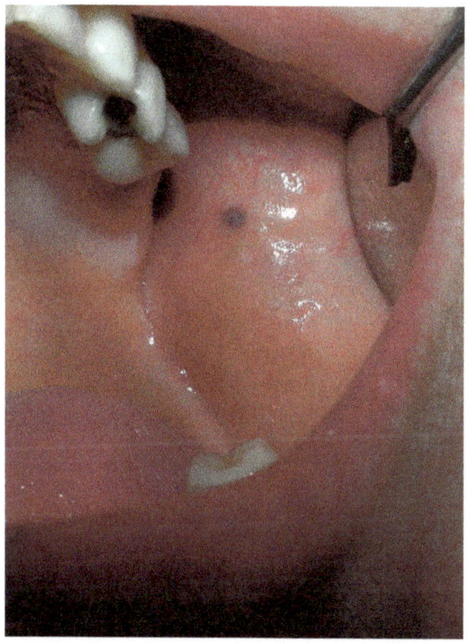

FIGURE 2: Clinical photographs of the 2 × 2 mm pigmented lesion of the right buccal mucosa. Histopathological examination was consistent with amalgam tattoo in both lesions (see Figure 1).

By contrast, amalgam tattoos (formerly called localized argyria) is one of the most frequent causes of exogenous pigmentation in the oral mucosa and is not uncommon to present as two or more lesions [5, 13–15], as seen in the present case. Amalgam consists of an alloy of liquid mercury with varying amounts of silver, tin, copper, and zinc. Amalgam tattoos are usually caused by amalgam splinters inadvertently implanted into the mucosa during dental restorations [5, 7, 13, 15] but may also be caused by diffusion through the teeth [15]. As amalgam has been the most commonly used material for dental fillings until the 1980s, there is still a large amount of prosthetic work being done on existing amalgam fillings. Thus the prevalence of amalgam tattoos remains high as the general population continues to have existing amalgam fillings replaced by the newer composite fillings. Depending on the depth in the tissue, the deposits of amalgam in the mucosa may be visible and present macroscopically as a localised pigmented area. Clinically, this phenomenon presents as grey, blue, or black, nonblanching macules in the oral mucosa [5, 13, 15]. Their appearance can be difficult to discern from other pigmented elements of the oral mucosa including mucosal melanoma.

Histologically, deposits of amalgam are seen as granules along blood vessels and collagen fibres or as solid fragments in the tissue. There may be an associated foreign-body reaction [7, 13].

Amalgam tattoos are harmless and asymptomatic. They can be safely diagnosed by the finding of radio-opaque granules on X-ray, but large particles of amalgam must be present in order for this method to be useful [5–7, 13]. Many endogenous and exogenous conditions can cause pigmentation of the oral mucosa; see Table 1. Pigmented lesions of the mucosa should always be biopsied if the diagnosis is uncertain [2, 5, 6, 8, 13].

4. Conclusion

As amalgam fillings still are ubiquitous and amalgam tattoos remain one of the most common causes of intraoral pigmentation, we consider amalgam tattoos to be an important differential diagnostic consideration, when assessing patients suspect for mucosal melanoma of the oral cavity. Information regarding previous prosthetic dental work should be included in the patient's medical history, and an X-ray showing metal deposits in the mucosa can safely rule out mucosal melanoma. But when in doubt, we recommend a diagnostic biopsy for histopathological examination.

Conflict of Interests

The authors declare that they have no conflict of interests.

References

[1] H. Gavriel, G. McArthur, A. Sizeland, and M. Henderson, "Review: Mucosal melanoma of the head and neck," *Melanoma Research*, vol. 21, no. 4, pp. 257–266, 2011.

[2] M. Gorsky and J. B. Epstein, "Melanoma arising from the mucosal surfaces of the head and neck," *Oral Surgery, Oral Medicine, Oral Pathology, Oral Radiology, and Endodontics*, vol. 86, no. 6, pp. 715–719, 1998.

[3] N. Seetharamu, P. A. Ott, and A. C. Pavlick, "Mucosal melanomas: a case-based review of the literature," *Oncologist*, vol. 15, no. 7, pp. 772–781, 2010.

[4] A. G. Shuman, E. Light, S. H. Olsen et al., "Mucosal melanoma of the head and neck: predictors of prognosis," *Archives of Otolaryngology, Head and Neck Surgery*, vol. 137, no. 4, pp. 331–337, 2011.

[5] D. Eisen, "Disorders of pigmentation in the oral cavity," *Clinics in Dermatology*, vol. 18, no. 5, pp. 579–587, 2000.

[6] A. Kauzman, M. Pavone, N. Blanas, and G. Bradley, "Pigmented lesions of the oral cavity: review, differential diagnosis, and case presentations," *Journal of the Canadian Dental Association*, vol. 70, no. 10, pp. 682–683, 2004.

[7] D. Krahl, A. Altenburg, and C. C. Zouboulis, "Reactive hyperplasias, precancerous and malignant lesions of the oral mucosa," *Journal of the German Society of Dermatology*, vol. 6, no. 3, pp. 217–232, 2008.

[8] A. Buchner, P. W. Merrell, and W. M. Carpenter, "Relative frequency of solitary melanocytic lesions of the oral mucosa," *Journal of Oral Pathology and Medicine*, vol. 33, no. 9, pp. 550–557, 2004.

[9] R. R. Clark and T. Shoaib, "Sentinel lymph node biopsy: a new perspective in head and neck mucosal melanoma?" *Melanoma Research*, vol. 17, no. 1, p. 59, 2007.

[10] I. Stárek, P. Koranda, and P. Beneš, "Sentinel lymph node biopsy: a new perspective in head and neck mucosal melanoma?" *Melanoma Research*, vol. 16, no. 5, pp. 423–427, 2006.

[11] R. R. Clark, T. Shoaib, D. S. Soutar et al., "Sentinel lymph node biopsy in oral malignant melanoma—a possible means of investigating the clinically node-negative neck," *European Journal of Plastic Surgery*, vol. 28, no. 6, pp. 403–407, 2006.

[12] D. G. Pfister, K. K. Ang, D. M. Brizel et al., "Mucosal melanoma of the head and neck," *J Natl Compr Canc Netw*, vol. 10, no. 3, pp. 320–338, 2012.

[13] A. Burchner and L. S. Hansen, "Amalgam pigmentation (amalgam tattoo) of the oral mucosa. A clinicopathologic study of 268 cases," *Oral Surgery Oral Medicine and Oral Pathology*, vol. 49, no. 2, pp. 139–147, 1980.

[14] A. Buchner, "Amalgam tattoo (amalgam pigmentation) of the oral mucosa: clinical manifestations, diagnosis and treatment," *Refuat Hapeh Vehashinayim*, vol. 21, no. 3, pp. 25–92, 2004.

[15] B. M. Owens, W. W. Johnson, and N. J. Schuman, "Oral amalgam pigmentations (tattoos): a retrospective study," *Quintessence International*, vol. 23, no. 12, pp. 805–810, 1992.

Multiple Dental and Skeletal Abnormalities in an Individual with Filippi Syndrome

Meera Sandhu, Pooja Malik, and Rooposhi Saha

Pedodontics and Preventive Dentistry, ITS Center for Dental Studies and Research, C-4, ITS-CDSR, Campus, Muradnagar, Ghaziabad 201206, India

Correspondence should be addressed to Meera Sandhu; meerapedo@yahoo.co.in

Academic Editors: Y.-K. Chen, I. El-Hakim, C. Evans, M. A. Polack, and J. J. Segura-Egea

Filippi syndrome is an autosomal recessive condition characterized by variable soft tissue syndactyly of the fingers and toes, microcephaly, pre- and postnatal growth retardation, mildly abnormal craniofacial appearance, and mental retardation. We report on a child with Filippi syndrome who shows syndactyly of fingers, severe postnatal growth retardation, postnatal microcephaly, and moderate to severe mental retardation. In addition, there is a mildly dysmorphic face along with ocular and a number of dental abnormalities. Radiologically, hands demonstrate bony syndactyly, without any hypoplasia of bones. This phenotype can easily be classified in the group of craniodigital syndromes, but it is difficult to make a more clearly defined diagnosis, based on other minor anomalies, because of the presence of overlapping features. On the basis of various pathognomic features, we conclude that our patient could be an additional case of Filippi syndrome. Moreover, newly recognised features in this patient may be due to variability in phenotypic expression.

1. Introduction

Filippi syndrome is a rare disorder involving finger and toe abnormalities, a small head, characteristic face, and physical and mental retardation. The number of digits involved and the extent of webbing between digits are variable as are many of the other features. In 1985, Filippi [1] reported a new syndrome with mental retardation, postnatal short stature, unusual faces, syndactyly, and severe microcephaly in two brothers and their younger sister originating from Italy. Here, we report a further observation of Filippi syndrome, with severe skeletal anomalies.

2. Case Report

An eighteen-year-old female reported with the chief complaint of missing teeth in the lower front jaw region. She gave a history of trauma 1 year ago in which she lost her front teeth. No other significant history in terms of medications or family was obtained. She gives a history of a surgical attempt of separating the joined fingers, during which half of her ring finger of the left hand was lost due to postsurgical infection. The prenatal, natal, and post natal history was also nonsignificant. She also had mild to moderate mental retardation. On general examination, she was seen to have an abnormally short stature with a height of 4 feet 6 inches and weight of 30 kgs. She also had a loss of vision in the left eye and was wearing eye prosthesis (Figure 1). She was also seen to have syndactyly in relation to middle, ring, and little fingers of both hands (Figure 2). On intraoral examination, she had good oral hygiene and missing right and left mandibular central incisors (Figure 3).

Relative microdontia with respect the crown root length was shorter than normal measurements (as measured on a radiovisuography), by approximately 8 mm, in mandibular right and left first molars and first premolars (Figure 4) and also in maxillary first molars (Figure 5) bilaterally. The soft tissue and other oral mucosal structures did not reveal any abnormality. Various investigations like orthopantomogram, lateral, and posteroanterior (PA) view of skull and hand wrist X-rays were taken to confirm the findings. The PA view (Figure 6) of skull was found to be normal. The orthopantomogram revealed the congenital absence of all the third molars and a generalised horizontal bone loss (Figure 7). In addition to the aforesaid, enlarged pulp

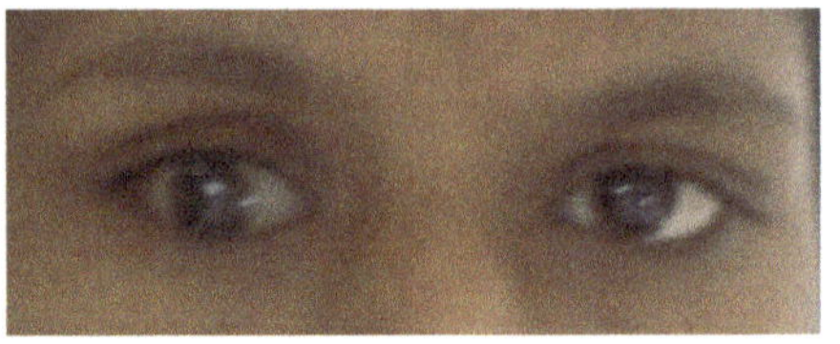

FIGURE 1: Left eye with an eye prosthesis.

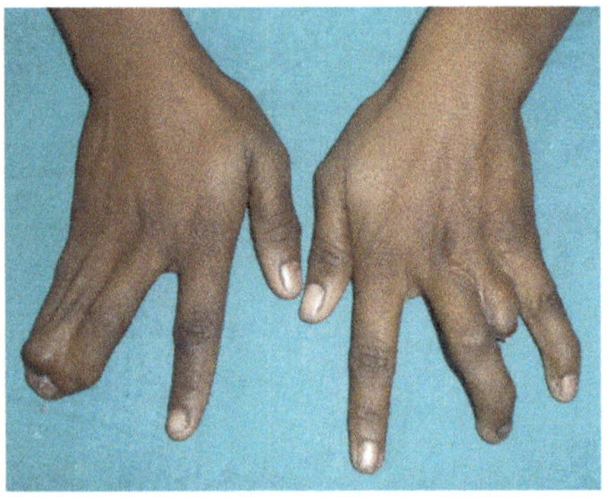

FIGURE 2: Hands showing syndactyly of fingers.

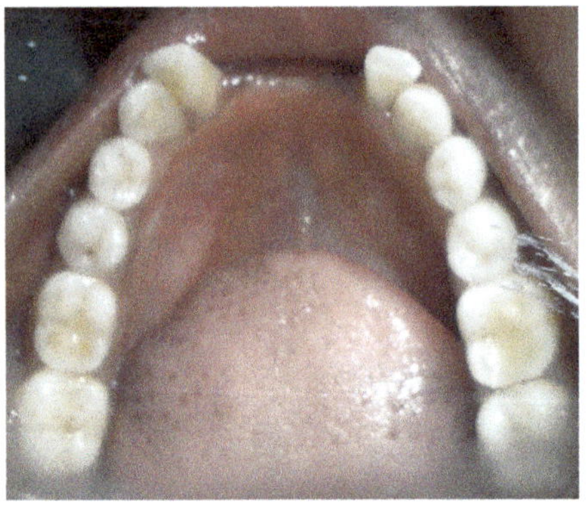

FIGURE 3: Pretreatment mandibular arch showing missing central incisors.

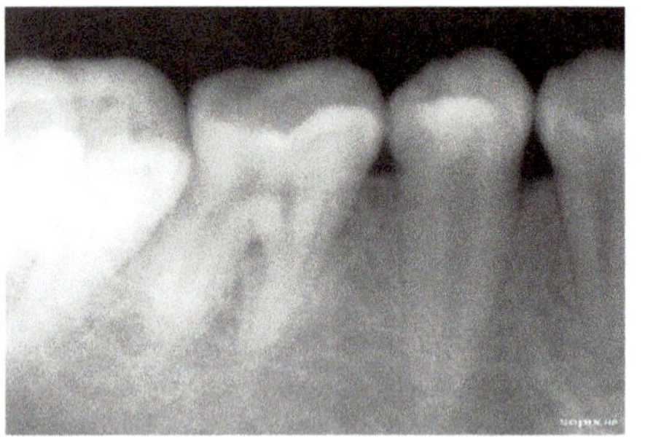

FIGURE 4: Short crown root length of mandibular I molar and premolar.

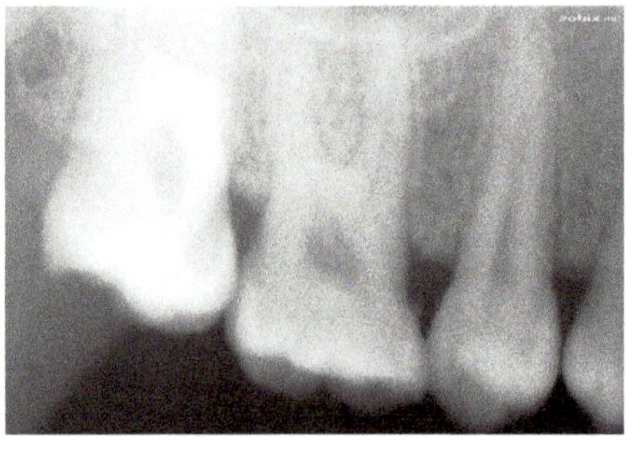

FIGURE 5: Short crown root length of maxillary I molar.

TABLE 1: Dental findings in this report.

Congenital absence of all third molars
Horizontal bone loss in spite of good oral hygiene
Shortened crown root length in multiple teeth
Enlarged pulp chambers in molars

chambers with respect to the maxillary right and left second molars (Figure 8) were also observed. Hand wrist X-ray revealed bony union of the middle, ring, and little fingers of both hands (Figure 9).

3. Discussion

Filippi syndrome is a very rare disorder involving finger and toe abnormalities, a small head, characteristic face, and physical and mental retardation. The number of digits involved and extent of webbing between digits are variable as are many of the other features. The main characteristics in our patient were post natal growth retardation, bony syndactyly of the fingers, and moderate mental retardation. Other features noted were a number of dental findings like congenitally missing teeth, bone loss inspite of good oral hygiene, short crown root length of certain teeth, and an enlargement of pulp chambers (Taurodontism) (Table 1). In addition, in the present case, a congenital loss of vision has also been reported. These multiple congenital anomalies and mental retardation, (MCA/MR Syndromes) very much resemble these described by Filippi [1] and reported in other families by Meinecke [2]. However, other skeletal anomalies, such as dislocation of the elbows with hypoplasia of the radial heads and speech abnormalities, were not present in our case (Table 2).

Occurrence of the disease in both sexes and consanguinity add to the view that an autosomal recessive mode of inheritance is likely in Filippi syndrome [3]. Lorenz et al. [4], Scott et al. [5], and Zerres et al. [6] independently reported

TABLE 2: Clinical features in six patients with Filippe syndrome.

Sex	Filippi [1]			Meinecke [2]		This report
	M	M	F	M	F	F
Mental retardation	+	+	+	+	+	+
Short stature	+	+	+	+	+	+
Syndactyly (Hands)	+	+	−	+	+	+
Elbow dislocation	−	−	−	−	−	−
Delayed bone age	+	−	?	?	−	−
Dental findings	−	−	−	−	−	+
Visual disturbances	−	−	−	−	−	+

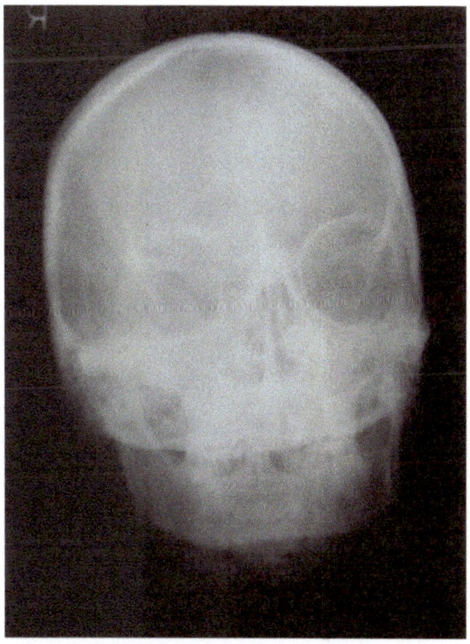

FIGURE 6: PA view of skull.

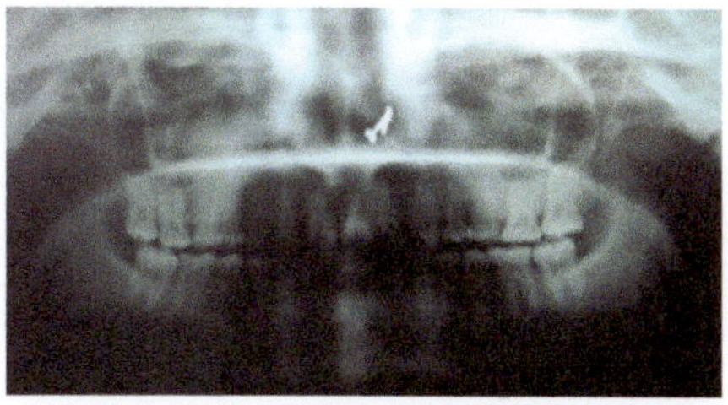

FIGURE 7: Orthopantomogram.

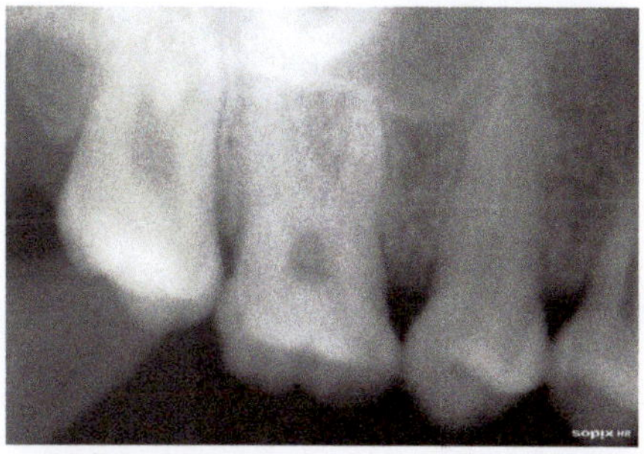

FIGURE 8: Maxillary second molar with an enlarged pulp chamber.

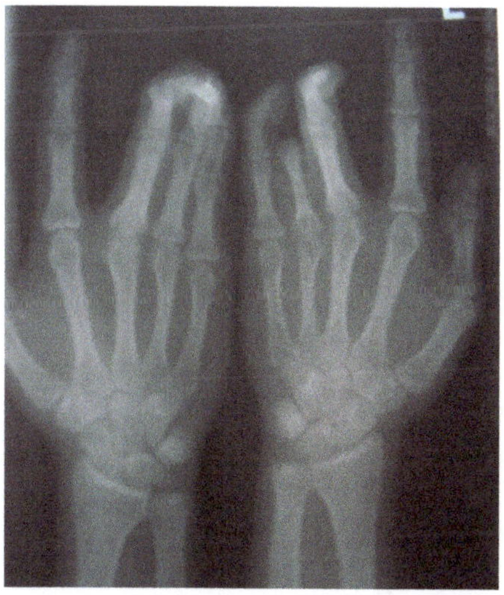

FIGURE 9: Hand wrist X-ray showing bony union of 3 fingers.

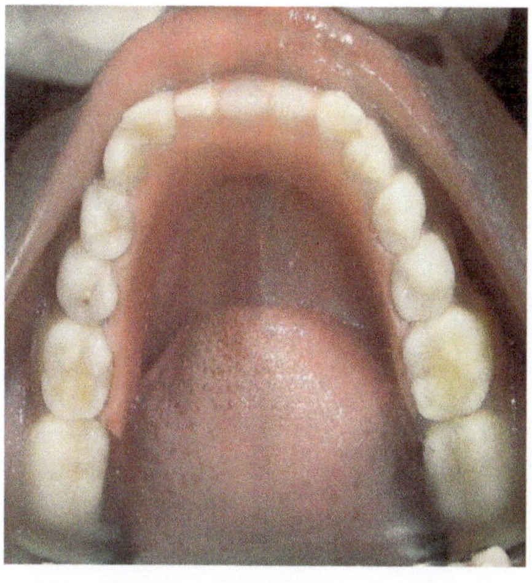

FIGURE 10: Posttreatment mandibular arch showing removable partial denture.

two distinct MCA/MR syndromes with microcephaly, syndactyly, and short stature. However, in both cases, the facial appearance is very different from the dysmorphism observed in Filippi syndrome. Thus, Filippi syndrome appears to be an independent and possibly homogeneous genetic condition.

In this case, the patient's missing teeth were replaced using a removable partial denture (Figure 10) and recalled for regular follow up checkups.

References

[1] G. Filippi, "Unusual facial appearance, microcephaly, growth and mental retardation, and syndactyly. A new syndrome?" *American Journal of Medical Genetics*, vol. 22, no. 4, pp. 821–824, 1985.

[2] P. Meinecke, "Short stature, microcephaly, characteristic face, syndactyly and mental retardation: the Filippi syndrome. Report on a second family," *Genetic Counseling*, vol. 4, no. 2, pp. 147–151, 1993.

[3] D. Héron, T. B. de Villemeur, A. Munnich, and S. Lyonnet, "Filippi syndrome: a new case with skeletal abnormalities," *Journal of Medical Genetics*, vol. 32, no. 8, pp. 659–661, 1995.

[4] P. Lorenz, G. K. Hinkel, C. Hoffmann, and E. Rupprecht, "The craniodigital syndrome of Scott: report of a second family," *American Journal of Medical Genetics*, vol. 37, no. 2, pp. 224–226, 1990.

[5] C. R. Scott, J. I. Bryant, and C. B. Graham, "A new craniodigital syndrome with mental retardation," *The Journal of Pediatrics*, vol. 78, no. 4, pp. 658–663, 1971.

[6] K. Zerres, M. Rietschel, E. Rietschel, F. Majewski, and P. Meinecke, "Postnatal short stature, microcephaly, severe syndactyly of hands and feet, dysmorphic face, and mental retardation: a new syndrome?" *Journal of Medical Genetics*, vol. 29, no. 4, pp. 269–271, 1992.

24

Misdiagnosis of Extensive Maxillofacial Infection and Its Relationship with Periodontal Problems and Hyperglycemia

Cristian Statkievicz, Leonardo P. Faverani, Pedro Henrique Silva Gomes-Ferreira, Gabriel Ramalho-Ferreira, and Idelmo Rangel Garcia-Junior

Department of Surgery and Integrated Clinic, Aracatuba Dental School, Universidade Estadual Paulista (UNESP), 16015-050 Araçatuba, SP, Brazil

Correspondence should be addressed to Cristian Statkievicz; c.statkievicz@gmail.com

Academic Editor: Giuseppe Colella

Background. Complex dental infections can reach distant areas of the alveolar process, invading the secondary fascial spaces. *Objectives.* This case report aims to show a misdiagnosis of odontogenic infection and a great need for dentist in the hospital environment. *Case Report.* A male patient presented facial asymmetry and trismus, while the facial CT examination showed a hyperdense mass involving the left masseteric, pterygomandibular, and superficial temporal regions. The patient was then referred to oral oncology center by emergency physician with cancer suspicion. After 15 days, the patient returned to the same emergency room and was attended by the surgical and maxillofacial trauma team, presenting tachycardia, tachypnea, dysphagia, and trismus. During anamnesis, the patient reported being an uncontrolled diabetic. In intraoral exam, a poor oral condition and generalized periodontitis were observed. *Results.* Correct diagnosis of odontogenic infection was established and adequately treated. *Conclusions.* Symptomatology bland may mask the severity of an infection; every increase in volume associated with trismus, poor oral hygiene with or without hyperglycemia should be heavily investigated for the presence of an infectious process. It emphasizes the importance of a dentist working with the physician in emergency room.

1. Introduction

Maxillofacial infections are usual in patients of all ages, representing a substantial risk to life when reaching deep facial spaces [1]. The signs and symptoms are evident due to proximity between nerves, muscles, and ligaments, which quickly impairs the function of affected region, leading to pain and trismus [2]. Although well-defined, facial anatomy presents peculiar ways for infection spreading, which, when invaded, communicate with each other being able to store large amounts of pus, what may cause upper airways compression and/or face asymmetry, requiring a fast and accurate treatment [3].

In general, the computed tomography (CT) assists in the identification of infection limits, which is vital for a precise diagnosis [1] and provides the surgeon conditions for appropriate surgical drainage, along with cause removal. These two steps are the basis for therapy, supported by the administration of specific antibiotics [4, 5].

Infectious processes within the oral cavity are generally associated with an inadequate oral hygiene, periodontal disease, and caries [6], being exponentially aggravated in immunosuppressed and especially diabetic patients [7]. Therefore, the dentist or doctor must keep odontogenic infection under suspicion when a painful edema is observed in face or neck [2]. Thus, a specialized consultation with a dentist or an oral and maxillofacial surgeon can avoid serious complications and save lives [2].

Although it is hard to determine whether an infection will get worse at the moment the patient is admitted for treatment [6], the triad anamnesis, physical examination, and image tests should be performed thoroughly. Thus, this study aims to highlight, through a case report, the importance of

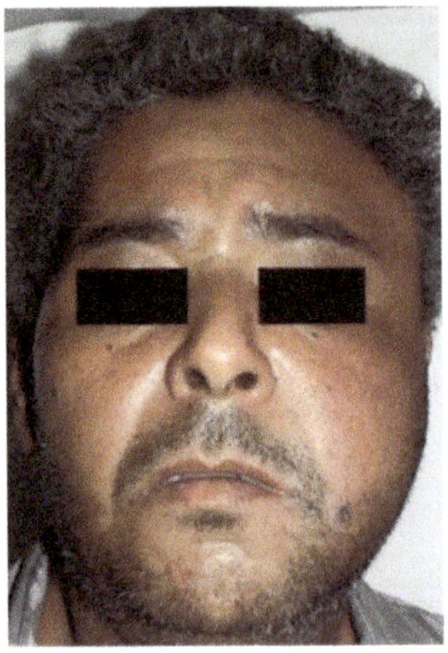

Figure 1

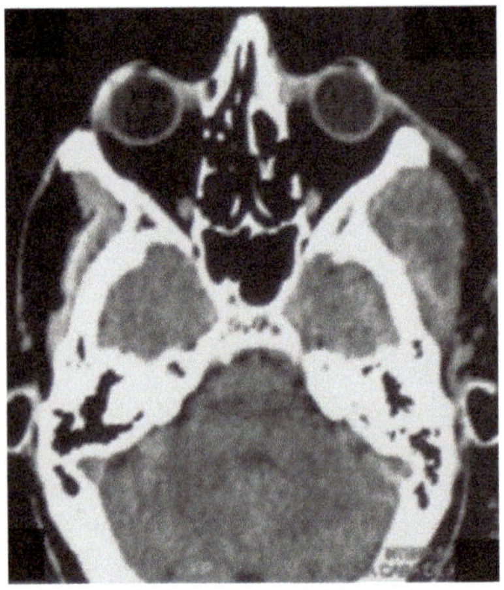

Figure 2

dentists or oral and maxillofacial surgeons in the diagnosis and treatment of maxillofacial infections.

2. Case History

A 46-year-old male patient attended the emergency room of the *Santa Casa de Misericordia de Araçatuba* Hospital, *SP*, complaining about facial pain and swelling (Figure 1). On physical examination, left hemiface asymmetry and trismus were observed, while the facial CT examination showed a hyperdense mass involving the left masseteric, pterygomandibular, and superficial temporal regions (Figures 2 and 3). The patient was then referred to oral oncology center with cancer suspicion. However, he did not attend the oral oncology center.

After 15 days, the patient returned to the same emergency room and was attended by the surgical and maxillofacial trauma team, presenting tachycardia, tachypnea, dysphagia, sore throat and breathing difficulty, trismus, and edema with floatation point in the temporal region. During anamnesis, the patient reported being uncontrolled diabetic, so a quick

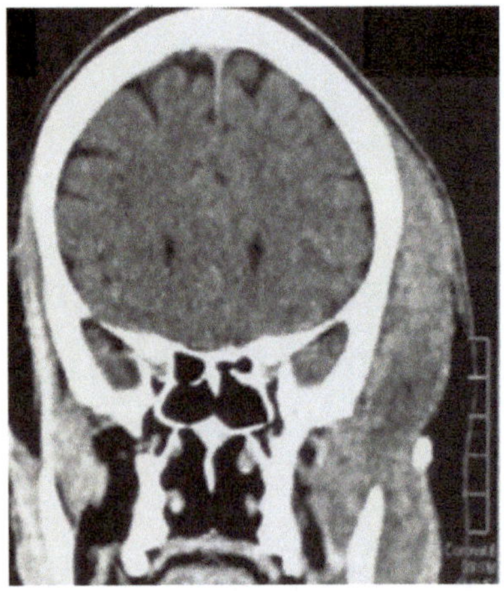

Figure 3

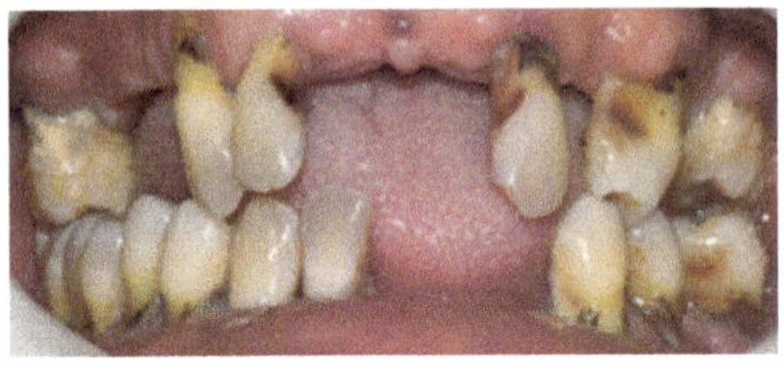

Figure 4

glucose test was performed noting a 600 mg/dL glucose level. In intraoral exam, a poor oral condition and generalized periodontitis were observed (Figure 4). The diagnosis was a complex odontogenic infection involving the masseteric, pterygomandibular, and superficial temporal spaces, confirmed by computed tomography.

The treatment started immediately with intravenous antibiotic prophylaxis with 2 g sodium cephalothin (Keflin, União Química, Brasilia, DF, Brazil) and 500 mg metronidazole (Sanofi-Aventis Pharmaceuticals Ltd., Sao Paul, SP, Brazil) and administration of 10 IU insulin. The surgical procedure was conducted under general anesthesia and initiated by the location of floatation point in temporal region (Figure 5), where an aspiration punction for antibiogram culture and surgical drainage of superficial temporal space by Gillies technique with installation of a Penrose drain were performed (Figure 6). Two oral incisions were performed to access the masseteric and pterygomandibular spaces. Then, because of periodontal conditions and social-cultural aspect of the patient, a serial extraction was indicated (Figures 7 and 8). On the second day after surgery, the patient presented a good general condition and good mouth opening. The antibiotic therapy was 1 g ceftriaxone and was continued for 48 hours after symptom remission. The patient was referred to a dentist for rehabilitation with total prosthesis (Figure 9).

3. Discussion

Dental infection starts with pulp necrosis, which is disseminated to tissues through the apical foramen, reaching

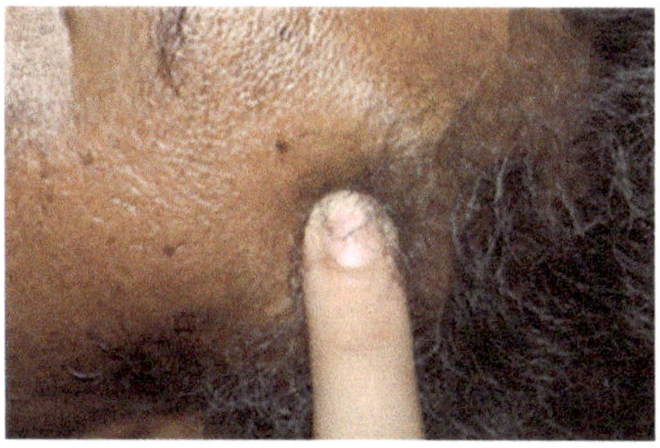

Figure 5

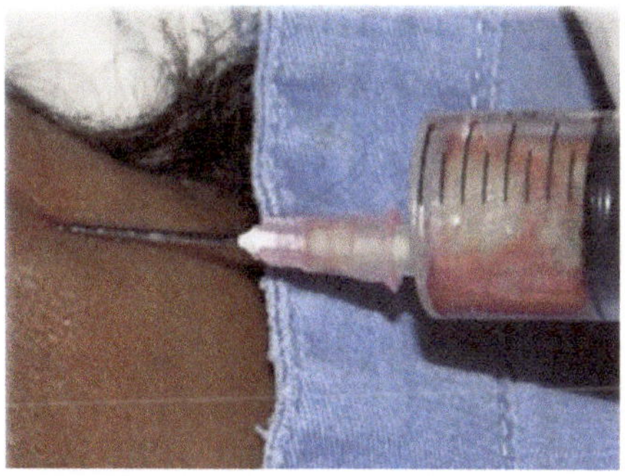

Figure 6

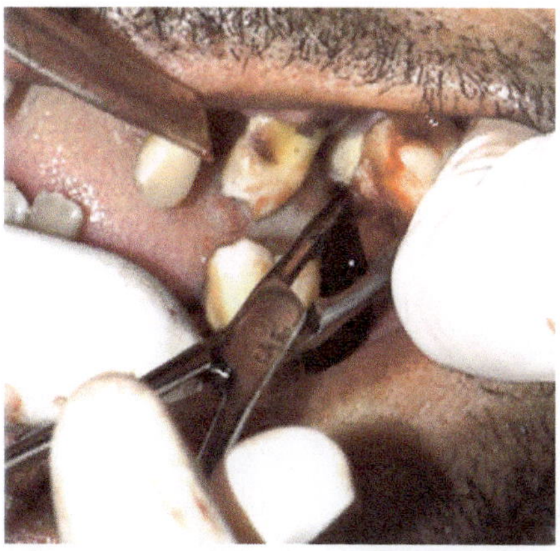

Figure 7

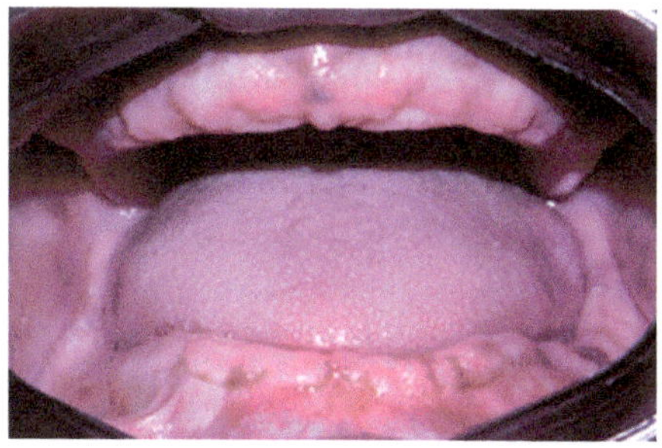

Figure 8

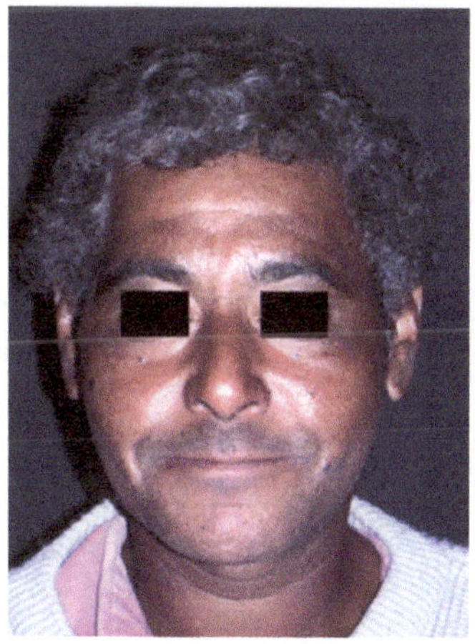

Figure 9

areas distant from the infection focus [8]. In a study with 185 patients suffering from deep neck infection, 50% of the cases were odontogenic [9], such as the case reported in our study. The current aspect of diagnosis and treatment of head and neck infections has improved due to technological advances in imaging and different types of antibiotics [10]. However, there is a low incidence of complications in patients with predisposing diseases for the development of infectious processes [5].

Uncontrolled diabetes mellitus can lead to high blood glucose levels, which contribute to a more aggressive infection course, owing to a deficiency in chemotaxis, phagocytosis, and bactericidal function. These factors predispose long periods of hospitalization increasing the risk of complications [7]. According to this report, a 600 mg/dL glycemic rate exacerbates infectious process and reduces pharmacological effect of antibiotics, making glycemic blood control a key factor in the cure of dental infection.

The clinical signs and symptoms of facial infection are remarkable, especially in superficial areas such as temporal and buccal space, clinically observed as a pronounced volumetric increase in the region [2]. However, some patients who exhibit milder signs may underestimate the case severity. Among the facial areas, when pterygomandibular space is affected, it should be treated aggressively, due to the possibility of contamination passing the edge of medial pterygoid muscle reaching the pharyngeal space [2].

Although not necessary in superficial infections, the CT scan is extremely valuable when the infection reaches deep spaces and when associated with an experienced clinical examination it is possible to identify clinically important pus cavities [1]. However, an evaluation performed by a nonspecialized professional can lead to misdiagnosis.

The cure of dental infections is usually achieved without major complications. Nevertheless, it is recommended that the dentist/doctor includes oral cavity as one of the main areas to be evaluated on physical examination in patients with painful edema in the head and neck region, investigating possible associated diseases that may be supporting the infection.

A problem in emergency attendance is the lack of knowledge from the side of the physician about dentistry comorbidities. Most misdiagnoses of head and neck infections happened due to first clinical examination failure; sometimes, it can be confused with tumor lesion. In this case, the first attendance led to wrong diagnosis and it could promote several complications, including death. Therefore, an oral and maxillofacial surgeon is essential to emergency room.

Conflict of Interests

The authors declare that there is no conflict of interests regarding the publication of this paper.

References

[1] A. Gonzalez-Beicos and D. Nunez, "Imaging of acute head and neck infections," *Radiologic Clinics of North America*, vol. 50, no. 1, pp. 73–83, 2012.

[2] T. R. Flynn, "The swollen face: severe odontogenic infections," *Emergency Medicine Clinics of North America*, vol. 18, no. 3, pp. 481–519, 2000.

[3] A. Wabik, B. K. Hendrich, J. Nienartowicz, M. Guziński, and M. J. Sąsiadek, "Odontogenic inflammatory processes of head and neck in computed tomography examinations," *Polish Journal of Radiology*, vol. 79, no. 1, pp. 431–438, 2014.

[4] J. S. Jundt and R. Gutta, "Characteristics and cost impact of severe odontogenic infections," *Oral Surgery, Oral Medicine, Oral Pathology and Oral Radiology*, vol. 114, no. 5, pp. 558–566, 2012.

[5] D. Opitz, C. Camerer, D.-M. Camerer et al., "Incidence and management of severe odontogenic infections—a retrospective analysis from 2004 to 2011," *Journal of Cranio-Maxillofacial Surgery*, vol. 43, no. 2, pp. 285–289, 2015.

[6] S. Ylijoki, R. Suuronen, H. Jousimies-Somer, J. H. Meurman, and C. Lindqvis, "Differences between patients with or without the need for intensive care due to severe odontogenic infections," *Journal of Oral and Maxillofacial Surgery*, vol. 59, no. 8, pp. 867–872, 2001.

[7] J. S. Chang, K. H. Yoo, S. H. Yoon et al., "Odontogenic infection involving the secondary fascial space in diabetic and non-diabetic patients: a clinical comparative study," *Journal of the Korean Association of Oral and Maxillofacial Surgeons*, vol. 39, no. 4, pp. 175–181, 2013.

[8] C. T. M. H. Saito, J. L. Gulinelli, H. F. Marão et al., "Occurrence of odontogenic infections in patients treated in a postgraduation program on maxillofacial surgery and traumatology," *The Journal of Craniofacial Surgery*, vol. 22, no. 5, pp. 1689–1694, 2011.

[9] T.-T. Huang, T.-C. Liu, P.-R. Chen, F.-Y. Tseng, T.-H. Yeh, and Y.-S. Chen, "Deep neck infection: analysis of 185 cases," *Head & Neck*, vol. 26, no. 10, pp. 854–860, 2004.

[10] I. C. Uluibau, T. Jaunay, and A. N. Goss, "Severe odontogenic infections," *Australian Dental Journal*, vol. 50, supplement, no. 4, pp. S74–S81, 2005.

25

Periodontal Regeneration Using Platelet-Derived Growth Factor in Infrabony Defects: A Series of Three Cases

Kaustubh Thakare,[1] M. L. Bhongade,[1] Preeti Charde,[1] Priyanka Jaiswal,[1] Nachiket Shah,[1] and Aniruddha Deshpande[2]

[1] *Department of Periodontology and Implantology, Sharad Pawar Dental College and Hospital, Maharashtra, Wardha 442001, India*
[2] *Department of Periodontology and Implantology, CSMSS Dental College and Hospital, Maharashtra, Aurangabad 431001, India*

Correspondence should be addressed to Preeti Charde; preeti.perio@gmail.com

Academic Editors: T. Kubota and T. Lombardi

The periodontal researchers and clinicians, in an effort to develop effective regenerative therapies, have sought to understand key events involved in the regeneration of periodontium. Polypeptide growth factors are a class of natural biological mediators which regulate key cellular events in tissue repair. Platelet-derived growth factor (PDGF) is the most thoroughly studied growth factor in periodontal regeneration. The present case series evaluate the effectiveness of platelet-derived growth factor (rh-PDGF-BB) in combination with beta-tricalcium phosphate (β-TCP) to achieve periodontal regeneration in 3 infrabony defects.

1. Introduction

Periodontal treatment modalities now strive to provide one or more of the following to enhance periodontal regeneration: appropriate matrices, biologic mediators, and/or precursor cells. Polypeptide growth factors are a class of natural biological mediators which regulate key cellular events in tissue repair. Platelet-derived growth factor (PDGF) is the most thoroughly studied growth factor in periodontics. Since the late 1980s, when it was first discovered that PDGF promoted regeneration of bone, cementum, and periodontal ligament (PDL) by Lynch et al. (1989) [1], nearly 100 studies have been published on its effect on PDL and alveolar bone cells and regeneration of periodontium in both animals and humans.

These studies have clearly demonstrated the mechanism of action of PDGF, showing the presence of cell surface receptors for PDGF on PDL and alveolar bone cells and elucidating PDGF's stimulatory effect on the proliferation and chemotaxis of osteoblast, PDL fibroblasts, and cementoblasts [2–4].

The presence of ideal scaffold plays a basic role in periodontal regeneration [5]. Filling the regenerative spaces with a biocompatible material may facilitate or accelerate the periodontal regeneration process by adding more solid surfaces on which the cells can initiate regeneration. Beta-tricalcium phosphate (β-TCP) is a purified, multicrystalline, and porous form of calcium phosphate with a Ca : Po_4 ratio similar to that of natural bone material. It provides matrix or scaffolding for periodontal regeneration and also facilitates the stabilization of the blood clot [6].

Therefore, the present case series was carried out to evaluate the effectiveness of platelet-derived growth factor (rh-PDGF-BB) in combination with beta-tricalcium phosphate (β-TCP) to achieve periodontal regeneration in 3 infrabony defects.

2. Case Presentations

After proper examination and diagnosis, 3 patients with infrabony defect were selected from the Department of Periodontology and Implantology. Initial therapy consisting of oral hygiene instructions, supra and subgingival scaling, and root planing under local anesthesia was performed. 6 weeks after the initial therapy, surgical therapy was initiated. Prior to surgery at baseline, clinical measurements including probing pocket depth (PPD), clinical attachment loss (CAL), and gingival recession (GR) were recorded with Florida Probe (Florida Probe Corporation, Gainesville, FL, USA) with a constant probing force of 15 gm (pressure −154 N/cm^2), tip diameter of 0.45 mm, precision of 0.2 mm and a probe length of 11 mm and William's graduated probe. At Baseline an intraoral periapical radiograph was taken of selected site with long cone (XCP Rinn, Dentsply) paralleling technique. Radiographic measurements were obtained by utilizing a film mount with millimeter grid scale (Nix Company Ltd., Tokyo, Japan). These are pocket-mount-type grids for intraoral film. Grid scale lines are printed at 1 mm intervals with bold lines at 5 mm intervals. The developed IOPA films were inserted in the mount to evaluate radiographic defect depth (DD), which is measured from the crest of bone to the base of bony defect. All the clinical and radiographic measurements were again recorded at 6 months post-operatively.

Case 1. A 35-year-old female patient presented with clinical and radiographic measurements on mesial surface of 46 (see Table 1).

Case 2. A 40-year-old male patient presented with clinical and radiographic measurements on mesial surface of 36 (see Table 2).

Case 3. A 38-year-old male patient presented with clinical and radiographic measurements on mesial surface of 36 (see Table 3).

2.1. Surgical Procedure. Immediately before the surgical treatment, the patients were made to rinse the mouth with 0.2% chlorhexidine gluconate solution for 1 minute. The Patients were draped to expose only the oral cavity. Asepsis was maintained throughout the entire procedure. The area subjected to surgery was anaesthetized by nerve block or infiltration anaesthesia, depending upon the surgical site, using local anaesthetic solution 2% solution xylocaine containing 1 : 100,000 epinephrine.

Conventional approach consisting in a periodontal access flap was initiated by intracrevicular (sulcular) incisions using Bard-Parker number 12 and 15 surgical blades on the buccal and lingual aspects. A tooth each mesial and distal to the defect associated tooth were included in the flap.

Full-thickness (mucoperiosteal) flap was reflected using a periosteal elevator (24 G Hu-Friedy, USA) to expose alveolar bone in area of osseous defect. The osseous defect was debrided off granulation tissue using hand instruments (Gracey Curettes, Hu-Friedy, USA) and ultrasonic instruments (EMS, Minipiezon), thus exposing the root surface, alveolar bone, and periodontal ligament. Intramarrow penetration was performed with a half-round bur, in case of insufficient bleedings from the walls of the lesion.

At this stage, the defects were treated with insertion of rh-PDGF-BB plus beta-tricalcium phosphate (GEM 21S, Growth-Factor-Enhanced Matrix, BioMimetic Therapeutics, Inc., Franklin, TN, USA). According to the manufacturer's directions, the beta-tricalcium phosphate particles were hydrated with 0.3 mg/mL rh-PDGF-BB and then gently packed into the osseous defects to the level of most coronal osseous wall. The mucoperiosteal flaps were positioned coronally to achieve primary coverage over the graft and sutured using interdental interrupted sutures (4–0, nonresorbable surgical sutures, braided black silk, Mersilk, Ethicon, Johnson Ltd.). The surgical site was dressed with periodontal surgical dressing (Coe-Pak, GC, Inc, ALSIP, IL, USA), on the buccal and lingual aspects.

Antibiotic coverage consisting in Amoxicillin 500 mg three times a day and analgesics consisting in combination of Ibuprofen 325 mg and Paracetamol 400 mg three times a day were prescribed for 5 days after surgical period. Patients were instructed to rinse twice daily with 0.2% chlorhexidine gluconate for 6 weeks. Periodontal dressing and sutures were removed 8–10 days after surgery. After this period, patients were reinstructed to resume mechanical oral hygiene measures, including careful brushing with soft toothbrush and interdental cleaning with an interdental brush) and to discontinue chlorhexidine.

In the present case series, at 6 months of followup after surgery, significant improvement was found in clinical parameters. Patients 1 and 2 showed 100% radiographic defect fill while as patient 3 showed 80% radiographic defect depth fill. *Clinical and radiographic measurements at 6 months of followup:*

Case 1: see Table 4.

Case 2: see Table 5.

Case 3: see Table 6.

TABLE 1

PPD	CAL	GR	DD
9.8 mm	12 mm	2.2 mm	4 mm

TABLE 2

PPD	CAL	GR	DD
6.2 mm	6.2 mm	0 mm	3 mm

TABLE 3

PPD	CAL	GR	DD
5.8 mm	5.8 mm	0 mm	5 mm

TABLE 4

PPD	CAL	GR	DD
3.2 mm	5.4 mm	2.2 mm	0 mm

TABLE 5

PPD	CAL	GR	DD
3 mm	3 mm	0 mm	0 mm

TABLE 6

PPD	CAL	GR	DD
2.8 mm	3.6 mm	0.8 mm	1 mm

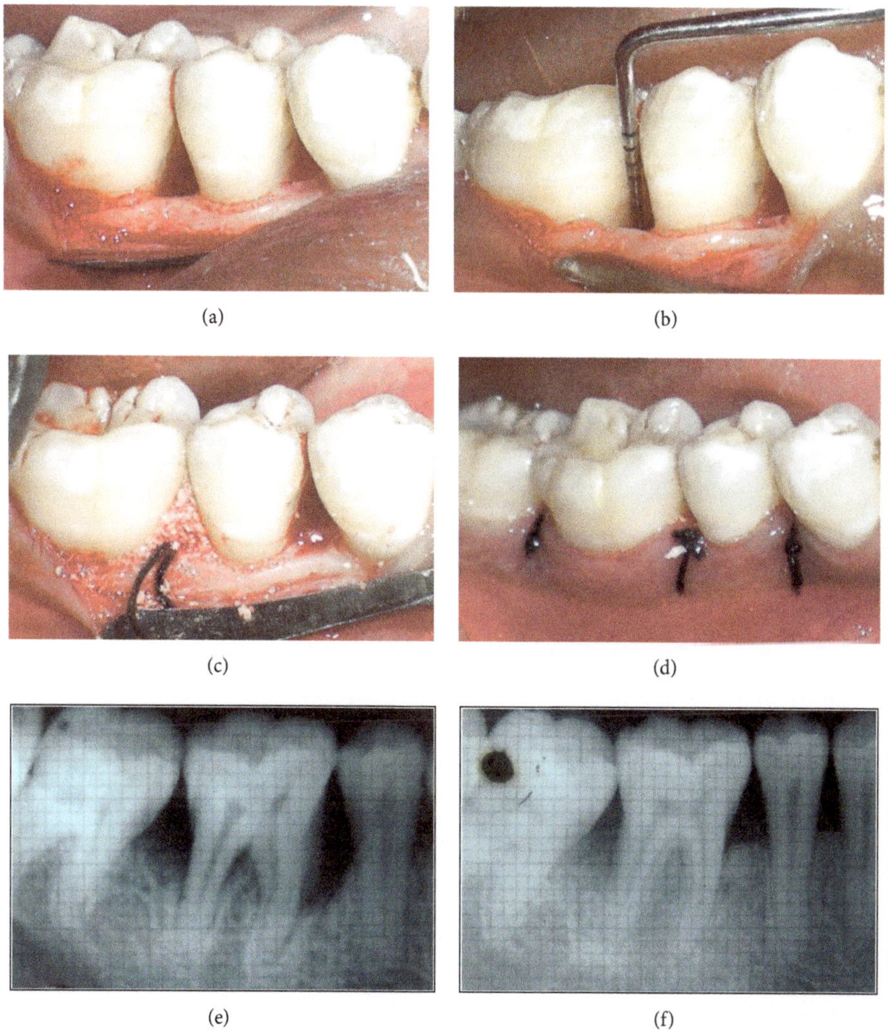

FIGURE 1: (a) Preoperative view. (b) Configuration and depth of defect. (c) Placement of rh-PDGF-BB in combination with β-TCP. (d) Suturing. (e) Preoperative radiograph. (f) Postoperative radiograph.

3. Discussion

Changes in the clinical attachment levels (CALs) following regenerative therapy are the most commonly used clinical outcome variable in regenerative studies. In the present case series, a significantly greater amount of mean CAL gain was observed at 6 months of followup. The results obtained in the present case series are comparable with other reported studies. Camelo et al. [7] studied the effectiveness of purified recombinant human platelet-derived growth factor (rh-PDGF-BB) mixed with a synthetic β-TCP matrix for the treatment of osseous defects and observed significant mean CAL gain of 3.8 mm for rh-PDGF-BB combined with β-TCP group compared to β-TCP alone group (3.2 mm). Camelo et al. [8] also reported a significant mean CAL gain at sites treated with rh-PDGF-BB in combination with β-TCP. In the present case series, a significantly greater amount of mean CAL gain could be related to the molecular characteristic of rh-PDGF-BB that enhances cell attachment and proliferation.

Reduction of pocket depth in order to limit the risk of local reinfection is a primary goal of periodontal therapy. Shallow pockets have a strong, negative predictive value for future disease progression, while deep pockets in treated areas are risk indicators for periodontal disease progression. In the present study, pocket depth reduction was significant in all three patients. These findings are in accordance with those of a study by Nevins et al. [9], where mean PPD reduction of 5.93 mm in sites treated with combination of rh-PDGF-BB with β-TCP (Figure 1).

During 6 months, the infrabony lesions in this study, responded well to rh-PDGF-BB combined with β-TCP treatment with regard to the reduction in radiographic defect depth. Radiographic bone measurement is a noninvasive, painless alternative to direct bone measurement. Therefore, in the present case series, radiographic monitoring of alveolar bone changes was carried out. These findings are in accordance with those of previous reported studies.

Nevins et al. [10] reported a gain in defect fill of 2.9 to 3.0 mm (57%) in sites treated with rh-PDGF-BB + β-TCP.

4. Conclusion

On the basis of the results of the present case series study and within the limitations of the study, it can be concluded that treatment with rh-PDGF-BB in combination with β-TCP resulted in a significantly higher CAL gain and PPD reduction and radiographic defect fill.

References

[1] S. E. Lynch, R. C. Williams, A. M. Polson et al., "A combination of platelet-derived and insulin-like growth factors enhances periodontal regeneration," *Journal of Clinical Periodontology*, vol. 16, no. 8, pp. 545–548, 1989.

[2] C. L. Strayhorn, J. S. Garrett, R. L. Dunn, J. J. Benedict, and M. J. Somerman, "Growth factors regulate expression of osteoblast-associated genes," *Journal of Periodontology*, vol. 70, no. 11, pp. 1345–1354, 1999.

[3] D. K. Dennison, D. R. Vallone, G. J. Pinero, B. Rittman, and R. G. Caffesse, "Differential effect of TGF-β1 and PDGF on proliferation of periodontal ligament cells and gingival fibroblasts," *Journal of Periodontology*, vol. 65, no. 7, pp. 641–648, 1994.

[4] N. E. Saygin, W. V. Giannobile, and M. J. Somerman, "Molecular and cell biology of cementum," *Periodontology 2000*, vol. 24, no. 1, pp. 73–98, 2000.

[5] R. K. Schenk, "Bone regeneration: biologic basis," in *Guided Bone Regeneration in Implant Dentistry*, D. Buser, C. Dahlin, and R. K. Schenk, Eds., pp. 49–100, Quintessence, London, UK, 1995.

[6] M. Szpalski and R. Gunzburg, "Applications of calcium phosphate—based cancellous bone void fillers in trauma surgery," *Orthopedics*, vol. 25, supplement 5, pp. s601–s609, 2002.

[7] M. Camelo, M. L. Nevins, R. K. Schenk, S. E. Lynch, and M. Nevins, "Periodontal regeneration in human class II furcations using purified recombinant human platelet-derived growth factor-BB (rhPDGF-BB) with bone allograft," *International Journal of Periodontics and Restorative Dentistry*, vol. 23, no. 3, pp. 213–225, 2003.

[8] M. Camelo, M. L. Nevins, R. K. Schenk et al., "Clinical, radiographic, and histologic evaluation of human periodontal defects treated with bio-oss and bio-gide," *International Journal of Periodontics and Restorative Dentistry*, vol. 18, no. 4, pp. 321–331, 1998.

[9] M. Nevins, J. Hanratty, and S. E. Lynch, "Clinical results using recombinant human platelet-derived growth factor and mineralized freeze-dried bone allograft in periodontal defects," *International Journal of Periodontics and Restorative Dentistry*, vol. 27, no. 5, pp. 421–427, 2007.

[10] M. Nevins, W. V. Giannobile, M. K. McGuire et al., "Platelet-derived growth factor stimulates bone fill and rate of attachment level gain: results of a large multicenter randomized controlled trial," *Journal of Periodontology*, vol. 76, no. 12, pp. 2205–2215, 2005.

26

Cysticercosis Involving Muscle of Mastication

Sarbjeet Singh,[1] V. Sreenivasan,[2] Kanika Garg,[2] Nikhel Dev Wazir,[3] Jaspal Singh Rajput,[4] and Pawandeep Sandhu Virk[5]

[1] *Department of Oral Medicine & Radiology, Institute of Dental Sciences, Sehora, Jammu 181132, India*
[2] *Department of Oral Medicine & Radiology, Subharti Dental College and Hospital, Meerut, Uttarpradesh 250002, India*
[3] *Department of Conservative & Endodontics, Institute of Dental Sciences, Sehora, Jammu 181132, India*
[4] *Department of Pedodontics, SGT Dental College, Hospital & Research Center, Gurgoan, Haryana 122505, India*
[5] *Department of Pedodontics, Desh Bhagat Dental College & Hospital, Muktsar, Punjab 152026, India*

Correspondence should be addressed to Sarbjeet Singh; saku500@yahoo.com

Academic Editors: S. S. De Rossi, L. Manuel Junquera Gutierrez, and E. F. Wright

Cysticercosis is a parasitic infection caused by the larval stages of the parasitic cestode, *Taenia solium*. It is a common disease in developing countries where it is also endemic. The central nervous system (CNS) is the most important primary site of infection and the disease can present with solitary or multiple space occupying lesions. Cases of cysticercosis presenting as isolated muscle mass (pseudotumours) without involvement of the CNS have also been recently described in the literature. We present two cases who presented to us with pain, swelling, and tenderness involving the temporalis muscle along with trismus. Ultrasonography and MRI findings were suggestive of cysticercosis involving the temporalis muscle which resolved after the albendazole therapy.

1. Introduction

Cysticerci are spherical milky white cysts containing fluid and a single invaginated scolex with hooklets [1]. When humans ingest eggs or gravid proglottids from the parasite *Taenia solium*, the covering of the eggs is digested in the stomach and the larval form (cysticercus cellulosae) of the parasite is hatched [1]. The larvae penetrate the mucosa, enters the blood vessels and lymphatics, and are distributed in the tissues all over the body but preferentially locate in the brain, muscle, skin, liver, lungs, and heart [1]. They are also found in oral and perioral tissues, particularly in the muscles of mastication, facial expression, the suprahyoid muscles, and the postcervical musculature as well as in the tongue, buccal mucosa, and lip [2–4]. Here we report two cases of cysticercosis affecting the temporalis muscle.

1.1. Case Report 1. A 50-year-old female patient presented to our department with complaint of pain and mild swelling on the right side of the face since the last 2 months. She gave a history that pain is aggravated while opening the mouth, chewing and on application of pressure on that area and was not relieved by NSAIDs. Her past medical history revealed history of typhoid fever 3 months back for which she had taken complete course of treatment.

On extraoral examination, maximal mouth opening was reduced to around 28 mm and a diffuse swelling around 1 × 1 cms in diameter was also observed in the right temporalis muscle which was soft to firm in consistency and was tender on palpation (Figure 1). Examination of the TMJ and other muscles of mastication revealed normal findings. On intraoral examination edentulous spaces were present involving the right and left mandibular posterior teeth.

On the basis of the history and examination findings, a clinical provisional diagnosis of myofascial pain was made and the patient was put on the treatment of muscle relaxants Tab Myospaz forte two times a day and topical application of voveran emuigel along with hot fomentation, soft diet, and bilateral chewing. The patient reported to us after 3 days but she did not have relief whatsoever. Reevaluation of the

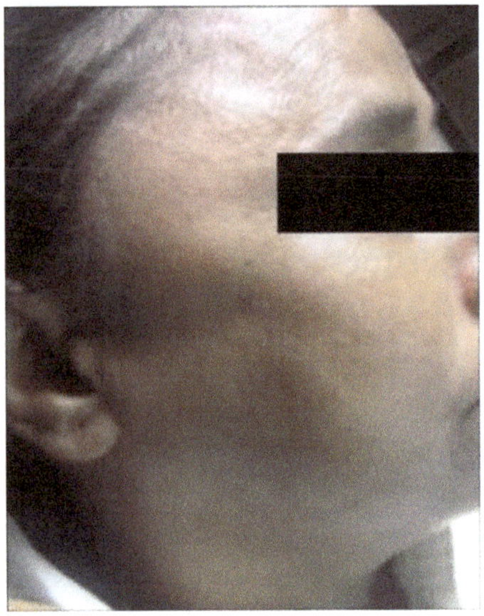

Figure 1

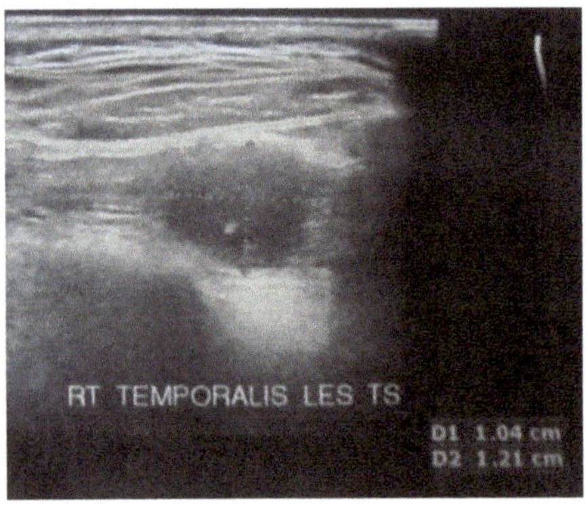

Figure 2

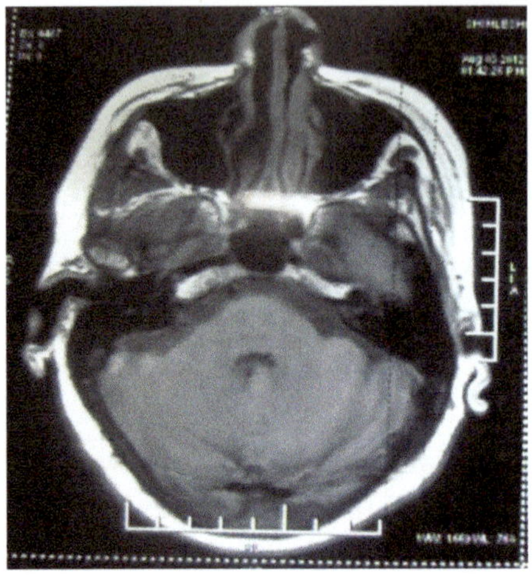

Figure 3

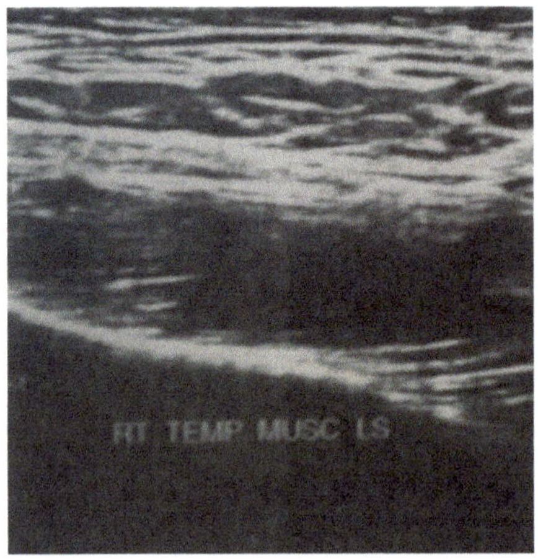

Figure 4

case was done and she was advised of blood investigations along with ultrasonogram (USG) and MRI involving the right side of the face. The findings of the blood investigations were normal. USG showed the presence of a well-defined anechoic lesion around 1.2 × 1 × 0.9 cms involving the right temporalis muscle with its long axis parallel to its fibres and 14 × 12 mm echogenic nidus was also seen within it (Figure 2). MRI revealed the presence of a rounded iso to mildly hyperintense lesion in the right temporalis muscle with an identifiable hypointense nidus on T1 and T2 and Fiesta-C images (Figure 3). The lesion also displayed T1 and T2 hypointense rim along with edema involving the right temporalis muscle. The features on both USG and MRI were suggestive of cysticercosis involving the right temporalis muscle.

For the treatment the patient was advised of anthelmintic albendazole 400 mg BD AND Crocin SOS for 4 weeks. Four-week follow-up of the patient showed significant reduction in the pain and the size of the swelling. Mild swelling stiltreatment was continued for another 5 days. USG examination after 4 weeks and 5 days showed coml persisted so the plete resolution of the lesion with no focal lesion identifiable in the right temporalis muscle (Figure 4). The swelling and pain had also subsided completely (Figure 5).

1.2. Case Report 2. A 42-year-old man complained of a gradually increasing swelling over the right temple region. The patient also complained of associated difficulty in speaking or chewing food. On examination, there was a well-defined, firm, and tender swelling of 2 × 1.5 cm involving the temporalis muscle on the right side (Figure 6). This time the patient was provisionally diagnosed as cysticercosis involving the temporalis muscle. A high-resolution sonographic examination of the temporal swelling was done. Sonography showed a well-defined, 1.5 × 1.8 cm, hypoechoic lesion with a small hyperechoic speck suggesting a scolex (Figure 7). Hence, the possibility of cysticercosis was considered. MRI (Figure 8) revealed the presence of a rounded hyperintense lesion in the right temporalis muscle with an identifiable hypointense nidus on T1 and T2 and Fiesta-C images. The features on both USG and MRI were suggestive of cysticercosis involving the right temporalis muscle. The patient was prescribed

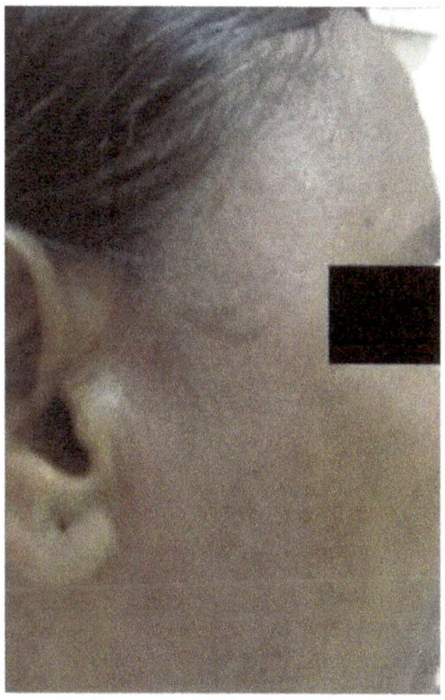

Figure 5

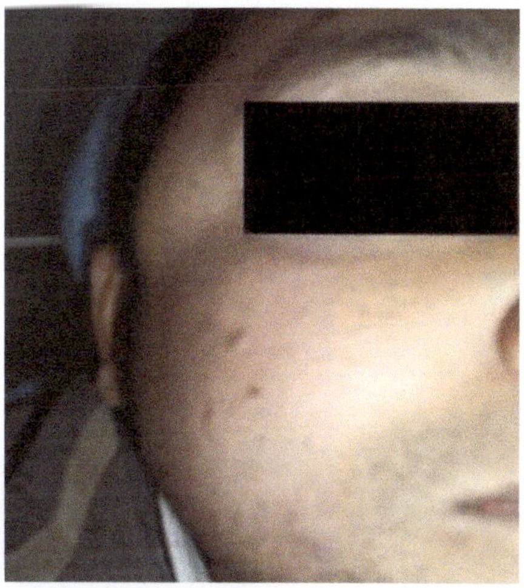

Figure 6

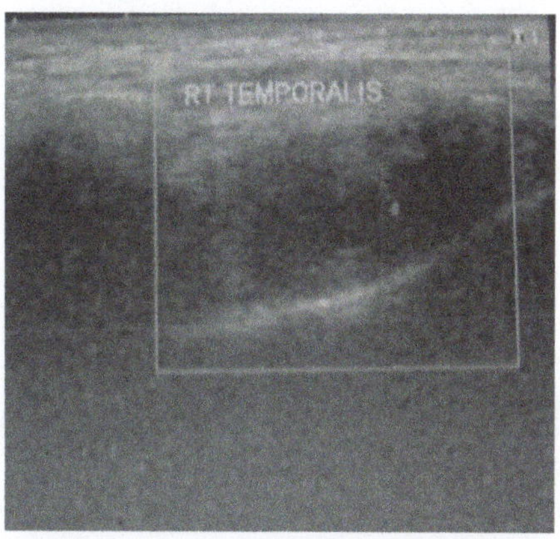

Figure 7

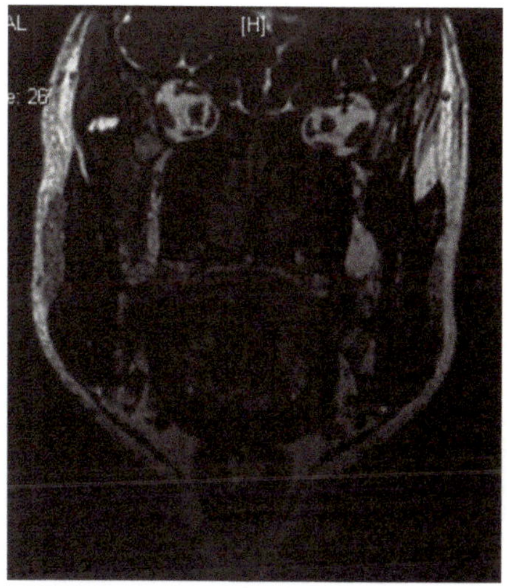

Figure 8

Tab albendazole 400 mg BD along with Crocin SOS for 4 weeks. The patient completely recovered and was completely asymptomatic after 4 weeks.

2. Discussion

Tapeworm infection is common in developing countries where the combination of rural society, crowding, and poor sanitation allows greater contact between humans and pigs and thus more opportunities for fecal contamination of food and water [1, 2].

Normally, humans are the definitive hosts for *T. solium*, the life cycle of which begins with ingestion of viable larvae in inadequately cooked pork. The cyst wall is destroyed by gastric secretion, releasing 1 scolex that passes into the small intestine, where it becomes fixed. Embryonated eggs and gravid proglottids are released in the feces, deposited on the soil, and later ingested by the intermediate host, the pig. Ingestion of unwashed green leafy vegetables like cabbage is also one of the sources of infection. The animal's gastric secretions destroy the egg wall, and after the passage into the duodenum, the larvae release from the eggs, penetrate the intestinal wall, and are carried by blood or lymph to various tissues. In the pig, the muscle tissue is particularly involved. Once in the muscle, the larvae develop into cysticerci [4]. The cystic structure contains a small, invaginated scolex and neck resembling the adult form. Ingestion of undercooked pork by humans once again initiates the parasitic cycle. If humans ingest eggs from adult tapeworm segments passed in human feces, they can become intermediate hosts. Humans can acquire the infection by ingesting water or food contaminated with human feces, by oral transmission via the hands of carriers of adult worms, or by internal regurgitation of eggs into the stomach after reverse peristalsis. The clinical course of cysticercosis depends on the number of cysts, the particular tissue infected, and the reaction of tissues to the organism [3]. The larvae may migrate to any organ and may remain viable for many years [4]. The organism most

TABLE 1

	Author/year	Muscles affected	No. of cases
(1)	Reddi et al. [5]/2001	Masseter	1
(2)	Sidhu et al. [6]/2002	Masseter	1
(3)	Sethi et al. [7]/2007	Temporalis	1
(4)	Mittal et al. [8]/2008	Masseter	1
(5)	Gokarn et al. [9]/2011	Masseter	1
(6)	Kumar et al. [10]/2011	Temporalis	1
(7)	Kumar et al. [11]/2011	Masseter	1
(8)	Present cases	Temporalis	2

often invades the central nervous system, eye, subcutaneous tissue, skeletal muscle, and heart, but occasionally the lungs, liver, and kidneys may be affected. Skeletal involvement may cause transient tenderness and either muscular atrophy or hypertrophy [3].

The literature review of the cases involving cysticercosis affecting muscles of mastication shows just two reports of cysticercosis affecting temporalis muscle and 5 case reports affecting the masseter muscle (Table 1).

All the cases presented with muscle tenderness and swelling similar to our cases. Diagnostic tests include radiologic imaging (particularly computerized tomography and MRI), serology, and tissue biopsy. Medical treatment with Albendazole and praziquantel ($50\,\mathrm{mg{\cdot}kg^{-1}{\cdot}d^{-1}}$ in 3 divided doses for 14 days and $75\,\mathrm{mg{\cdot}kg^{-1}{\cdot}d^{-1}}$ for 10 days) has been recommended for neurocysticercosis and subcutaneous cysticercosis [8]; however, praziquantel has no effect on calcified parasites. Preventive measures are important and include the thorough cooking of pork and all vegetables and early detection and complete removal of the worm.

Conflict of Interests

There are no financial or other relations that could lead to a conflict of interests.

References

[1] A. C. Chandler, *Introduction to Parasitology*, John Wiley & Sons, New York, NY, USA, 1958.

[2] G. Timosca and L. Gavrilita, "Cysticercosis of the maxillofacial region. A clinicopathologic study of five cases," *Oral Surgery, Oral Medicine and Oral Pathology*, vol. 37, no. 3, pp. 390–400, 1974.

[3] J. Kinnman, C. H. Chi, and J. H. Park, "Cysticercosis in otolaryngology," *Archives of Otolaryngology*, vol. 102, no. 3, pp. 144–147, 1976.

[4] E. H. Tschen, E. A. Tschen, and E. B. Smith, "Cutaneous cysticercosis treated with metrifonate," *Archives of Dermatology*, vol. 117, no. 8, pp. 507–509, 1981.

[5] S. P. Reddi, M. J. Morales, and R. R. Addante, "Solitary lesion in the masseter muscle," *Journal of Oral and Maxillofacial Surgery*, vol. 59, no. 1, pp. 71–75, 2001.

[6] R. Sidhu, R. Nada, A. Palta, H. Mohan, and S. Suri, "Maxillofacial cysticercosis: uncommon appearance of a common disease," *Journal of Ultrasound in Medicine*, vol. 21, no. 2, pp. 199–202, 2002.

[7] P. K. Sethi, N. K. Sethi, J. Torgovnick, and E. Arsura, "Cysticercosis of temporalis muscle: an unusual cause of temporal headaches. A case report," *Journal of Headache and Pain*, vol. 8, no. 5, pp. 315–316, 2007.

[8] A. Mittal, D. Das, N. Iyer, J. Nagaraj, and M. Gupta, "Masseter cysticercosis—a rare case diagnosed on ultrasound," *Dentomaxillofacial Radiology*, vol. 37, no. 2, pp. 113–116, 2008.

[9] A. Gokarn, S. Gokarn, and V. Rathod, "Ultrasonography for masseter muscle cysticercosis," *Indian pediatrics*, vol. 48, no. 2, pp. 141–143, 2011.

[10] V. Kumar, A. Gulati, and B. Mehra, "Cysticercosis of the temporalis muscle causing temporal headache in a pregnant woman," *International Journal of Gynecology and Obstetrics*, vol. 114, no. 1, p. 79, 2011.

[11] B. D. Kumar, B. Dave, and S. M. Meghana, "Cysticercosis of masseter," *Indian Journal of Dental Research*, vol. 22, no. 4, p. 617, 2011.

27

Replacement of Missing Anterior Teeth in a Patient with Chronic Mouth Breathing and Tongue Thrusting

Satheesh B. Haralur and Ali Saad Al-Qahtani

Department of Prosthodontics, College of Dentistry, King Khalid University, Abha 61417, Saudi Arabia

Correspondence should be addressed to Satheesh B. Haralur; hb_satheesh@yahoo.com

Academic Editors: M. A. Compagnoni, R. V. Lo Vasco, and K. Michalakis

The loss of anterior teeth has serious functional, esthetic disabilities, in addition to compromising the patients' quality of life. Various etiologies can be attributed to the anterior tooth loss, including trauma, caries, and periodontal diseases. The chronic mouth breathing due to nasal adenoids is known to enhance the gingival and periodontal diseases. The dental literature proves the association of nasal breathing, tongue thrusting, and anterior open bite. Arch shape and tooth position are primarily determined by the equilibrium of the forces from tongue and perioral musculature. Increased force from tongue musculature in the tongue thrusting patient leads to flaring of anterior teeth, making them susceptible for periodontal and traumatic tooth loss. Replacement of the anterior teeth in this patient will also help in restoration of anterior guidance, which is critical for the health of temporomandibular joint, posterior teeth, and musculature.

1. Introduction

Loss of anterior teeth has major detrimental social implications for the sufferer and significantly affects the normal social integration. Loss of anterior teeth is from multifactorial origin ranging from trauma, periodontal disease, dental caries, and persisting oral habits. If preventive treatment is not provided at an early age, they continue to persist up to adult age. Potential detrimental effects and management of these persisting oral habits are often overlooked by the oral health professionals. The excessive lymphoid tissue proliferation with chronic allergy and infection lead to obstruction of the nasal airway, resulting in chronic mouth breathing [1]. Studies have shown the strong correlation between mouth breathing as an etiological factor for tongue thrusting and anterior dental open bite [2]. The long existing malocclusion leads to having the tongue filling the space and results in loss of lip and muscle tonus. The disturbed balance between the force of the tongue and oral musculature leads to anterior migration of teeth. The exposed, flared teeth are highly susceptible for traumatic damage. The mouth breathing is also considered as one of the predisposing factors for initiation of periodontal disease [3, 4]. The chronic mouth breathing patient with high incidence of periodontal disease tend to lose the anterior teeth in their early age. Anterior dental open bite and loss of anterior teeth impede the emission of dental-alveolar sounds [5, 6]. The absence of anterior guidance prolongs the disocclusion time and predisposes the patients for temporomandibular disorders [7]. There is a paucity of dental literature regarding the effect of chronic mouth breathing and tongue thrusting and its prosthetic management. The well designed prosthesis can completely rehabilitate the aesthetic, functional, and phonetic debilitation. The objective of this case report is to explain the clinical prosthetic rehabilitation of the chronic mouth breathing and tongue thrusting patients with loss of maxillary and mandibular anterior teeth.

2. Case Presentation

A 35-year-old male patient visited the King Khalid University dental clinic for the replacement of both maxillary and mandibular anterior missing teeth. The patient was extremely unhappy with existing transitional, removable partial denture due to its poor stability, especially during speech

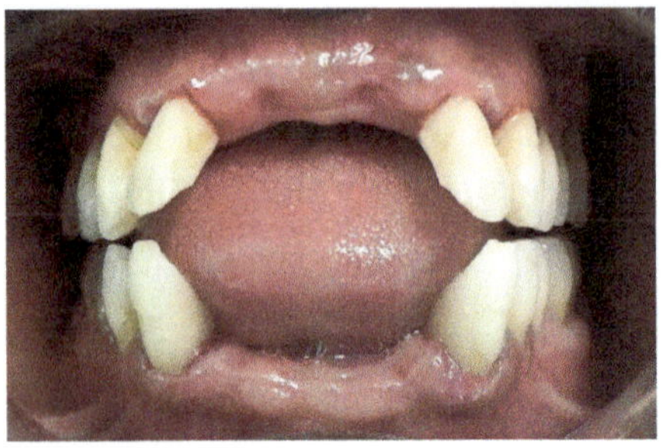

FIGURE 1: Patient presenting with loss and flaring of teeth and tongue occupying the space.

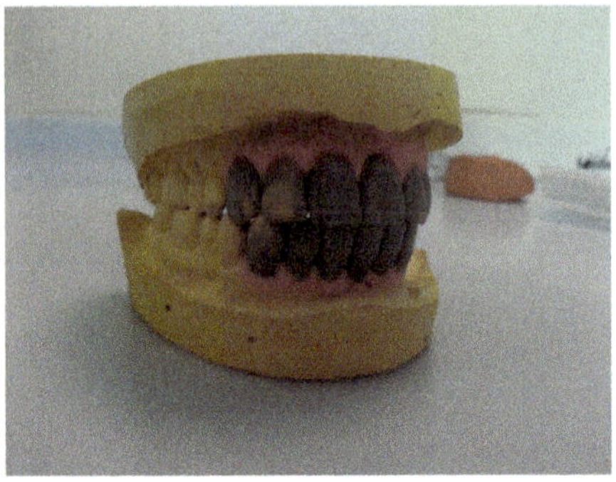

FIGURE 2: Diagnostic wax up of the diagnostic cast.

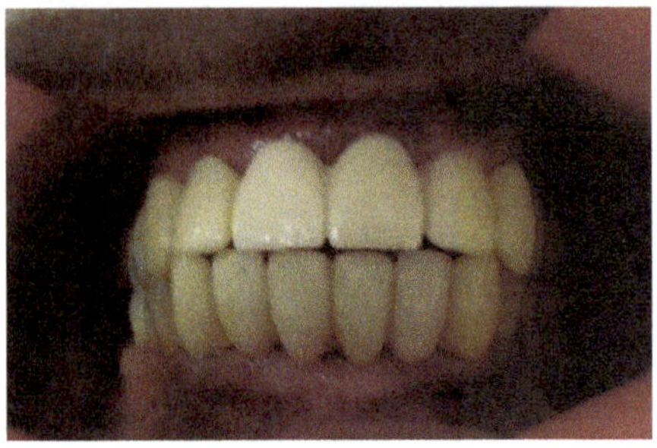

FIGURE 3: Refined and finalized provisional restoration.

and mastication. He gave a history of teeth extraction six months before due to mobility. He also reported on chronic mouth breathing due to enlarged adenoids and blocked nasal breathing, which was surgically treated a year back. The patient gave a graphic history of continued, progressive labial flaring of anterior teeth that subsequently became mobile to be extracted. On examination, it was observed that the patient had lost both maxillary central incisors and all four mandibular incisors (Figure 1). The adjacent maxillary lateral incisors showed slight labial flaring and grade 1 mobility; intraoral periapical X-ray confirmed approximately 20–25% alveolar bone loss. Routine TMJ examination showed no signs of pathology. The patency of nasal airways were checked by requesting to close the lip together and occluding one naris with the index finger alternatively. Ask the patient to breathe normally through open naris. The tongue movements were within normal limits. The evaluation of swallowing process without the removable prosthesis showed slight space between posterior teeth and minor hyperactivity of orbicularis oris and mentalis muscles. On complete evaluation of clinical signs symptoms along with clinical examination, it was diagnosed as loss of maxillary and mandibular anterior teeth due to combined effect of periodontal diseases, chronic mouth breathing, and tongue thrusting.

The treatment objectives were to replace the missing maxillary and mandibular central incisors along with rehabilitation of tongue thrusting habit. Treatment options to replace the missing anterior teeth was discussed with the patient, including the implant supported fixed prosthesis. The tooth that supported conventional fixed partial denture was selected according to the patient desire. The potential abutments were evaluated by the clinical and radiological examination to ascertain periodontal and pulpal health. The intentional root canal treatment was performed on maxillary right lateral incisors to gain common path of insertion. The bilateral canines and lateral incisors were the abutment for maxillary central incisors, while bilateral canines were selected as abutments for mandibular incisors [8]. The absence of gross soft or bony defect in the corresponding residual ridge of missing teeth was also favorable for tooth that supported fixed partial denture.

The diagnostic casts were made from irreversible hydrocolloid impression materials, with the help of face bow records mounted on a semiadjustable articulator. The existing removable denture had more teeth to compensate the slightly larger residual ridge space. To ascertain the esthetic outcome and patient response, the diagnostic wax up for the missing teeth structure was done (Figure 2). To obtain the acceptable esthetic proportion between the teeth, it was decided to distribute the excess edentulous area between abutment and pontics.

The autopolymerized acrylic denture base for the edentulous area was fabricated on dental cast; the modelling plastic compound was used to make the occlusal rim. The vertical height of the occlusal rims was adjusted according to the anatomic landmarks, visibility, and phonetics. The modelling plastic compound was softened and the patient was asked to perform all physiological muscle functions by sucking, swallowing, and phonetics. The recontoured modelling compound gave the exact tooth position and inclination according to the neutral zone [9].

Split putty indexing was made to guide the dental technician on the exact position and inclinations of pontics during fabrication of provisional restoration. The abutments were prepared for metal ceramic retainers; the definitive impression was made with heavy body-light body silicone impression materials. The poly ethyl methacrylate provisional fixed partial dentures were fabricated with indirect method. The provisional bridges were cemented with noneugenol temporary luting cement after minor correction for aesthetics, phonetics, and occlusion (Figure 3). The Patient was given an instruction to follow the tongue neuromuscular sensory stimuli by brushing and resistance to regain the desirable motor response [10]. The patient was recalled after 24 hours

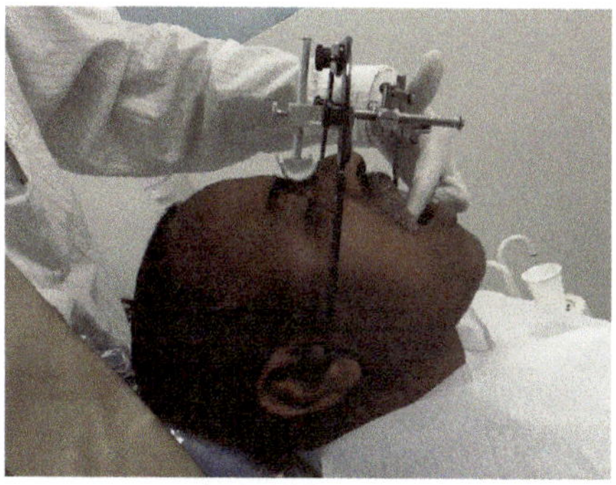

FIGURE 4: Face bow transfer for mounting working cast.

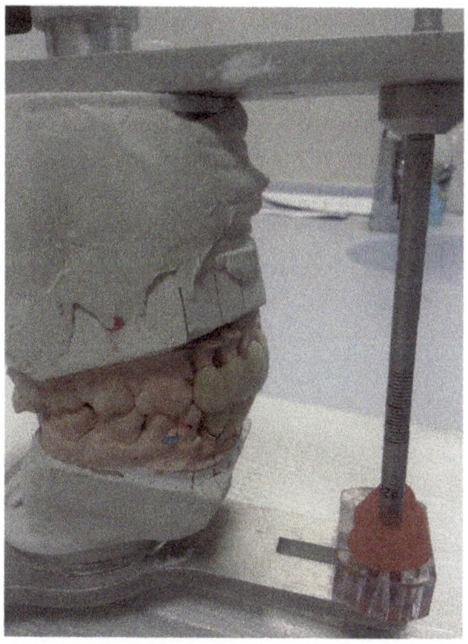

FIGURE 5: Customised incisal table.

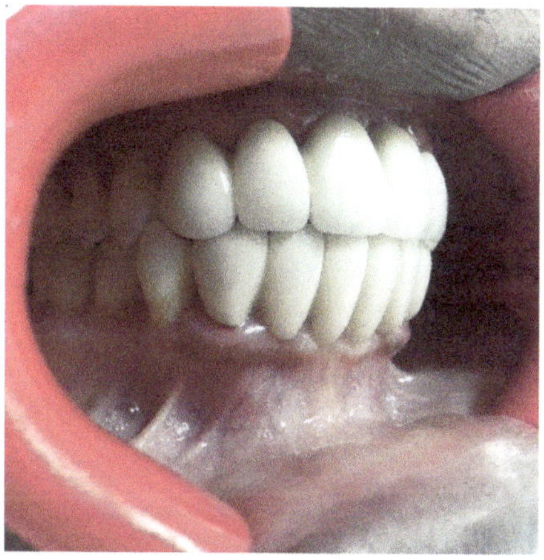

FIGURE 6: Final prosthesis.

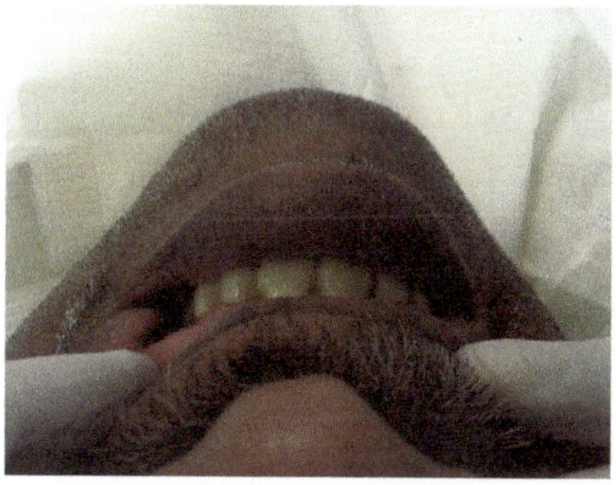

FIGURE 7: Establishment of proper lip position over the maxillary incisors.

to evaluate the patient opinion, gingival health, and comfort. The patient was given a scheduled appointment for six weeks to evaluate the overall satisfaction of esthetics, phonetics, and function. The continuous required minor adjustments were made to the provisional bridge during evaluation period. The provisional restorations with acceptable anterior guidance, esthetics, phonetics, and comfort were replicated to minute detail in permanent restoration.

The alginate impression with the cemented provisional restoration was made, and dental cast was mounted on the semiadjustable articulator with face bow transfer (Figure 4). The autopolymerized acrylic customized incisal guidance table was prepared on the semiadjustable articulator from the mounted casts (Figure 5). The customized incisal table enabled the dental technician to replicate the exact anterior guidance in the final restorations. The putty indexing of the provisional restorations was used to remake the labial contour, shape, and inclination in the final metal ceramic fixed partial denture. The final prosthesis was cemented with the glass-ionomer type-I luting cement after required occlusion refinements (Figures 6, 7, and 8).

The patient was recalled after one week to evaluate the residual cement, gingival health, and occlusal integrity. The patient was monitored during the first three months with a two-week-interval, followed by a month intervening three months. The patient showed a remarkable improvement in speech and controlling the tongue thrusting. He was highly satisfied with the aesthetic outcome of the prosthesis.

3. Discussion

The loss of anterior teeth compromises the patient's quality of life, its replacement will help to restore the functions of mastication, speech, and aesthetics. Evaluation of the history and disease course to understand the reason for tooth loss is vital to treatment outcome. Upper airway obstruction that lead chronic mouth-breathing may cause anterior open bite. The studies reported the existence of the strong association between chronic mouth breathing, dental anterior open bite, and tongue thrusting [10, 11]. Though some researchers believe the tongue merely occupies the space created by the malocclusion [12]. The studies have also reported that the tongue thrust leads to significant increase in maxillary anterior teeth proclination [13]. The increased incidence of gingival inflammation and periodontitis is observed in the chronic mouth breather, hastening tooth loss [3, 4, 14, 15]. The associated lip incompetency creates significant imbalance in

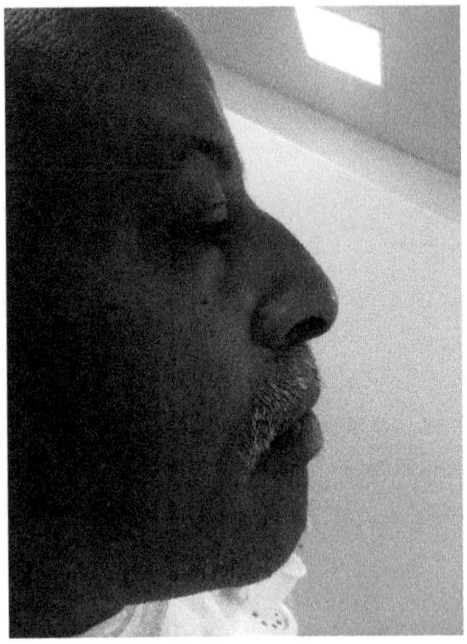

FIGURE 8: Reestablished lip support and lip competency.

force between the tongue and perioral musculature, resulting in progressive flaring of incisors [16]. The prosthetic rehabilitation should carefully consider all the involved factors to address them individually.

Persistent tongue thrusting lead to failure of orthodontics, malocclusion, and instable removable prosthesis. The replacement of the teeth in the neutral zone will help in stabilizing the tooth position and restore proper lip support. It will also help in eliminating the detrimental lateral force from tongue musculature on the supporting abutment [17, 18]. The neutral zone determination is followed mainly in poorly supported complete denture fabrication. It is important to reestablish the tooth position in neutral zone during simultaneous replacement of maxillary and mandibular incisors in a patient with tongue thrusting. The reestablishment of incisor vertical overlap help to restore the missing anterior guidance. The research has shown that the optimum anterior guidance is vital for the health of both posterior teeth and temporomandibular joint [7, 19]. The replacement of missing anterior teeth morphological characteristics and their relation to oral structure are also important for rehabilitation of phonetics. The quality of the prosthesis, especially the reduced stability, can compromise the speech production; prolonged use of improper prosthesis harm the adjustment to the new prosthesis [20]. The tongue dysfunction habits are required to be treated for the long term positive prognosis of the prosthesis [21]. The tongue is remarkable in its ability to adapt to changes in the surroundings; the neuromuscular facilitation stimulation enable the faster tongue adaptation. Brushing and pressure application act as sensory stimuli to reduce the flaccidity of the tongue. The well designed prosthesis and meticulous followup care will completely rehabilitate patients with tongue thrusting with anterior tooth loss.

Conflict of Interests

The authors declare that there is no conflict of interests regarding the publication of this paper.

References

[1] W. G. Watson, "Open-bite-A multifactorial event," *American Journal of Orthodontics*, vol. 80, no. 4, pp. 443–446, 1981.

[2] G. M. Greenlee, G. J. Huang, S. S.-H. Chen, J. Chen, T. Koepsell, and P. Hujoel, "Stability of treatment for anterior open-bite malocclusion: a meta-analysis," *American Journal of Orthodontics and Dentofacial Orthopedics*, vol. 139, no. 2, pp. 154–169, 2011.

[3] B. M. Pennel and J. G. Keagle, "Predisposing factors in the etiology of chronic inflammatory periodontal disease," *Journal of Periodontology*, vol. 48, no. 9, pp. 517–532, 1977.

[4] N. E. Ahmad, A. E. Sanders, R. Sheats et al., "Obstructive sleep apnea in association with periodontitis: a case-control study," *Journal of Dentistry and Oral Hygiene*, vol. 87, no. 4, pp. 188–199, 2013.

[5] H. Tanaka, "Speech patterns of edentulous patients and morphology of the palate in relation to phonetics," *The Journal of Prosthetic Dentistry*, vol. 29, no. 1, pp. 16–28, 1973.

[6] K. M. Sansone, H. N. Filho, G. Berretin-Félix, and A. G. Brasolotto, "Oral myofunctional and vocal characteristics in subjects subjected to oral rehabilitation with osseointegrated implants," *Clinical Oral Implants Research*, vol. 17, no. 3, pp. 328–330, 2006.

[7] C. H. Schuyler, "The function and importance of incisal guidance in oral rehabilitation. 1963," *The Journal of Prosthetic Dentistry*, vol. 86, no. 3, pp. 219–232, 2001.

[8] M. Lulic, U. Brägger, N. P. Lang, M. Zwahlen, and G. E. Salvi, "Ante's (1926) law revisited: a systematic review on survival rates and complications of fixed dental prostheses (FDPs) on severely reduced periodontal tissue support," *Clinical Oral Implants Research*, vol. 18, supplement 3, pp. 63–72, 2007.

[9] V. E. Beresin and F. J. Schiesser, "A study of the importance of the neutral zone in complete dentures," *The Journal of Prosthetic Dentistry*, vol. 66, no. 5, p. 718, 1991.

[10] M. L. Falk, M. Wells, and S. Toth, "A subcortical approach to swallow pattern therapy," *American Journal of Orthodontics*, vol. 70, no. 4, pp. 419–427, 1976.

[11] A. S. Cayley, A. P. Tindall, W. J. Sampson, and A. R. Butcher, "Electropalatographic and cephalometric assessment of tongue function in open bite and non-open bite subjects," *European Journal of Orthodontics*, vol. 22, no. 5, pp. 463–474, 2000.

[12] B. Ingervall and R. Schmoker, "Effect of surgical reduction of the tongue on oral stereognosis, oral motor ability, and the rest position of the tongue and mandible," *American Journal of Orthodontics and Dentofacial Orthopedics*, vol. 97, no. 1, pp. 58–65, 1990.

[13] S. Alexander and P. Sudha, "Genioglossis muscle electrical activity and associated arch dimensional changes in simple tongue thrust swallow pattern," *Journal of Clinical Pediatric Dentistry*, vol. 21, no. 3, pp. 213–222, 1997.

[14] M. C. Haytac and I. A. Oz, "Atypical streptococcal infection of gingiva associated with chronic mouth breathing," *Quintessence International*, vol. 38, no. 10, pp. E577–E582, 2007.

[15] J. J. Keller, C.-S. Wu, Y.-H. Chen et al., "Association between obstructive sleep apnoea and chronic periodontitis: a

population-based study," *Journal of Clinical Periodontology*, vol. 40, no. 2, pp. 111–117, 2013.

[16] W. J. Straub, "Malfunction of the tongue. Part I. The abnormal swallowing habit: its cause, effects, and results in relation to orthodontic treatment and speech therapy," *American Journal of Orthodontics*, vol. 46, no. 6, pp. 404–424, 1960.

[17] P. Kursoglu, N. Ari, and S. Calikkocaoglu, "Using tissue conditioner material in neutral zone technique," *The New York State Dental Journal*, vol. 73, no. 1, pp. 40–42, 2007.

[18] V. E. Beresin and F. J. Schiesser, "The neutral zone in complete dentures. 1976," *The Journal of Prosthetic Dentistry*, vol. 95, no. 2, pp. 93–101, 2006.

[19] E. H. Williamson and D. O. Lundquist, "Anterior guidance: its effect on electromyographic activity of the temporal and masseter muscles," *The Journal of Prosthetic Dentistry*, vol. 49, no. 6, pp. 816–823, 1983.

[20] L. Molly, O. Nackaerts, K. Vandewiele, E. Manders, D. Van Steenberghe, and R. Jacobs, "Speech adaptation after treatment of full edentulism through immediate-loaded implant protocols," *Clinical Oral Implants Research*, vol. 19, no. 1, pp. 86–90, 2008.

[21] C.-F. Cheng, C.-L. Peng, H.-Y. Chiou, and C.-Y. Tsai, "Dentofacial morphology and tongue function during swallowing," *American Journal of Orthodontics and Dentofacial Orthopedics*, vol. 122, no. 5, pp. 491–499, 2002.

28

Periodontal Plastic Microsurgery in the Treatment of Deep Gingival Recession after Orthodontic Movement

Sérgio Kahn,[1] Walmir Júnio de Pinho Reis Rodrigues,[2] and Marcos de Oliveira Barceleiro[3]

[1] *Department of Periodontics, Veiga de Almeida University (UVA), Rua Ibituruna 108, Tijuca, 20271-021 Rio de Janeiro, RJ, Brazil*
[2] *School of Dentistry, Serra dos Órgãos University Center (UNIFESO), Avenida Alberto Torres 111, Alto, 25964-004 Teresópolis, RJ, Brazil*
[3] *Department of Dentistry, School of Dentistry, Fluminense Federal University (UFF), Rua Silvio Henrique Braune 22, Centro, 28625-650 Nova Friburgo, RJ, Brazil*

Correspondence should be addressed to Sérgio Kahn; sergiokahn@terra.com.br

Academic Editors: A. I. Abdalla, B. T. Amaechi, and K. H. Zawawi

Gingival recession is a condition that affects a large portion of the young and adult population and negatively affects the aesthetic aspects of the smile. Many factors are related to its development, including orthodontic movement beyond the osseous limits. Many treatment options have been proposed to cover the exposed root surface. The aim of this article was to describe three cases where a subepithelial connective tissue graft was performed, using a microsurgical technique, in the treatment of deep gingival recession after orthodontic treatment. This technique resulted in successful root coverage and keratinized tissue gain, improving the gingival esthetic pattern.

1. Introduction

Gingival recession can be defined as the location of marginal periodontal tissues apical to the cementoenamel junction [1]. This condition is prevalent in the young and adult populations [2]. The prevalence, extension, and severity of gingival recession have been observed to increase with age, affecting 79% of adults >40 years old in a representative sample of the Brazilian population [3]. It occurs in patients with either good or poor oral hygiene [4] and has multiple etiological factors [5] like traumatic tooth brushing [6], dehiscence, smoking, biological width invasion, inflammation, occlusal trauma, piercings [7], and orthodontic movement.

Although controversial, the scientific evidence demonstrates that gingival recession can develop in patients who undergo orthodontic movement [8, 9]. Furthermore, some studies have confirmed a positive correlation between the increase of severity and extension of gingival recession and orthodontic treatment [10].

The main factors related to the occurrence of gingival recession related to orthodontic movement are tooth movement beyond the osseous limits of the alveolar process and excessive tooth proclination during treatment, especially in adult patients [11, 12].

Thin gingival biotypes and the gingival inflammation associated with biofilm were observed as the risk factors for the development of gingival recession associated with orthodontic treatment [13].

There are several options for the treatment of gingival recession, including the free gingival graft [14], the sliding flap [15], the double pedicle flap [16], the subepithelial connective tissue graft [17], the enamel matrix derivative, the acellular dermal matrix, and growth factors [18–20].

The scientific evidence shows that the subepithelial connective tissue graft promotes higher levels of root coverage, high predictability and provides more gingival thickness [18–20].

As new techniques and materials are developed, new surgical approaches are necessary to minimize the surgical trauma and overcome the limitations related to the manual ability and natural vision of the surgeons. The incorporation of a surgical microscope to periodontal plastic surgery provides better illumination and adequate magnification to

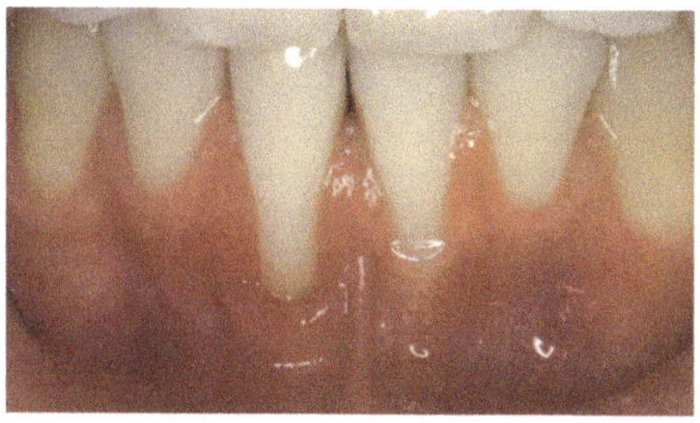

FIGURE 1: Initial aspect of patient 1 showing Miller Class III localized gingival recessions at the mandibular central incisors.

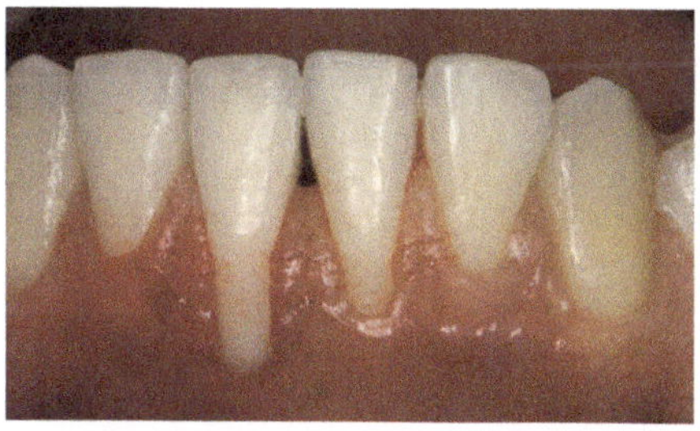

FIGURE 2: First and second incisions.

increase the precision of a surgeon's surgical skill. Thus, minimally invasive techniques were developed to minimize tissue trauma and allow primary wound closure [21–23].

The aim of this study is to report three cases where a subepithelial connective tissue graft was performed using a microsurgical approach to treat deep gingival recession after orthodontic treatment.

2. Case Reports

Three patients from a private dental clinic with aesthetic complaints related to deep gingival recession were included in this report. All patients were healthy and nonsmokers and signed an informed consent. The details about each patient are described as follows.

Patient 1: 27-year-old white female, having previous orthodontic treatment over a period of 5 years, presenting with a thin gingival biotype [24] and Miller [25] Class III gingival recession at the mandibular central incisors (Figure 1).

Patient 2: 26-year-old white female, who started orthodontic treatment approximately 3 years earlier, presenting with a thick gingival biotype [24] and Miller [25] Class III gingival recession at the left mandibular central incisor (Figure 10).

Patient 3: 26-year-old white male, who started orthodontic treatment approximately 2 years earlier, presenting with a thin gingival biotype [24] and Miller [25] Class II gingival recession at the right mandibular central incisor (Figure 17).

2.1. Initial Therapy. All patients were submitted to a plaque control program, which included oral hygiene instructions, scaling and root planning using an ultrasonic device, and crown polishing.

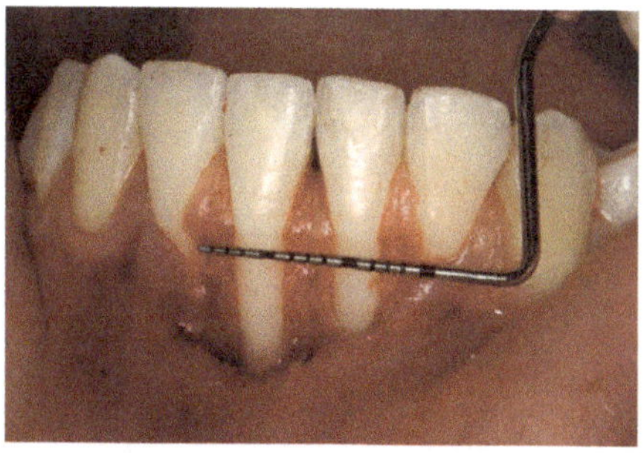

FIGURE 3: Measurement of recipient site after performing a partial thickness flap.

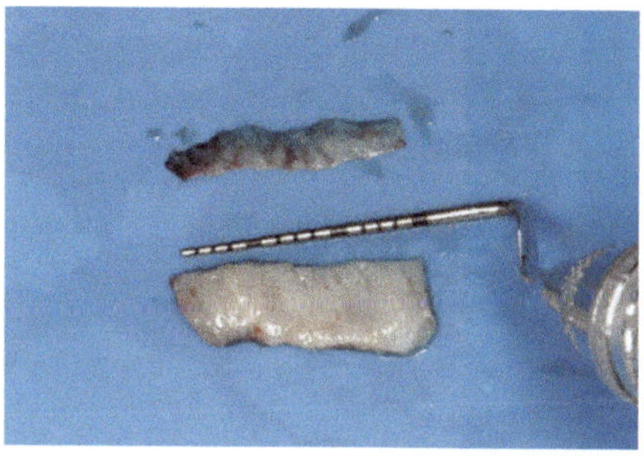

FIGURE 4: Connective tissue graft after the removal of the epithelium.

2.2. Surgical Therapy. All surgical procedures were performed by a single operator. A single 8 mg dose of dexamethasone was given to each patient one hour before surgery. Extraoral antisepsis was performed with a degerming agent and intraoral antisepsis was performed with a 0.12% chlorhexidine rinse. Mepivacaine (2.0%) with 1:100.000 epinephrine was used as an anesthetic solution.

All cases were performed using the microsurgical approach for root coverage, as described by De Campos et al. [22]. Initially, the exposed root surface was planned with a McCall 13/14 curette, followed by finishing burs. Citric acid gel (pH 1) was applied for 3 minutes. The surface was then washed for 45 seconds with a physiologic solution.

Both papillae adjacent to the recession were incised at buccal aspect. The first papillary incisions were horizontal at the level of the cementoenamel junction. The second papillary incisions were oblique and made at an apical level from those previously performed (Figures 2, 11 and 18). A third intrasulcular incision was performed to connect the papillary incisions. A partial thickness flap was performed from the second incision, allowing the removal of the gingival epithelium between the two incisions using Castroviejo scissors.

The recipient site was measured (Figure 3) using a periodontal probe and these measurements were transferred to the donor site. A palatal connective tissue graft was harvested from the area distal to the canine and anterior to the mesial aspect of the first molar on the same side of the surgery. The epithelium at the graft was removed (Figures 4 and 12).

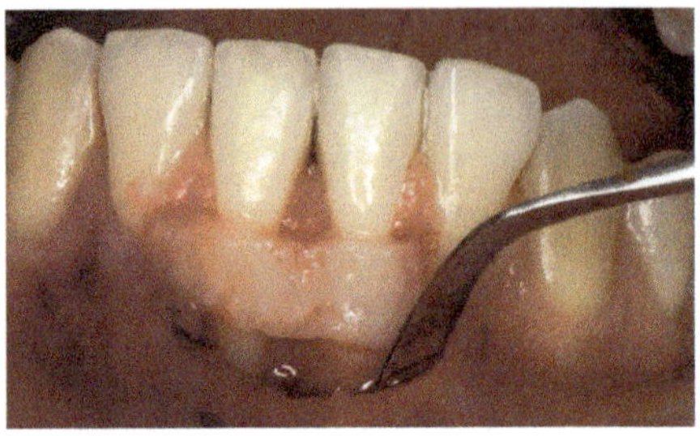

FIGURE 5: Graft stabilization at recipient site.

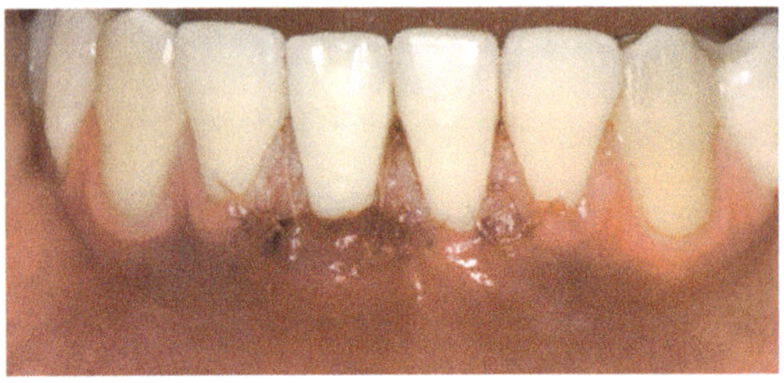

FIGURE 6: Microsutures.

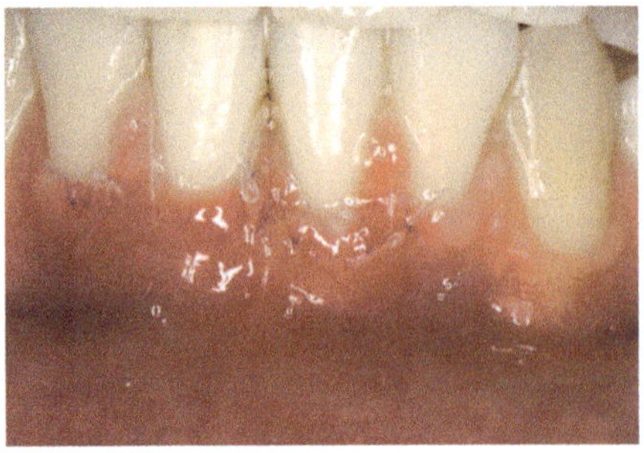

FIGURE 7: Seven-day follow-up of recipient site.

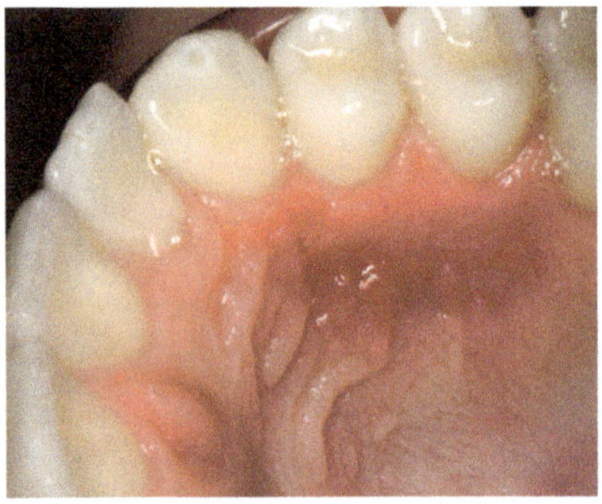

FIGURE 8: Seven-day follow-up of donor site.

After stabilizing the graft in the correct position (Figures 5, 13, and 19) using 6-0 vicryl sutures, the microsutures for flap approximation and coaptation were performed using 6-0 and 8-0 vicryl sutures, respectively (Figures 6, 14, and 20). The palate was then sutured with a continuous basting suture using a 4-0 silk thread. A thin layer of periodontal dressing was applied at both surgical sites.

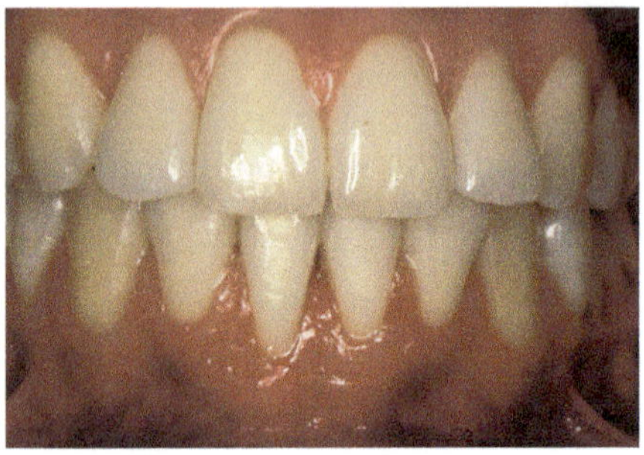

FIGURE 9: Thirty-day follow-up.

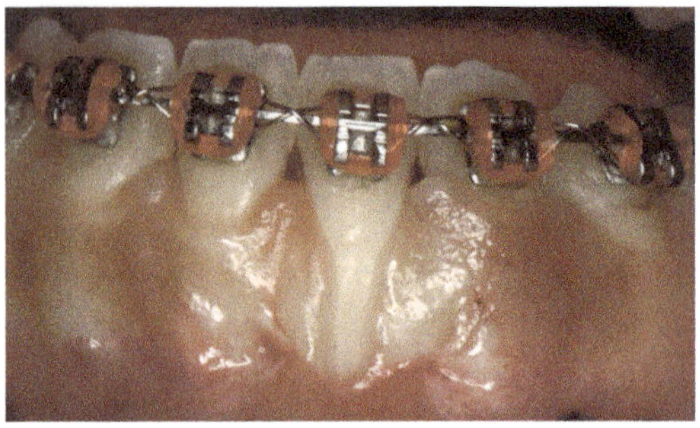

FIGURE 10: Initial aspect of patient 2 showing Miller class III localized gingival recession at the mandibular central left incisor.

2.3. Postoperative Care. The patients were instructed to use Amoxicillin 500 mg t.i.d. for 7 days, Dexamethasone 4 mg b.i.d. in the first 24 hours and sodium dipyrone 1 g q.i.d. in the first 48 h. Furthermore, tooth brushing was discontinued around the surgical sites for three weeks and plaque control was provided by rinsing with a 0.12% chlorhexidine solution twice a day. After this period, the patients were instructed to use a unituft brush to clean the site. After 7 days, the periodontal dressing and sutures were removed (Figures 7, 8, and 15) and the patients were called for follow-up visits (Figures 9 and 16). During the follow-up visits, Patient 3 presented with incomplete root coverage after the initial surgical procedure. A second surgical procedure was performed to provide complete root coverage (Figures 21, 22, 23, and 24).

3. Discussion

Orthodontic movement is one of the important factors in the development of gingival recession. However, the scientific evidence related to this topic is scarce and controversial, since many studies use a limited sample and lack well-established evaluation criteria [11].

The results of several studies have demonstrated a higher prevalence and severity of gingival recession after orthodontic treatment. Nevertheless, some authors have observed that gingival recession related to orthodontic treatment affects a small portion of patients, and although there was an increase in severity, it did not result in severe clinical consequences [8, 10, 13].

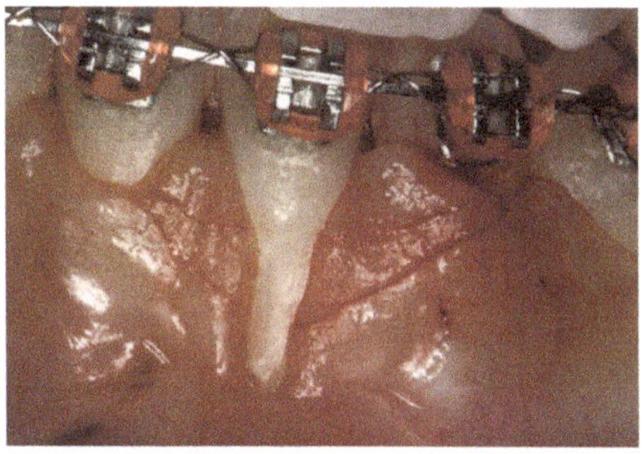

FIGURE 11: First and second incisions.

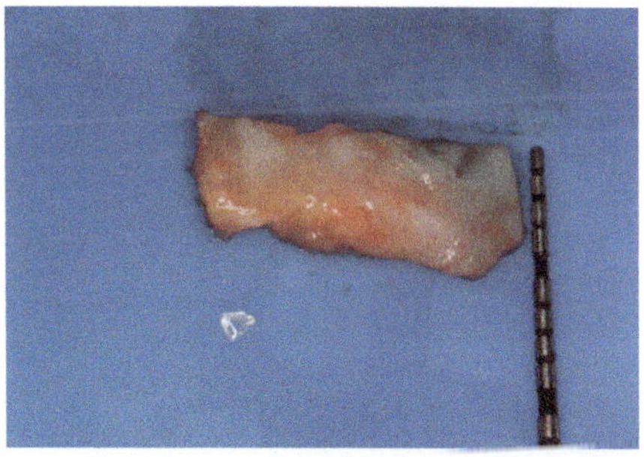

FIGURE 12: Connective tissue graft after the removal of the epithelium.

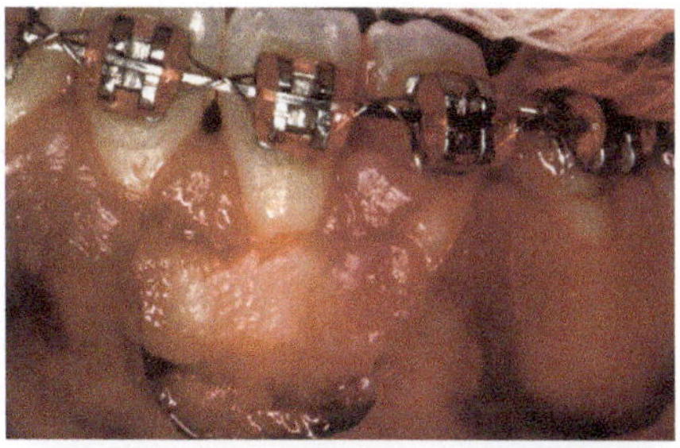

FIGURE 13: Graft stabilization at recipient site.

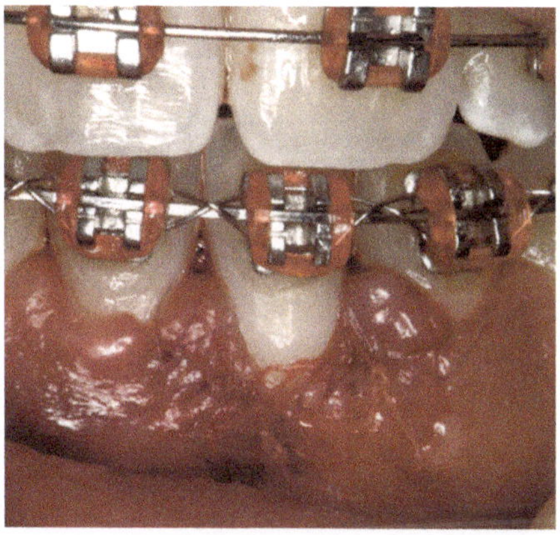

FIGURE 14: Microsutures.

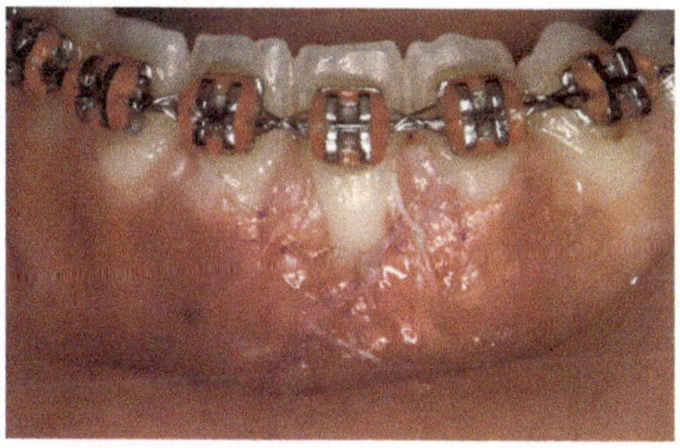

FIGURE 15: Seven-day follow-up of recipient site.

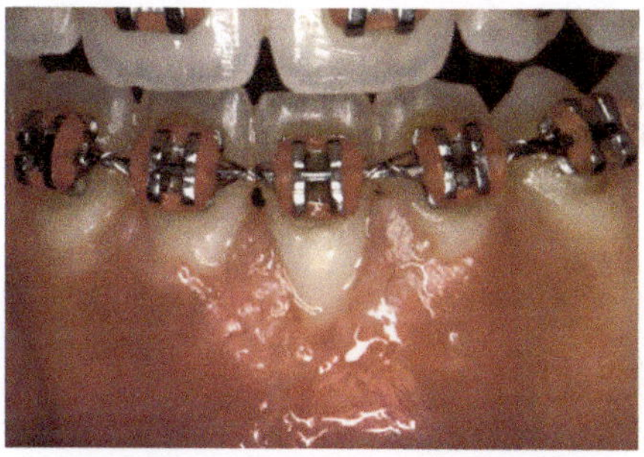

FIGURE 16: Thirty-day follow-up.

It was observed that the proclination of incisors is related to the development of recession [11, 12]. However, Vasconcelos et al. [9] found that retroclination was also related to an increase in the severity of gingival recession. On the other hand, Djeu et al. [26] did not find a correlation between the proclination of mandibular central incisors and gingival recession.

With regards to gingival thickness, Yared et al. [12] observed that free gingival margins with a thickness <0.5 mm presented greater and more severe recession associated with mandibular central incisors. However, one study using a human sample found that the mean amount of initial keratinized gingiva did not predispose the mandibular incisors and canines to gingival recession [27]. An animal study found that central incisor sites submitted to gingival grafts showed less gingival recession and maintenance of gingival thickness after vestibular orthodontic movement [28].

Kao and Pasquinelli [24] classified the periodontal biotype as thin or thick. Thin biotypes present a thin underlying bone, characterized by bony dehiscence and fenestration, which reacts to insults and disease with gingival recession. The presence of a thin biotype was identified as a possible predictor of gingival recession in a study by Melsen and Allais [13]. The present study reported two cases, 1 and 3, which had thin biotypes, since a highly scalloped soft tissue and bony architecture and a minimal amount of attached gingiva were observed.

The surgical manipulation of thin gingival biotypes imposes some challenges for the surgeons, since there is a higher possibility of flap dilacerations and/or perforations, which can interfere in the final result of the surgical treatment. Thus, it is possible that the incorporation of microsurgical techniques using appropriate illumination and magnification for more precise flap elevation and sutures can lead to primary wound closure [21–23].

According to Miller's [25] classification, complete root coverage can be anticipated in Classes I and II, partial root

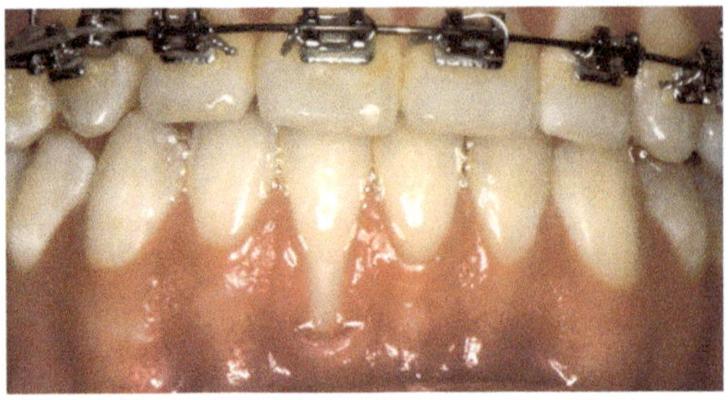

FIGURE 17: Initial aspect of patient 3 showing Miller Class II localized gingival recession at the mandibular central right incisor.

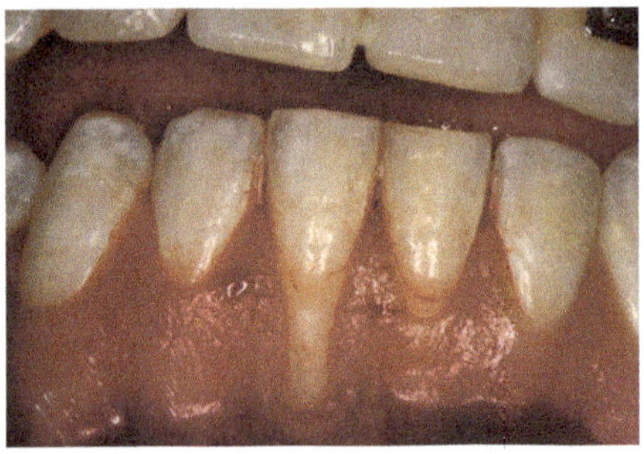

FIGURE 18: First and second incisions.

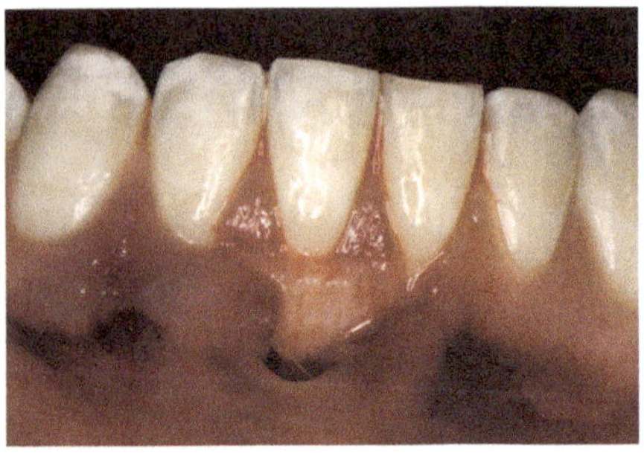

FIGURE 19: Graft stabilization at recipient site.

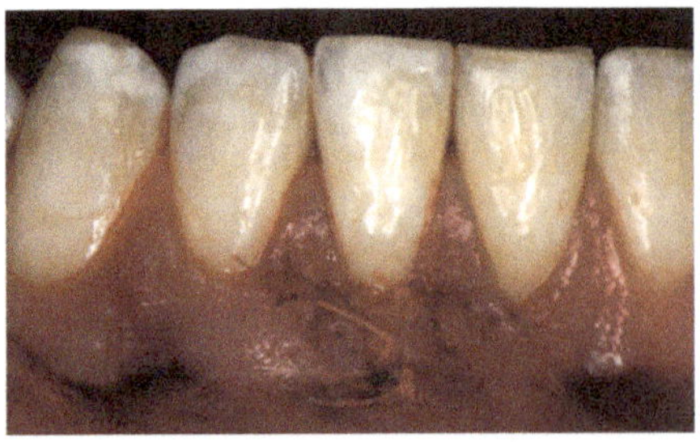

FIGURE 20: Microsutures.

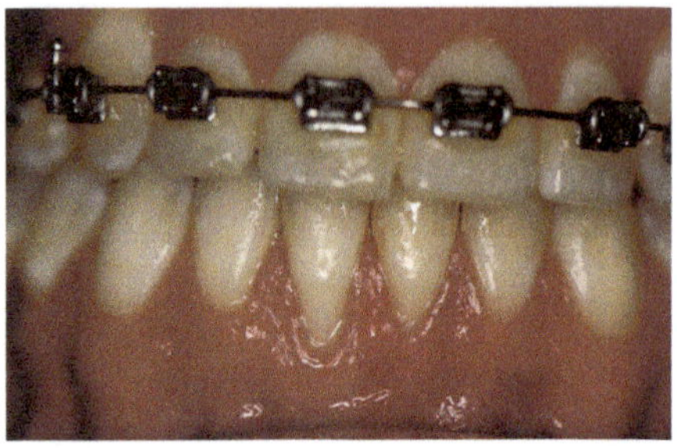

FIGURE 21: Follow-up visit. Patient 3 presented incomplete root coverage.

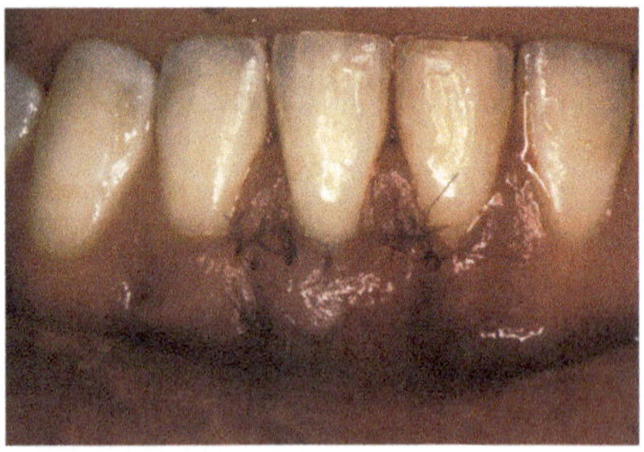

FIGURE 22: Second surgical procedure to achieve complete root coverage.

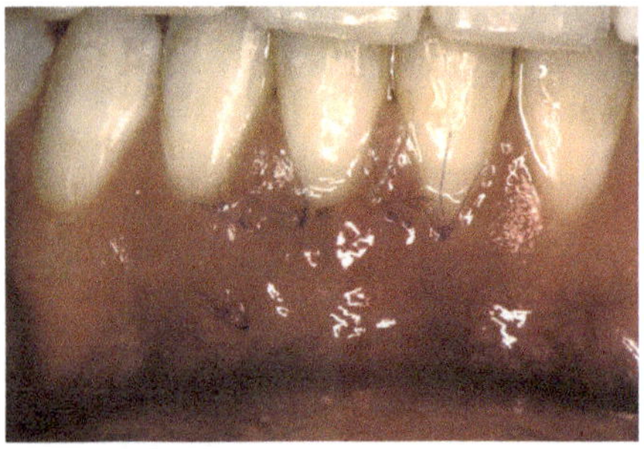

FIGURE 23: Seven-day follow-up of recipient site.

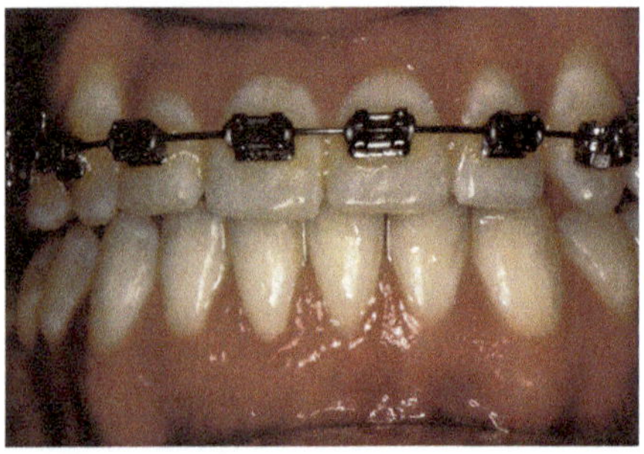

FIGURE 24: Thirty-day follow-up after the second intervention.

coverage is expected in Class III and root coverage is not anticipated in Class IV. The presented cases were classified as Class II or III, and satisfactory root coverage was achieved in all cases. Patient 3 had a Miller Class II recession and was submitted to a second surgical procedure, since complete root coverage was not achieved with the first procedure and the gingival margin remained disharmonious. The reasons for this fact can be related to the initial recession depth as well as to the quality of the soft and hard tissue [18].

Within the limits of this study, a subepithelial connective tissue graft using a microsurgical approach resulted in successful root coverage and increased keratinized tissue, improving the gingival esthetic pattern in cases where deep gingival recession was associated with orthodontic movement.

Conflict of Interests

The authors declare that there is no conflict of interests regarding the publication of this paper.

Funding

This study was self-supported by the authors.

References

[1] The American Academy of Periodontology, *Glossary of Periodontal Terms*, The American Academy of Periodontology, Chicago, Ill, USA, 2001.

[2] P. B. Raetzke, "Covering localized areas of root exposure employing the "envelope" technique," *Journal of Periodontology*, vol. 56, no. 7, pp. 397–402, 1985.

[3] C. Susin, A. N. Haas, R. V. Oppermann, O. Haugejorden, and J. M. Albandar, "Gingival recession: epidemiology and risk indicators in a representative urban Brazilian population," *Journal of Periodontology*, vol. 75, no. 10, pp. 1377–1386, 2004.

[4] H. Löe, A. Anerud, and H. Boysen, "The natural history of periodontal disease in man: prevalence, severity, and extent of gingival recession," *Journal of Periodontology*, vol. 63, no. 6, pp. 489–495, 1992.

[5] A. Borghetti and V. Monnet-Corti, *Chirurgie Plastique Parodontale*, Éditions CDP, Paris, France, 2000.

[6] P. S. Rajapakse, G. I. McCracken, E. Gwynnett, N. D. Steen, A. Guentsch, and P. A. Heasman, "Does tooth brushing influence the development and progression of non-inflammatory gingival recession? A systematic review," *Journal of Clinical Periodontology*, vol. 34, no. 12, pp. 1046–1061, 2007.

[7] A. Sardella, M. Pedrinazzi, C. Bez, G. Lodi, and A. Carrassi, "Labial piercing resulting in gingival recession. A case series," *Journal of Clinical Periodontology*, vol. 29, no. 10, pp. 961–963, 2002.

[8] L. Q. Closs, B. Grehs, D. B. Raveli, and C. K. Rösing, "Occurrence, extension, and severity of gingival margin alterations after orthodontic treatment," *World Journal of Orthodontics*, vol. 9, no. 3, pp. e1–e6, 2008.

[9] G. Vasconcelos, K. Kjellsen, H. Preus, V. Vandevska-Radunovic, and B. F. Hansen, "Prevalence and severity of vestibular recession in mandibular incisors after orthodontic treatment: a case-control retrospective study," *The Angle Orthodontist*, vol. 82, no. 1, pp. 42–47, 2012.

[10] S. Slutzkey and L. Levin, "Gingival recession in young adults: occurrence, severity, and relationship to past orthodontic treatment and oral piercing," *The American Journal of Orthodontics and Dentofacial Orthopedics*, vol. 134, no. 5, pp. 652–656, 2008.

[11] I. Joss-Vassalli, C. Grebenstein, N. Topouzelis, A. Sculean, and C. Katsaros, "Orthodontic therapy and gingival recession: a systematic review," *Orthodontics & Craniofacial Research*, vol. 13, no. 3, pp. 127–141, 2010.

[12] K. F. G. Yared, E. G. Zenobio, and W. Pacheco, "Periodontal status of mandibular central incisors after orthodontic proclination in adults," *The American Journal of Orthodontics and Dentofacial Orthopedics*, vol. 130, no. 1, pp. 6.e1–8.e1, 2006.

[13] B. Melsen and D. Allais, "Factors of importance for the development of dehiscences during labial movement of mandibular incisors: a retrospective study of adult orthodontic patients," *The American Journal of Orthodontics and Dentofacial Orthopedics*, vol. 127, no. 5, pp. 552–561, 2005.

[14] H. Björn, "Free transplantation of gingiva propria," *Swedish Dental Journal*, vol. 22, pp. 684–689, 1963.

[15] J. Grupe and R. Warren, "Repair of gingival defects by a sliding flap operation," *Journal of Periodontology*, vol. 27, no. 2, pp. 290–295, 1956.

[16] R. J. Harris, "The connective tissue and partial thickness double pedicle graft: a predictable method of obtaining root coverage," *Journal of Periodontology*, vol. 63, no. 5, pp. 477–486, 1992.

[17] B. Langer and L. J. Calagna, "The subepithelial connective tissue graft. A new approach to the enhancement of anterior cosmetics," *The International Journal of Periodontics & Restorative Dentistry*, vol. 2, no. 2, pp. 22–33, 1982.

[18] L. Chambrone, F. Sukekava, M. G. Araújo, F. E. Pustiglioni, L. A. Chambrone, and L. A. Lima, "Root-coverage procedures for the treatment of localized recession-type defects: a Cochrane systematic review," *Journal of Periodontology*, vol. 81, no. 4, pp. 452–478, 2010.

[19] T. W. Oates, M. Robinson, and J. C. Gunsolley, "Surgical therapies for the treatment of gingival recession. A systematic review," *Annals of Periodontology*, vol. 8, no. 1, pp. 303–320, 2003.

[20] M. Roccuzzo, M. Bunino, I. Needleman, and M. Sanz, "Periodontal plastic surgery for treatment of localized gingival recessions: a systematic review," *Journal of Clinical Periodontology*, vol. 29, supplement 3, pp. 178–194, 2002.

[21] J. M. Belcher, "A perspective on periodontal microsurgery," *The International Journal of Periodontics and Restorative Dentistry*, vol. 21, no. 2, pp. 191–196, 2001.

[22] G. V. de Campos, S. Bittencourt, A. W. Sallum, F. H. Nociti Júnior, E. A. Sallum, and M. Z. Casati, "Achieving primary closure and enhancing aesthetics with periodontal microsurgery," *Practical Procedures & Aesthetic Dentistry*, vol. 18, no. 7, pp. 449–454, 2006.

[23] D. A. Shanelec, "Periodontal microsurgery," *Journal of Esthetic and Restorative Dentistry*, vol. 15, no. 7, pp. 402–407, 2003.

[24] R. T. Kao and K. Pasquinelli, "Thick vs. thin gingival tissue: a key determinant in tissue response to disease and restorative treatment," *Journal of the California Dental Association*, vol. 30, no. 7, pp. 521–526, 2002.

[25] P. D. Miller Jr., "A classification of marginal tissue recession," *The International Journal of Periodontics & Restorative Dentistry*, vol. 5, no. 2, pp. 8–13, 1985.

[26] G. Djeu, C. Hayes, and S. Zawaideh, "Correlation between mandibular central incisor proclination and gingival recession during fixed appliance therapy," *The Angle Orthodontist*, vol. 72, no. 3, pp. 238–245, 2002.

[27] L. Q. Closs, P. Branco, S. D. Rizzatto, D. B. Raveli, and C. K. Rösing, "Gingival margin alterations and the pre-orthodontic treatment amount of keratinized gingiva," *Brazilian Oral Research*, vol. 21, no. 1, pp. 58–63, 2007.

[28] H. D. Holmes, M. Tennant, and M. S. Goonewardene, "Augmentation of faciolingual gingival dimensions with free connective tissue grafts before labial orthodontic tooth movement: an experimental study with a canine model," *The American Journal of Orthodontics and Dentofacial Orthopedics*, vol. 127, no. 5, pp. 562–572, 2005.

29

An Odontoma Found in the Wake of Maxillary Sinusitis Onset

Megumi Sotobori, Kohei Marukawa, Masatoshi Higuchi, Ryuichi Nakazawa, Akinori Moroi, Yuri Ishihara, Ran Iguchi, Akihiko Kosaka, Hiroumi Ikawa, and Koichiro Ueki

Division of Medicine, Department of Oral and Maxillofacial Surgery, Interdisciplinary Graduate School of Medicine and Engineering, University of Yamanashi, 1110 Shimokato Chuo, Chuo-shi, Yamanashi 409-3898, Japan

Correspondence should be addressed to Megumi Sotobori; msotobori@yamanashi.ac.jp

Academic Editors: A. I. Abdalla, A. C. B. Delbem, A. Kasaj, and A. Milosevic

Sinusitis of dental origin is a relatively frequent entity, and odontomas are considered to be the most common odontogenic tumors of the oral cavity. Eruption and infection of odontomas are extremely rare. Here, we report an interesting case where odontoma was found in the wake of the maxillary sinusitis onset.

1. Introduction

Although sinusitis of dental origin is a relatively frequent entity [1], maxillary dental infections, apical leakage, migration of a tooth or root during extraction, or the presence of ectopic tooth or cyst in the sinus can also cause sinusitis [2–4]. Reports relating to odontoma are few. A case of a large compound odontoma in the right maxillary sinus causing acute maxillary sinusitis is reported [5]. Griffith and Imperato [5] say that seven large antral odontomas were identified previously; however, none had typical findings of acute sinusitis.

On the other hand, the occurrence of complex odontomas is not considered to be rare in the jaws [6–11]. Most of them are asymptomatic and are discovered during routine radiographic investigations [6, 8, 10, 12]. Moreover, they are usually associated with disturbances of neighboring teeth eruption [12, 13]. Little has been reported on odontoma related to normal tooth germs instead of supernumerary tooth germs. So, we report a patient who had odontoma associated with the second permanent molar found in the wake of the onset of maxillary sinusitis.

2. Case Report

A 12-year-and-7-month-old female pediatric patient presented with suspicious left odontogenic maxillary sinusitis and no noteworthy personal history. She complained of persistent nasal congestion and tenderness in the left molars. As a disease history, she had pain and swelling of the left cervical lymph node for one month. Symptoms were improved by intravenous infusion of antibiotics by a pediatrician who pointed out the left maxillary sinusitis by CT imaging. On suspecting odontogenic maxillary sinusitis, the patient was referred to our hospital. There was no sign of eruption of the second upper left molar; however, there was tenderness in a considerable part of the gum. Normal X-ray of the skull showed an opaque image of teeth surrounding the impaction of the second molars in the upper left maxillary sinus area (Figure 1). Computed tomography revealed an opaque image of the maxillary sinus and thickening of the maxillary sinus mucosa (Figures 2 and 3). We performed resection of the lesion under general anesthesia. When peeling the mucoperiosteal flap, slight bulging and thinning of the buccal cortical bone were

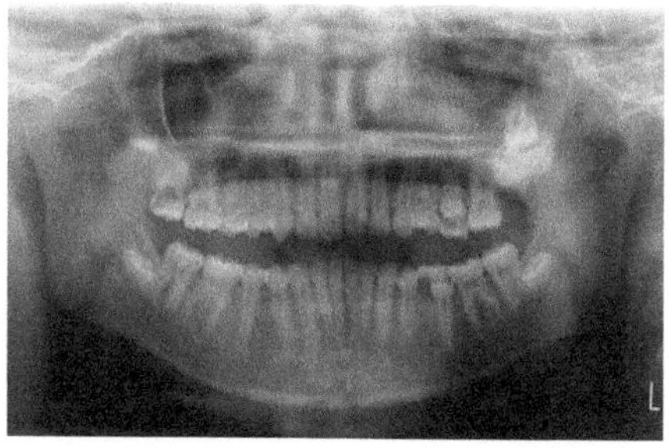

FIGURE 1: Initial panoramic radiograph.

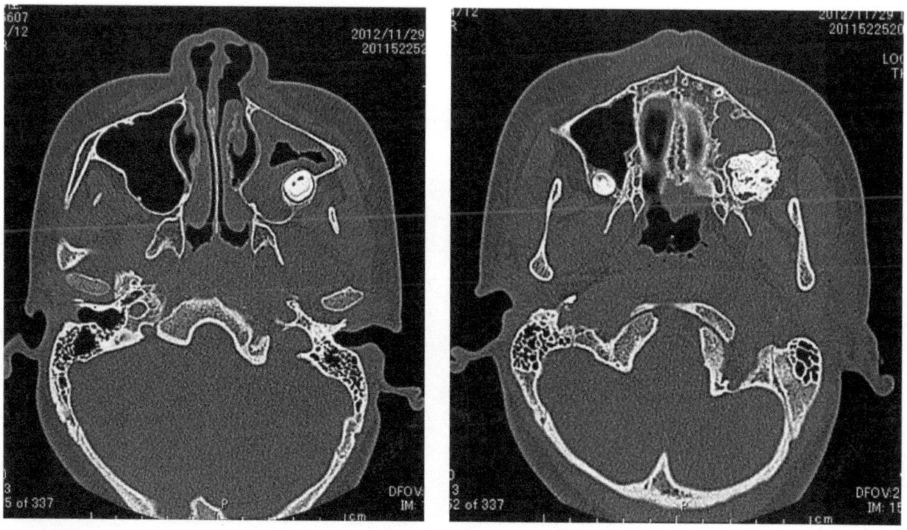

(a) (b)

FIGURE 2: Axial CT view of the lesion.

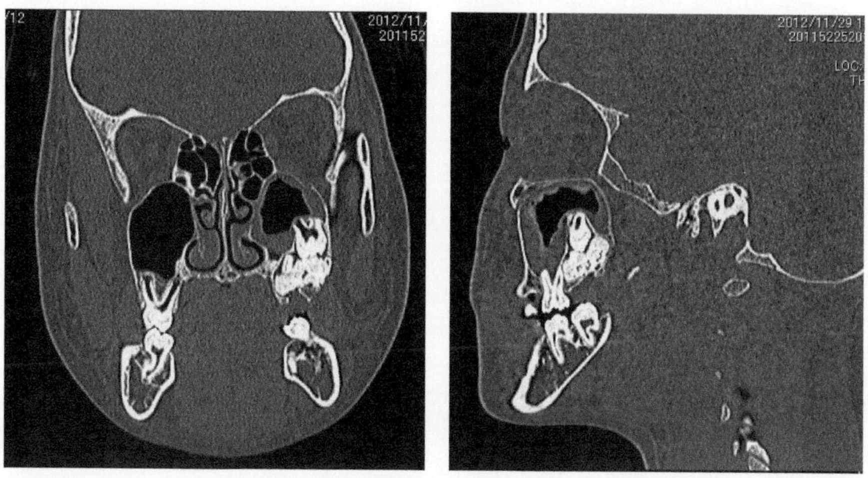

(a) (b)

FIGURE 3: CT view of the lesion. (a) Coronal view. (b) Sagittal view.

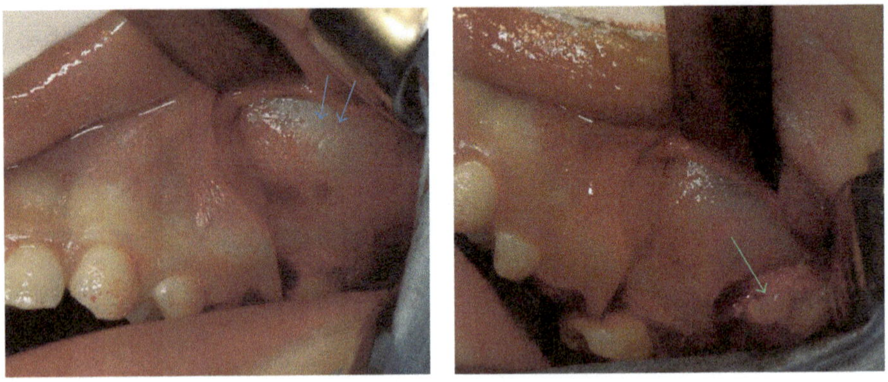

(a) (b)

FIGURE 4: Operative findings. (a) The blue arrows show bulging and thinning of the buccal cortical bone. (b) The green arrows show a solid dental-like mass that has been impacted.

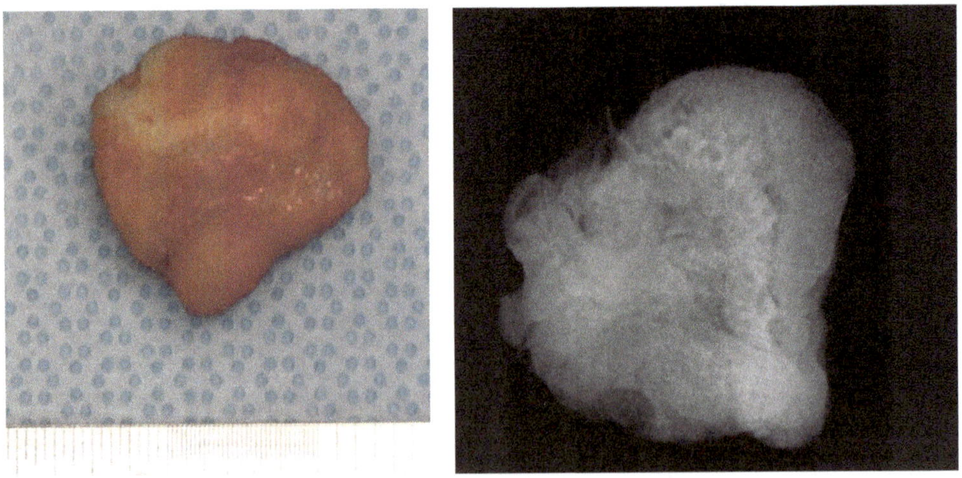

(a) (b)

FIGURE 5: View of the excised lesion. (a) Macroscopic findings. (b) X-ray finding.

noted (Figure 4(a)). Removal of the thinning bone revealed solid masses similar to dental hardening (Figure 4(b)). The lesion was removed easily as there was no adhesion to the surrounding bone and soft tissues. Moreover, there was no root exposure of the upper left first molar. The surgical specimens were 24 × 21 × 16 mm large tooth-like solid and second molar (Figures 5(a) and 5(b)). Pathologic examination revealed compound odontoma (Figures 6(a) and 6(b)). The postoperative course was good; all permanent teeth except the upper left second molar have erupted normally and with no complications or recurrence (Figure 7). Thickening of the maxillary sinus mucosa and an opaque image were not seen in the CT photo taken at 6 months after surgery (Figures 8 and 9).

3. Discussion

The presence of an odontoma in the sinus is exceptional [1]. Further, large odontomas involving the maxillary sinus are quite uncommon [5]. Griffith and Imperato [5] stated that there is no previous report of a large antral odontoma with the typical findings of acute sinusitis. His case of large compound odontoma in the right maxillary had severe pain and pressure. The patient was treated with antibiotics and resulted in complete remission of symptoms for several months, but the symptoms later recurred and the patient failed to respond to the symptomatic therapy. Sanders et al. [14] stated that there are only five reports of odontomas in the antrum producing symptoms of maxillary sinusitis. His case

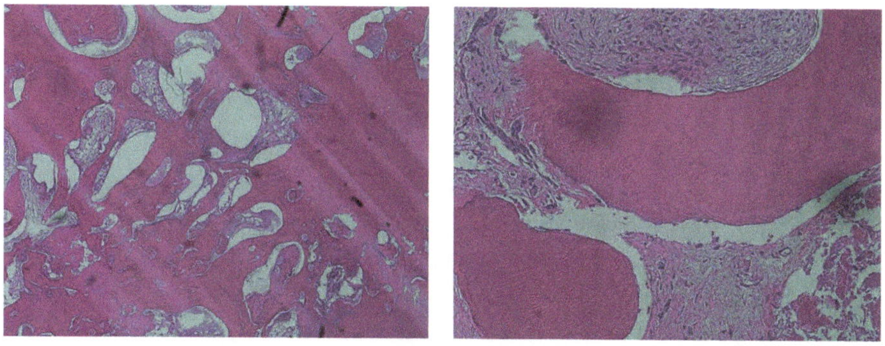

(a) (b)

Figure 6: Pathological examination (hematoxylin-eosin staining). Hard tissues like dentin or enamel are mixed randomly. (a) Original magnification ×4; (b) ×20.

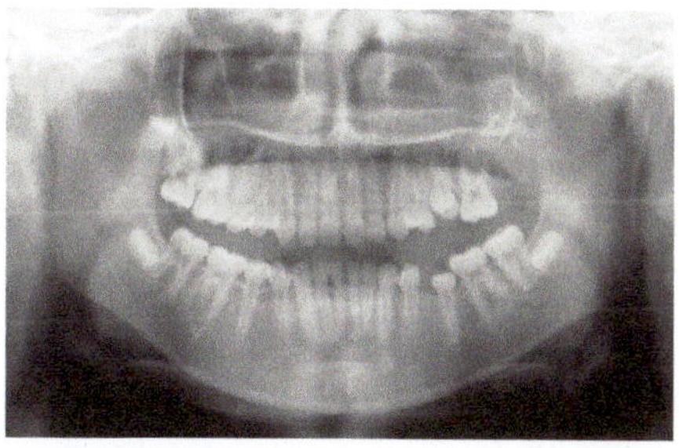

Figure 7: Postoperative panoramic radiograph.

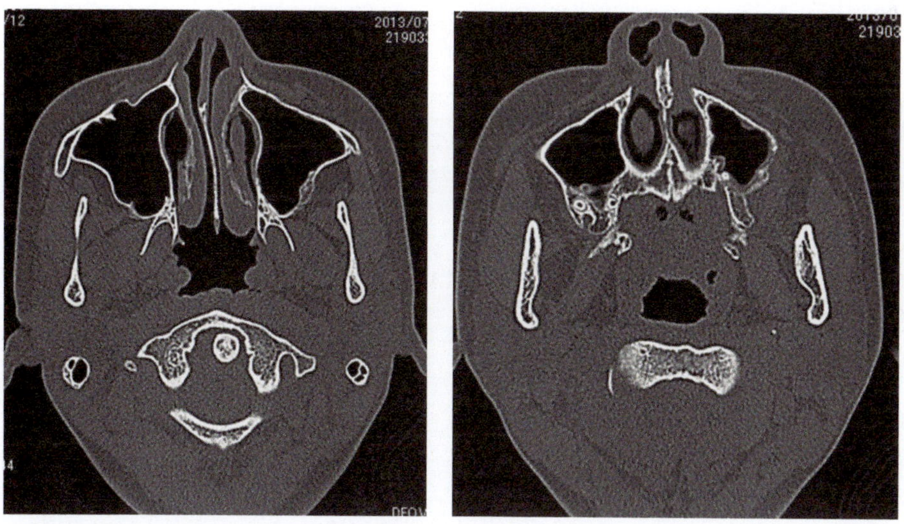

(a) (b)

Figure 8: Axial CT view of the lesion.

of odontoma of the right maxilla had right sinus congestion and pain. In our case, the patient complained of typical findings of persistent nasal congestion and tenderness or swelling in the left molars. Image findings also suggested maxillary sinusitis.

Odontomas are the most common odontogenic tumors [6–8, 10–13, 15] and are benign, slow growing, and nonaggressive [12, 13]. Most of them are asymptomatic and discovered during routine radiographic investigations [6, 8, 10, 12, 13, 16]. This case was found with odontoma in the wake of maxillary

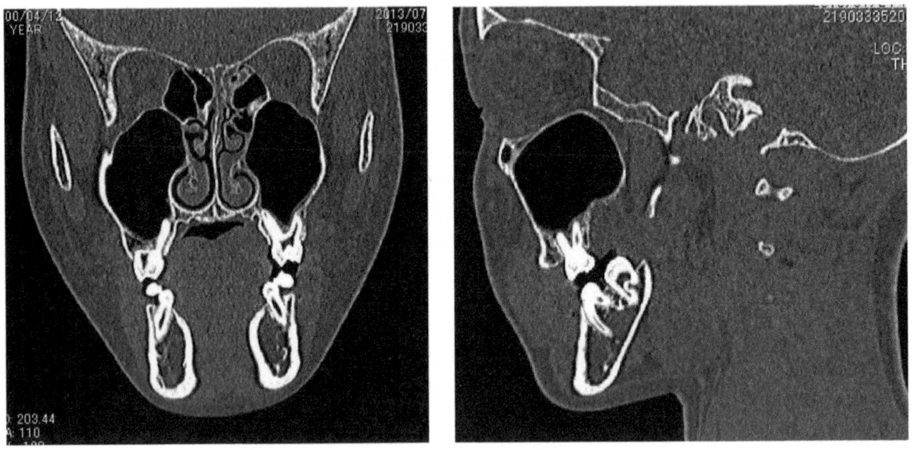

(a) (b)

Figure 9: CT view of the lesion. (a) Coronal view. (b) Sagittal view.

sinusitis symptoms such as pain and swelling. On the other hand, patients who develop odontoma secondary to long-term chronic maxillary sinusitis have also been reported [1]. Also, most of the odontomas related with supernumerary tooth germ and little odontomas are related to normal tooth germ, as follows. A 15-year-old female having maxillary anterior region's odontoma had normal eruption of the permanent teeth and completion of the root [12]. A 4-year-old female having an odontoma in the maxillary anterior region had normal eruption of the primary teeth and developed permanent tooth buds [15]. A 22-year-old male having an odontoma that extended into 2/3rd of the maxillary sinus had first and second molars that were impacted and lying above the odontoma [7]. Both the case of the 10-year-old boy with odontoma in the right maxillary anterior region [6] and that of the 14-year-old male with odontoma between the roots of 13 and 14 [17] are not associated with the normal tooth germs.

Eruption and infection of odontoma are uncommon [7, 10–12, 16], and odontomas are usually associated with tooth eruption disturbances [6, 12, 16]. Tozoglu et al. reported a case of complex odontoma that erupted into the oral cavity as a rare case [11]. Agrawal et al. stated that an unusual case of infected complex odontoma with eruption of odontoma in the oral cavity and perforation of the cheeks had a tooth that was impacted and that was the first report of such a case [16]. Though several cases of infected odontomas have been reported as rare [16, 18], infected odontoma with no eruption has not been reported yet. This case of infected odontoma in the maxillary sinus with no eruption is extremely rare.

References

[1] J. C. Del Hierro, M. R. González, M. D. Portela, E. G. Del Castillo, and J. C. Serrano, "Compound odontoma as a cause of chronic maxillary sinusitis," *Acta Otorrinolaringologica Espanola*, vol. 59, no. 7, pp. 359–361, 2008.

[2] O. Badarne, M. J. Koudstaal, J. F. van Elswijk, and E. B. Wolvius, "Odontogenic maxillary sinusitis based on overextension of root canal filling material," *Nederlands Tijdschrift voor Tandheelkunde*, vol. 119, no. 10, pp. 480–483, 2012.

[3] N. A. Patel and B. J. Ferguson, "Odontogenic sinusitis: an ancient but under-appreciated cause of maxillary sinusitis," *Current Opinion in Otolaryngology and Head and Neck Surgery*, vol. 20, no. 1, pp. 24–28, 2012.

[4] H. Chemli, M. Mnejja, M. Dhouib, F. Karray, A. Ghorbel, and M. Abdelmoula, "Maxillary sinusitis of odontogenic origin: surgical treatment," *Revue de Stomatologie et de Chirurgie Maxillo-Faciale*, vol. 113, no. 2, pp. 87–90, 2012.

[5] C. R. Griffith and A. A. Imperato, "Large antral odontoma as the cause of acute maxillary sinusitis: report of case," *Journal of the American Dental Association*, vol. 94, no. 1, pp. 107–110, 1977.

[6] S. Sreedharan and I. S. Krishnan, "Compound odontoma associated with impacted maxillary incisors," *Journal of Indian Society of Pedodontics and Preventive Dentistry*, vol. 30, no. 3, pp. 275–278, 2012.

[7] K. V. Arunkumar, Vijaykumar, and N. Garg, "Surgical management of an erupted complex odontoma occupying maxillary sinus," *Annals of Maxillofacial Surgery*, vol. 2, no. 1, pp. 86–89, 2012.

[8] T. Cabov, M. Krmpotić, J. Grgurević, B. Perić, D. Jokić, and S. Manojlović, "Large complex odontoma of the left maxillary sinus," *Wiener klinische Wochenschrift*, no. 21-22, pp. 780–783, 2005.

[9] M. Mupparapu, S. R. Singer, and J. Rinaggio, "Complex odontoma of unusual size involving the maxillary sinus: report of a case and review of CT and histopathologic features," *Quintessence International*, vol. 35, no. 8, pp. 641–645, 2004.

[10] S. Govindrajan, J. Muruganandhan, S. Shamsudeen, N. Kumar, M. Ramasamy, and S. Prasad, "Complex composite odontoma with characteristic histology," *Case Reports in Dentistry*, vol. 2013, Article ID 157614, 5 pages, 2013.

[11] S. Tozoglu, U. Yildirim, and M. C. Buyukkurt, "An erupted complex odontoma," *The New York State Dental Journal*, vol. 76, no. 5, pp. 52–53, 2010.

[12] D. Mehta, N. Raval, S. Udhani, V. Parekh, and C. Modi, "An unusual case report of erupted odontoma," *Case Reports in Dentistry*, vol. 2013, Article ID 570954, 3 pages, 2013.

[13] M. Soltan and A. Kacker, "Complex odontoma of the nasal cavity: a case report," *Ear, Nose and Throat Journal*, vol. 87, no. 5, pp. 277–279, 2008.

[14] B. Sanders, R. Halliday, and B. McKelvy, "Odontoma of the antrum presenting as maxillary sinusitis," *Journal of Oral Medicine*, vol. 31, no. 3, pp. 60–62, 1976.

[15] A. Mathew, P. Shenai, L. Chatra, K. Veena, P. Rao, and R. Prabhu, "Compound odontoma in deciduous dentition," *Annals of Medical and Health Sciences Research*, vol. 3, no. 2, pp. 285–287, 2013.

[16] B. Agrawal, H. Gharote, P. Nair, and S. Shrivastav, "Infected complex odontoma: an unusual presentation," *BMJ Case Reports*, 2012.

[17] M. Yadav, P. Godge, S. M. Meghana, and S. R. Kulkarni, "Compound odontoma," *Contemporary Clinical Dentistry*, vol. 3, suppement 1, pp. S13–S15, 2012.

[18] F. G. Repass, "Infected compound composite odontoma, report of case," *Journal of Oral Surgery*, vol. 4, no. article 245, 1946.

30

Management of a Severely Submerged Primary Molar: A Case Report

Iman Parisay,[1] Fatemeh Kebriaei,[2] Bentolhoda Varkesh,[2] Milad Soruri,[2] and Roya Ghafourifard[2]

[1] *Pediatric Dentistry, Dental Material Research Center, School of Dentistry, Mashhad University of Medical Sciences, Mashhad, Iran*
[2] *Department of Pediatric Dentistry, School of Dentistry, Shahid Sadoughi University of Medical Sciences, Yazd, Iran*

Correspondence should be addressed to Bentolhoda Varkesh; dr_hoda_v@yahoo.com

Academic Editors: M. Ashkenazi, C. Evans, H. C. Gungor, and M. A. Polack

Ankylosis is a condition frequently associated with primary molars, wherein the ankylosed primary teeth remain in a fixed position, while the adjacent teeth continue to erupt, moving occlusally. In this case report, a five-year-old boy, who had a retained and submerged left lower second primary molar, was presented. Luxation of ankylosed primary molar was considered as a treatment approach. After four months, the tooth erupted to the occlusal level, and there was evidence of further development of a permanent successor in radiographic evaluation. After one year, tooth mobility, bone formation, and development of a permanent successor were in good condition.

1. Introduction

Dental infraocclusion is defined as teeth below the occlusal plane. In the literature, the terms submergence and infraocclusion are often used to refer to an ankylosis [1, 2].

The frequency of ankylosed teeth has been reported to be between 1.3% and 38.5% [3]. The mandibular first primary molars are the most frequently affected teeth, followed by second mandibular and maxillary primary molars [3].

The exact cause of teeth ankylosis is still unknown, but several theories have been proposed [3, 4] such as familial pattern, traumatic injury to Hertwig's epithelial root sheath, deficiency in bone growth, a problem in local metabolism and inflammation, localized infection, and chemical or thermal irritations.

Ankylosis is classified as slight, moderate, or severe according to the place of the occlusal level of the infraoccluded tooth [5]. If the infraocclusion is less than 2 mm, it shows slight ankylosis, while moderate submergence shows the occlusal surface of the ankylosed tooth to the contact area. Severe ankylosis shows infraocclusion below the contact area of the adjacent teeth [5].

Diagnosing ankylosed teeth is not difficult and is usually based on clinical signs and radiographic findings. Clinically, ankylosed teeth have a sharp, solid sound on a percussion test in comparison to a cushion sound in normal teeth [2].

Obliteration of the periodontal ligament space is noted radiographically. The roots are less radiopaque, and as the ankylosis progresses, they are less distinguished from surrounding bone. Areas of fusion of cementum and bone, as well as periodontal ligament remnants that are fibrotic with very few cells, have been observed histologically. No mucopolysaccharidase activity, which is essential for the normal process of root resorption during eruption of permanent successor, is seen [6].

Ankylosis of deciduous molars has a negative impact on normal occlusal development and may cause problems such as

(a) significant tipping of adjacent teeth to the area of the submerged tooth, which may cause a reduction in arch length, especially when severe ankylosis of second primary molars occurs in early mixed dentition [5, 7];

(b) ectopic eruption or impaction of successor premolar;

(c) The increase in caries and periodontal disease susceptibility [3].

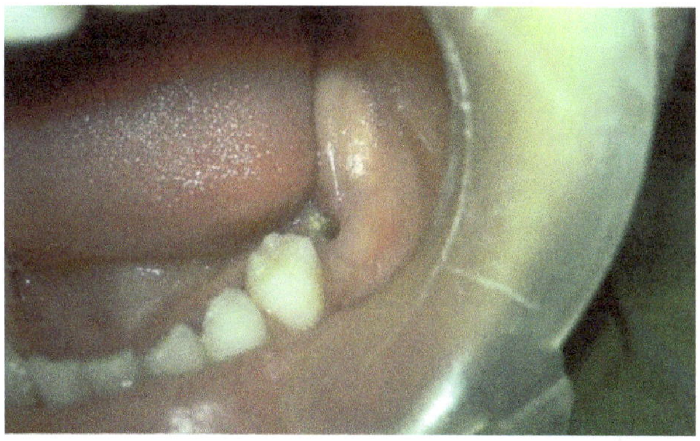

Figure 1: Intraoral view of the left second submerged primary mandibular molar.

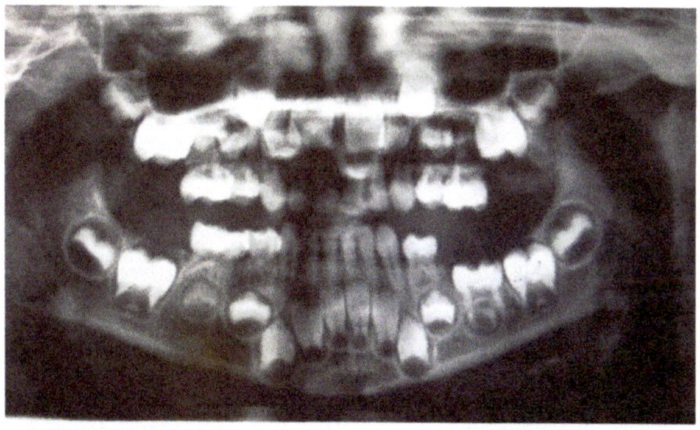

Figure 2: Radiographic view of the left second submerged primary mandibular molar.

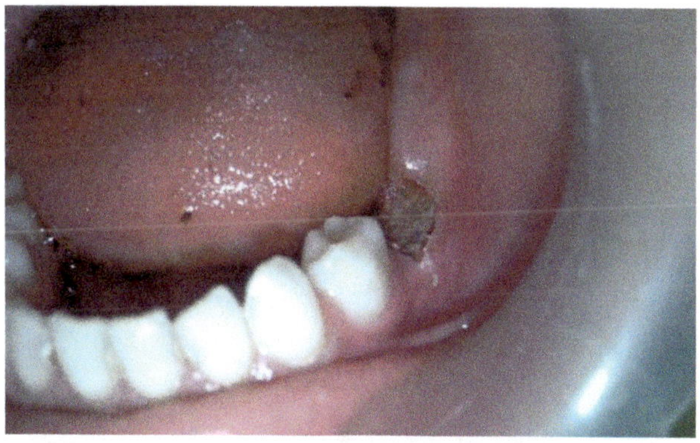

Figure 3: The surgical site was packed with reinforced zinc oxide eugenol.

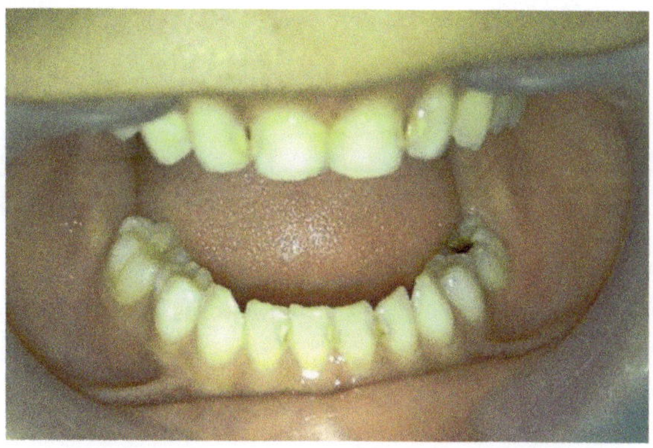

Figure 4: The tooth position four months after luxation.

Hence, early diagnosis of infraoccluded primary molars is extremely important to prevent the previously mentioned problems.

There are several treatment procedures according to the age of the patient, the amount of tilting of adjacent teeth, and the condition of the permanent successor as follows:

(i) monitoring the ankylosed tooth [7];

(ii) early extraction and space maintenance [5];

(iii) restoration of occlusal height [8];

(iv) luxation [3].

Here is a report of a case with ankylosis of the second primary molar in late primary dentition with a new treatment approach.

2. Case Report

A five-year-old boy was referred to the Pediatric Dentistry Department of Shahid Sadoughi University of Medical Sciences by his general dentist to assess his infraoccluded primary mandibular molar.

The patient had no relevant medical history of any systemic disease and his family reported no drug use.

Intraoral examination revealed multiple carious lesions in his maxillary anterior teeth and a severe infraoccluded left second primary mandibular tooth, the mesiolingual cusp of which was the only cusp that could be seen (Figure 1).

A subsequent radiographic examination revealed an ankylosed second primary molar along with less development of a successor tooth bud in comparison with the antimer. The second premolar dental follicle was completely situated between the roots of the ankylosed primary molar (Figure 2).

Considering the abnormal development of the patient's permanent successor tooth, emergency intervention seemed logical. In order to prevent serious damage to dental follicle, surgical extraction was not considered; therefore, conservative intervention was a preferred treatment approach. The occlusal table of the submerged tooth was exposed by removing covering gingiva, and the surgical site was packed with reinforced zinc oxide eugenol (Zonalin, Kemdent, UK) to provide a path for the tooth to erupt (Figure 3). A carious lesion was detected in the central pit of the occlusal surface.

After one week, the ankylosed tooth was luxated mesially and distally by a surgical elevator, and because of no clinical or radiographic evidence of tooth eruption, after one month, the tooth was luxated for a second time.

After four months, the primary tooth erupted and reached the occlusal level of the primary dentition (Figure 4). There was evidence of further developments of a permanent successor in radiographic evaluation.

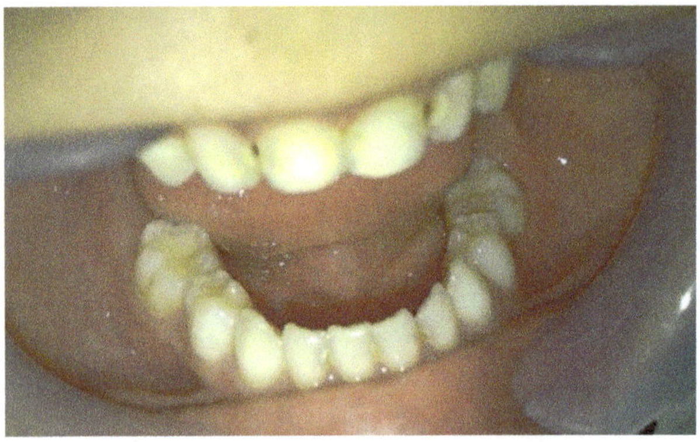

FIGURE 5: Restored tooth with resin composite.

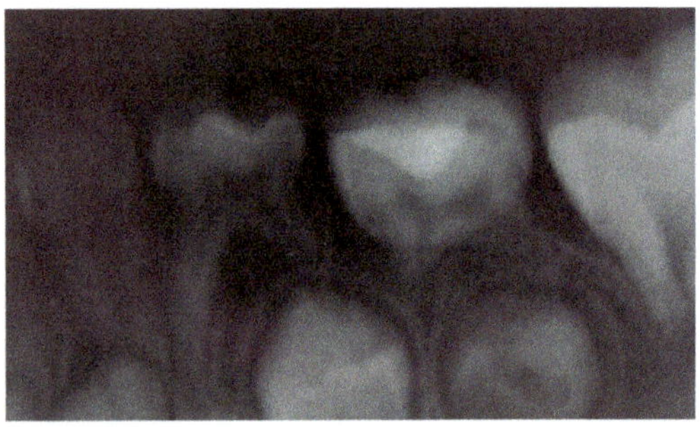

(a)

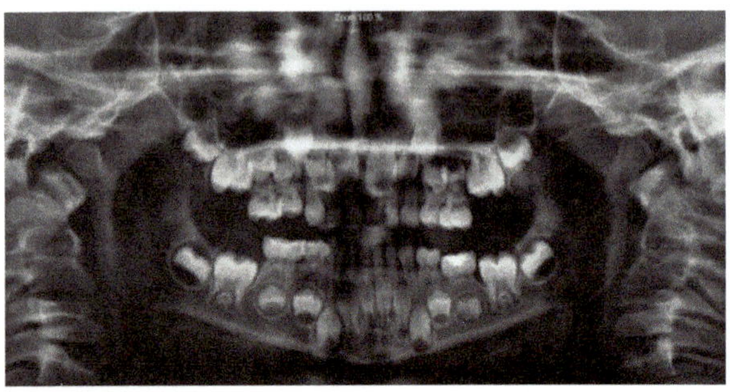

(b)

FIGURE 6: (a) Ten-month periapical view. (b) Ten-month panoramic view.

Following the complete eruption of the primary tooth, the carious lesion was restored with posterior resin composite (P60, 3M ESPE, USA) (Figure 5).

A favorable result was seen regarding tooth mobility, bone formation, and the development of a permanent successor in ten-month followup (Figure 6).

3. Discussion

In the management of an ankylosed tooth, early recognition and a thorough diagnosis are the most important factors for successful treatment [2].

Various treatment approaches have been proposed that depend on the age of the patient, the developmental stage of the root, the position of the tooth, the severity of infraocclusion, the number of the teeth affected, the severity of tilting of adjacent teeth, and the presence and location of the permanent successor [3].

It is often difficult to decide exactly the starting point of treatment. In the case of a cooperative patient with regular recall periods, a watchful waiting approach maybe the best. Moreover, if there is no evidence of unusual caries problems or loss of arch length, the dentist may choose to keep the tooth under observation [2].

A conservative treatment approach for ankylosed primary teeth is the continuous supervision of tooth eruption evidenced with periodic radiographic observation of normal root resorption [9, 10].

A tooth that is definitely ankylosed may surprisingly undergo root resorption at a given time and be normally shed. In this case, it may seem logical not to extract all the infraoccluded teeth but instead to follow rigorously, as there is a chance for it in the eruption path. However, in this patient, because of severe infraocclusion of the second primary molar and the risk of space loss in the near future while the first permanent molar erupts, immediate intervention was considered.

Another conservative treatment option was composite buildup or a stainless steel crown to prevent tipping of adjacent teeth and to restore the occlusion to the correct height, thereby preventing the tooth of the opposing arch from supraeruption. However, for this case, because the infraocclusion was severe, it was imprudent and even impossible to buildup the occlusal table with either composite resin or a stainless steel crown.

Extraction as an eventual treatment, preferably as early as possible [4, 5], is recommended by many authors. Other authors recommend this treatment only in the case of severely affected primary molars and where the evidence of possible future crowding is observed [11]. Early extraction is only advisable when there is occlusal disturbance with severe tipping of adjacent teeth and malposition of the permanent succedaneous combined with severe infraocclusion [7]. However, early extraction may be technically difficult and may result in root fractures or disturbance of the successor tooth bud [3, 12]. In this case, due to the five-year-old patient's fear of surgery and the parents' insistence on adopting a more conservative treatment as well as the possible complications of surgical extraction such as bone loss, this method was not considered, and so luxation was considered.

Luxation is a treatment option for ankylosed teeth, permitting the teeth to continue its eruption. The theory behind luxation of affected primary molars is that the bony union between the alveolus and the ankylosed teeth can be broken [3].

Biederman as well as Skolnick have reported the efficacy of a luxation technique in breaking bony ankylosis [13, 14]. If this technique is not immediately successful, then it can be repeated in six months [2].

Lygidakis et al. adopted surgical luxation and elevation as a treatment approach for a localized secondary eruption failure of the mandibular right first permanent molar [15]. This treatment included surgical luxation of the tooth, followed by elevation to the occlusal plane and stabilization to the adjacent teeth. A three-year followup showed a successful result without considering the clinical or radiological pathology of the area [15].

Although luxation to free ankylosed permanent teeth (not generally recommended) and the absence of a case report introducing luxation as a treatment approach for ankylosed primary molars have been attempted with limited success [8], in this present case, we decided to luxate the ankylosed tooth.

Despite the limited success of the luxation method in ankylosed permanent teeth [8], in this patient, the submerged primary molar reached the occlusal plane after luxation by elevator after four months.

4. Conclusion

Although the majority of ankylosed teeth with permanent successors shed normally, early and proper intervention to prevent occlusal discrepancies is advisable. There are several management methods in case of ankylosed primary molars, and from these methods, luxation can be considered a safe and effective treatment approach for the management of infraoccluded primary molars.

References

[1] Z. Kirziolu, H. Karayilmaz, and B. Baykal, "Value of computed tomography (CT) in imaging the morbidity of submerged molars: a case report," *European Journal of Dentistry*, vol. 1, no. 4, pp. 246–250, 2007.

[2] J. A. Dean, D. R. Aery, and R. E. McDonald, *Dentistry for the Child and Adolescent*, Mosby, St. Louis, Mo, USA, 9th edition, 2011.

[3] F. R. Jenkins and R. E. Nichol, "Atypical retention of infraoccluded primary molars with permanent successor teeth," *European Archives of Paediatric Dentistry*, vol. 9, no. 1, pp. 51–55, 2008.

[4] S. Ponduri, D. J. Birnie, and J. R. Sandy, "Infraocclusion of secondary deciduous molars—an unusual outcome," *Journal of Orthodontics*, vol. 36, no. 3, pp. 186–189, 2009.

[5] L. B. Messer and J. T. Cline, "Ankylosed primary molars: results and treatment recommendations from an eight-year longitudinal study," *Pediatric Dentistry*, vol. 2, no. 1, pp. 37–47, 1980.

[6] B. Suprabha and S. Pai, "Ankylosis of primary molar along with congenitally missing first permanent molar," *Journal of Indian Society of Pedodontics and Preventive Dentistry*, vol. 24, pp. 35–37, 2006.

[7] J. Kurol and B. Thilander, "Infraocclusion of primary molars and the effect on occlusal development, a longitudinal study," *European Journal of Orthodontics*, vol. 6, no. 4, pp. 277–293, 1984.

[8] F. J. Krakowiak, "Ankylosed primary molars," *Journal of Dentistry for Children*, vol. 45, no. 4, pp. 288–292, 1978.

[9] J. Kurol and L. Olson, "Ankylosis of primary molars-a future periodontal threat to the first permanent molars?" *European Journal of Orthodontics*, vol. 13, no. 5, pp. 404–409, 1991.

[10] G. K. Belanger, M. Strange, and J. R. Sexton, "Early ankylosis of a primary molar with self-correction: case report," *Pediatric Dentistry*, vol. 8, pp. 37–40, 1986.

[11] G. B. Winter, M. J. Gelbier, and J. R. Goodman, "Severe Infra-occlusion and failed eruption of deciduous molars associated with eruptive and developmental disturbances in the permanent dentition: a report of 28 selected cases," *British Journal of Orthodontics*, vol. 24, no. 2, pp. 149–157, 1997.

[12] G. M. Raghoebar, G. Boering, H. W. B. Jansen, and A. Vissink, "Secondary retention of permanent molars: a histologic study," *Journal of Oral Pathology and Medicine*, vol. 18, no. 8, pp. 427–431, 1989.

[13] W. Biederman, "Etiology and treatment of tooth ankylosis," *American Journal of Orthodontics*, vol. 48, no. 9, pp. 670–684, 1962.

[14] I. M. Skolnick, "Ankylosis of maxillary permanent first molar," *The Journal of the American Dental Association*, vol. 100, no. 4, pp. 558–560, 1980.

[15] N. A. Lygidakis, S. Bafis, and E. Vidaki, "Case report: surgical luxation and elevation as treatment approach for secondary eruption failure of permanent molars," *European Archives of Paediatric Dentistry*, vol. 10, supplement 1, pp. 46–48, 2009.

Spontaneous Eruption of Premolar Associated with a Dentigerous Cyst

Irla Karlinne Ferreira de Carvalho and Anibal Henrique Barbosa Luna

Paraiba Federal University (UFPB), 58091-900 João Pessoa, PB, Brazil

Correspondence should be addressed to Irla Karlinne Ferreira de Carvalho; irla_karlinne@hotmail.com

Academic Editor: Jose López-López

Dentigerous cyst (DC) is the second most common odontogenic cyst with greater incidence in young patients. It presents as a unilocular, asymptomatic radiolucency involving the crown of an impacted tooth, commonly noticed in X-rays to investigate absence, wrong tooth position, or delay in the chronology of eruption. Decompression/marsupialization (D/M) is the most implemented treatment, especially when preserving the tooth involved is advised. The aim of this study is to discuss the DC characteristics that contribute to spontaneous eruption of premolars, by reporting the case of a conservative treatment of DC. This eruption depends on factors such as age, angulation of inclusion, rate of root formation, depth of inclusion, and eruption space. This paper reports the case of a 10-year-old patient with a radiolucent lesion diagnosed as DC involving element 35, which erupted as a result of treatment. The patient was observed during 1 year and 6 months.

1. Introduction

Dentigerous cysts (DC), also denominated follicular cysts, are one of the two most common types of odontogenic cysts associated with impacted, included, or partially erupted teeth [1].

It is ranked the second most common odontogenic cyst, and the literature has shown an occurrence of approximately 24% among all the true cysts of the maxillae [2]. The majority of reports have shown a peak incidence of this cyst in the second and third decade of life, although some have reported the fifth decade [3].

A typical DC clinically presents as a unilocular, asymptomatic, radiolucent lesion involving the crown of an included or impacted tooth. Generally there is no pain or discomfort associated with it, unless it becomes secondarily infected [2]. The radiolucence generally arises at the cementoenamel junction of the tooth [3].

The large majority are discovered accidentally when radiographs are taken to investigate a failure of eruption or a poorly positioned tooth [2]. In the majority of cases, the diagnosis of a DC is simple. However, differential diagnosis must be made with alterations such as a dental follicle or a hyperplastic dental follicle and even an odontogenic keratocyst or unicystic ameloblastoma [3].

It is formed due to an alteration in the reduced epithelium of the enamel and develops from an accumulation of fluid between the reduced epithelium of the enamel and the crown of the developing tooth [2]. The teeth most frequently affected are the third molars, maxillary canines, and premolars [1].

Enucleation and decompression/marsupialization (D/M) are the forms of treatment most used for DC [4]; the only difference between them is by the use of a device in decompression to maintain communication of the lesion with the oral cavity. Some important criteria must be considered for the treatment plan, such as the size of the cyst, age, proximity to anatomic structures [5], clinical importance, and possibility of making use of the tooth involved.

In spite of the clinical peculiarities of each case and of the method of treatment chosen, these lesions have a favorable prognosis. Therefore, the aim is to report a case of conservative treatment of a dentigerous cyst in a pediatric patient.

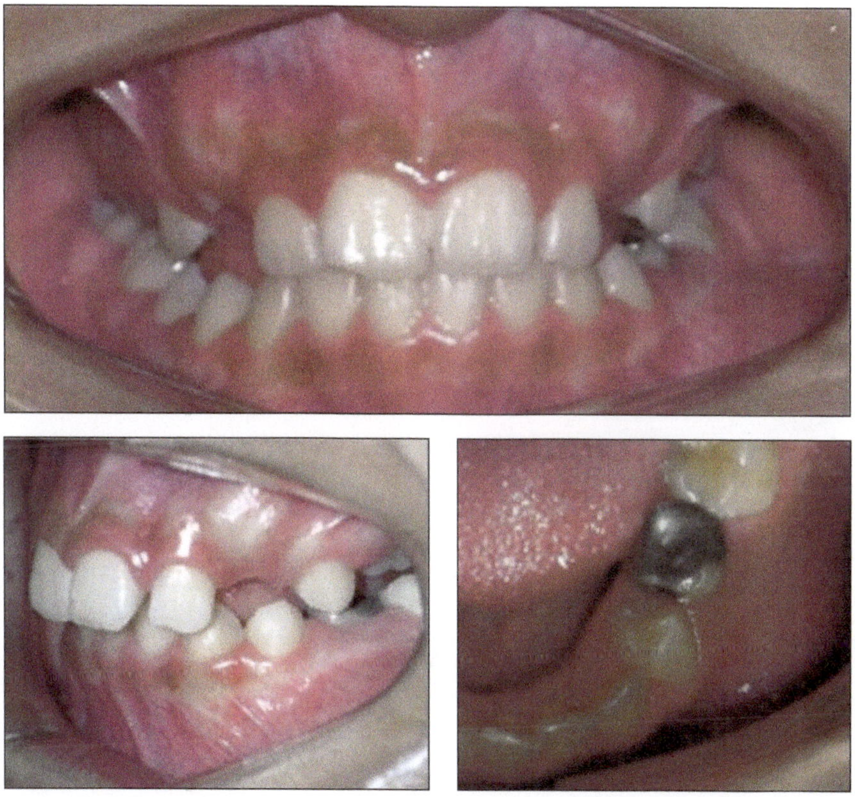

FIGURE 1: Swelling in the vestibular cortex of the left premolar area and retention of second primary molar, with large amalgam restoration.

2. Case Report

The patient, L. J. S., a 10-year-old boy, mulatto, presented to the Oral and Maxillofacial Clinic of the Lauro Wanderley University Hospital (HULW/UFPB), accompanied by his guardian, complaining of "pain when chewing on the left side." He presented no facial asymmetry on physical exam; however, on intraoral inspection, left second premolar was observed to be absent, with retention of left second primary molar with a large amalgam restoration showing a mesiodistal dimension of 10 mm. In addition, an increase in volume, firm on palpation and asymptomatic, was found, with a normal aspect of the oral mucosa in the region of the left mandibular body, leading to obliteration of the sulcus (Figure 1). The panoramic radiograph showed a unilocular, radiolucent lesion with well-defined margins and radiopaque halo in the mandibular body on the left side, involving second left premolar with a depth of inclusion of 14 mm. The lesion extended from the periapical region of left first premolar to the mesial root of left first molar, measuring 3.3 cm × 2.7 cm, suggesting the diagnosis of dentigerous cyst. It presented a 77.3° angle between the line that passes through the long axis of left second premolar and the plane bisecting the long axes of the adjacent teeth. There was a 17.5° angle formed between the line that follows the long axis of the mentioned tooth and the line that passes through the cementoenamel junction of the neighboring teeth (Figure 2).

The patient was submitted to incisional biopsy under local anesthesia. The serum-blood colored surgical aspirate confirmed the hypothesis of cystic lesion. The opportunity was taken to remove tooth, the left second primary molar, and install a transalveolar silicone drain, which was removed after 3 weeks (Figure 3). The anatomopathological exam was conclusive for a dentigerous cyst associated with the presence of inflammatory infiltrate. The patient was clinically and radiographically followed up for a period of 1 year and 6 months, until complete regression of the lesion and eruption of tooth 35 (Figures 4 and 5).

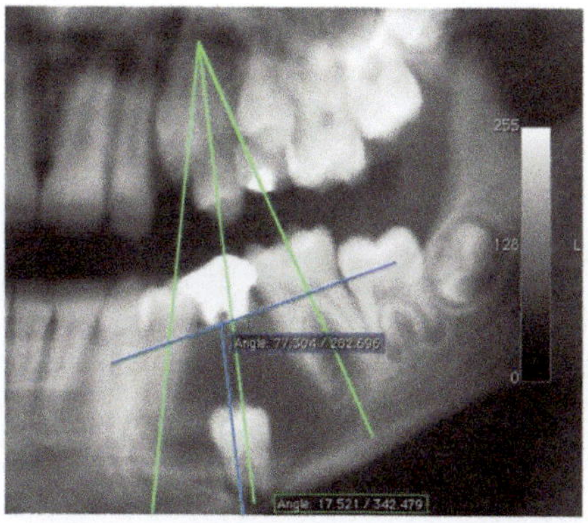

FIGURE 2: Angulation proposed in the studies of Fujii et al. [11] and Hyomoto et al. [10], to the value of 77.3°, in green. Angulation proposed by Yahara et al. [12], to the value of 17.5°, in blue.

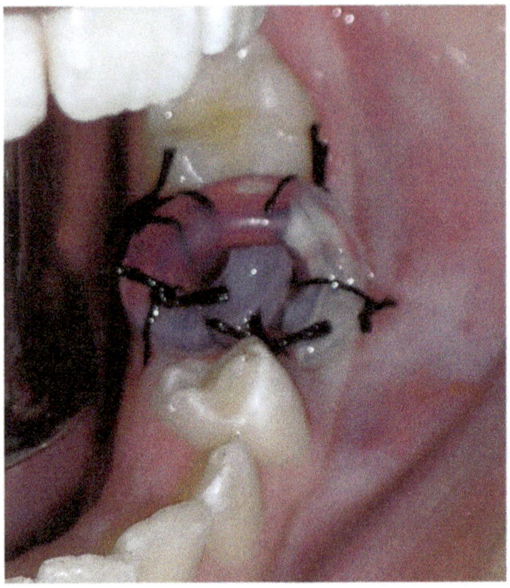

FIGURE 3: After extraction of second primary molar, the alveolus was communicated with the cyst, allowing the insertion of a decompression catheter.

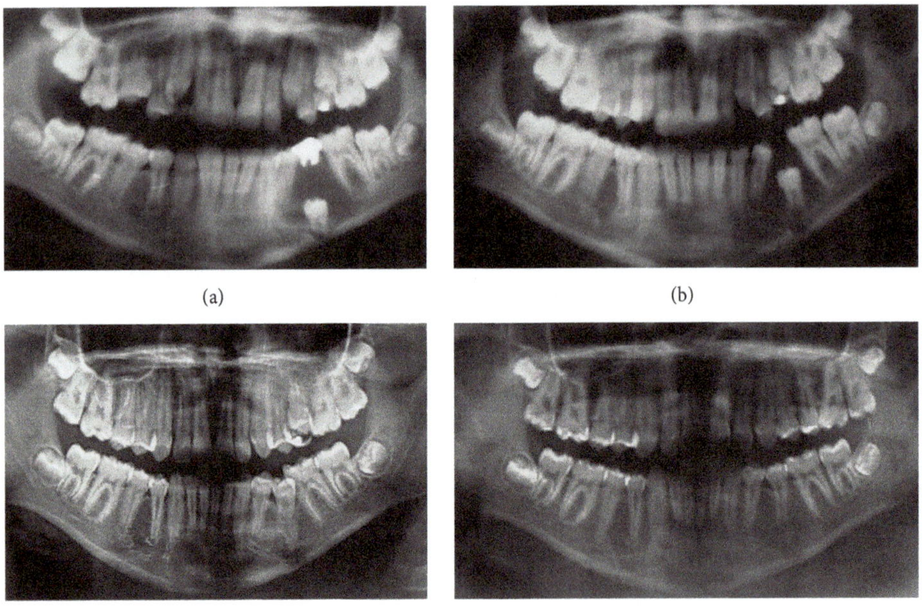

(a) (b) (c) (d)

FIGURE 4: Initial aspect of the lesion (a). Note the extensive restoration of teeth 75 and 35 with incomplete rhizogenesis. Note the regression of the lesion and eruption of tooth 35 at 4 (b), 6 (c), and 11 months (d) after D/M.

3. Discussion

The DC is the most frequently occurring cyst among the odontogenic cysts, with the exception of the radicular cyst. There are few demographic studies about the subject involving populations in Brazil. In a retrospective study conducted in the Oral Pathology Service of FO-UFMG, in a period of 51 years, 19,064 oral biopsies were found. Of these, 2,812 cases (14.7%) were diagnosed as odontogenic cysts, with the DC showing a prevalence of 25.3% of these cases, being more common in young patients between the second and third decade of life [6]. Therefore, in spite of odontogenic cysts presenting a low incidence in children, the DC is of important clinical significance in pediatric dentistry, because it affects a significant number of child patients [7].

The DC is normally detected by chance, because it is asymptomatic. Therefore, they are generally detected due to a delay in the chronology of eruption of the tooth involved, causing deformation in the alveolar bone and expansion of the cortical bone, attaining important dimensions as a result of the delay in their diagnosis. In these cases, surgical treatment with minimal lesion to anatomic structures is

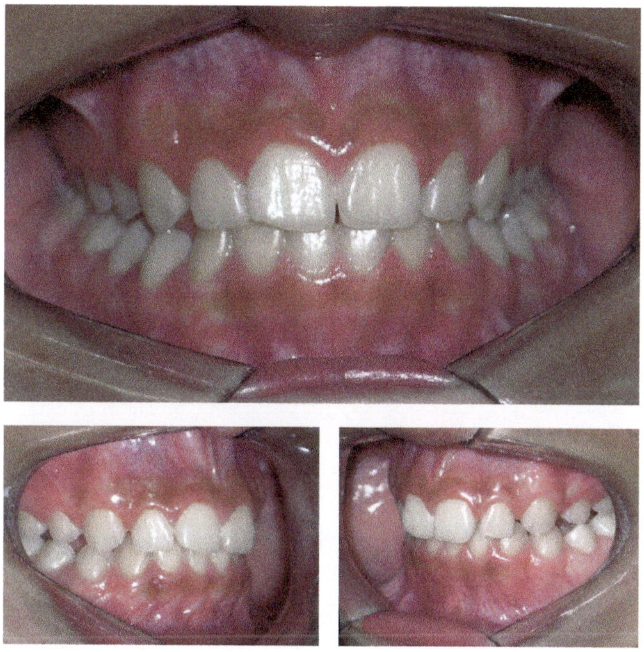

FIGURE 5: The patient was clinically followed up for a period of 1 year and 6 months, until complete regression of the lesion and eruption of tooth 35.

TABLE 1: Factors related to spontaneous eruption of premolars associated with DC.

Factors analyzed	Hyomoto et al., 2003 [10]	Fujii et al., 2008 [11]	Yahara et al., 2009 [12]
Age	The smaller, the greater the chances of eruption	Under 10 years old	Mean age 9.8 years
Depth of inclusion	4.4 mm*	Smaller than 5.1 mm*	The smaller, the greater the chances of eruption
Angulation of tooth	$20.4^\circ \pm 21.8^{\circ *}$	Smaller than $25^{\circ *}$	Close to $60.2^{\circ **}$
Space present for eruption	Does not influence	Larger than 1 cm	Does not influence
Rhizogenesis	1/2	Incomplete	Does not influence

*According to Hyomoto et al. [10] and Fujii et al. [11], it is considered the angle formed between the line that passes through the long axis of the included tooth and the plane bisecting the long axes of the neighboring teeth. The depth is considered as from the cementoenamel junction.
**According to Yahara et al. [12], it is the measurement of the angle formed between the line that crosses the long axis of the tooth involved and the line that passes through the cementoenamel junction of the neighboring teeth.

fundamental. Postoperative defects of the facial structures in individuals exposed to treatment for enucleation of the cyst may bring about functional and esthetic problems, in addition to producing psychological consequences [8]. Therefore, enucleation is reserved for smaller lesions, or those in which it is not possible to save the tooth involved.

The M/D technique minimizes the risk of complications such as the loss of tooth germs, lesions to blood vessels and nerves, and loss of bone structures of the face. It is a simple, conservative surgical procedure that favors the eruption of displaced teeth and in the majority of cases results in good occlusion. By virtue of the foregoing, it is the treatment option for extensive lesions [9] and is well accepted in the treatment of cooperative pediatric patients, particularly when there is the possibility of preserving the tooth involved in the lesion and to allow eruption, thus diminishing the functional and esthetic damage to the patient. In the clinical case presented, enucleation would have resulted in the extraction of tooth 35 and probable lesion of the inferior alveolar/mental nerves, as well as fragilization of the left mandibular body, predisposing the patient to an eventual mandibular fracture. The patient developed without paresthesia or bone defects in the perilesional area.

An interesting topic concerning the case refers to the possibility of eruption of premolars involved with DC. Studies such as the ones of Hyomoto et al. [10], Fujii et al. [11], and Yahara et al. [12] have analyzed the factors that interfere in the spontaneous eruption of mandibular premolars associated with this cyst, based on the findings in panoramic radiographs (Table 1). Hyomoto et al. [10] furthermore observed that in the presence of inflammatory infiltrate the included teeth tend to erupt more easily, suggesting that the larger the quantity of inflammatory cells, the greater the predictability of eruption of the tooth associated with the cyst. This case ratifies the findings of the abovementioned authors, as the gradual eruption of the tooth involved in the lesion was observed in the radiographic images, until its functional occlusion occurred. The patient was 10 years of age, with 10 mm space present for eruption and the lesion involving tooth 35 with incomplete rhizogenesis and presence of inflammatory infiltrate. As regards angulation of the tooth involved, both by the method used by Hyomoto et al. [10] and Fujii et al. [11] and by the method of Yahara et al. [12], the case presented was shown to be favorable to eruption of the tooth involved, as may be observed in Figure 2. These findings may explain the fact of the extensive depth of inclusion not being sufficiently important, of itself alone, to result in the failure of spontaneous eruption of tooth 35.

Therefore, the characteristics of the inclusion are of fundamental importance in order to enable one to opt for an adequate treatment plan, with M/E being a simple technique to perform, with low postoperative morbidity, and easily accepted by the patient and his/her family members.

Among the treatment modalities proposed for DC, enucleation must be used in smaller lesions, in which there are no risks of injuring important anatomic structures and causing functional and esthetic damage, or when tooth eruption is improbable. The logic of the use of M/D follows the principle of inversion.

Spontaneous eruption of premolars associated with DC depends on a series of factors. Age, depth of inclusion, angulation, and degree of rhizogenesis are factors universally used. The quantity of space present between the neighboring teeth and the presence of inflammatory infiltrate may also be considered. Studies have confirmed that there is great predictability of the eruption of mandibular premolars related to dentigerous cysts [10–12]. Therefore, one must know the factors that have a positive influence on this process, so that one avoids unnecessarily sacrificing teeth and all the sequelae resulting from this fact. The time of intervention and decision making by the clinician is essential in order to establish a favorable prognosis, deciding on which treatment modality is appropriate after individual analysis of each case.

Disclosure

The study was conducted at Paraiba Federal University, Campus I, Cidade Universitária S/N, 58091-900.

Competing Interests

The authors declare that they have no competing interests.

References

[1] W.-T. Qian, Z.-G. Ma, Q.-Y. Xie, X.-Y. Cai, Y. Zhang, and C. Yang, "Marsupialization facilitates eruption of dentigerous cyst-associated mandibular premolars in preadolescent patients," *Journal of Oral and Maxillofacial Surgery*, vol. 71, no. 11, pp. 1825–1832, 2013.

[2] V. Aher, P. Chander, R. Chikkalingaiah, and F. Ali, "Dentigerous cysts in four quadrants: a rare and first reported case," *Journal of Surgical Technique and Case Report*, vol. 5, no. 1, pp. 21–26, 2013.

[3] L. L. Zhang, R. Yang, L. Zhang, W. Li, D. MacDonald-Jankowski, and C. F. Poh, "Dentigerous cyst: a retrospective clinicopathological analysis of 2082 dentigerous cysts in British Columbia, Canada," *International Journal of Oral & Maxillofacial Surgery*, vol. 39, no. 9, pp. 878–882, 2010.

[4] F. M. Serra e Silva, R. Sawazaki, and M. de Moraes, "Eruption of teeth associated with a dentigerous cyst by only marsupialization treatment: a case report," *Journal of Dentistry for Children (Chicago, Ill.)*, vol. 74, no. 3, pp. 228–230, 2007.

[5] L. G. M. Vaz, M. T. V. Rodrigues, and F. J. Osny, "Dentigerous cyst: clinical and radiographic characteristics and criteria for treatment planning," *Revista Gaúcha de Odontológia*, vol. 58, no. 1, pp. 127–130, 2010.

[6] S. M. Grossmann, V. C. Machado, G. M. Xavier et al., "Demographic profile of odontogenic and selected nonodontogenic cysts in a Brazilian population," *Oral Surgery, Oral Medicine, Oral Pathology, Oral Radiology and Endodontology*, vol. 104, no. 6, pp. e35–e41, 2007.

[7] D. S. Barrozo, J. A. C. Hanemann, O. M. B. Araújo, and M. C. Pereira, "Cisto dentígero na infância: relato de caso e revisão de literatura," *Jornal Brasileiro de Odontopediatria & Odontologia do Bebê*, vol. 5, no. 27, pp. 364–369, 2002.

[8] J. Berdén, G. Koch, and C. Ullbro, "Case series: treatment of large dentigerous cysts in children," *European Archives of Paediatric Dentistry*, vol. 11, no. 3, pp. 140–145, 2010.

[9] S. D. A. Berti, A. B. Pompermayer, P. H. Couto Souza, O. M. Tanaka, V. P. D. Westphalen, and F. H. Westphalen, "Spontaneous eruption of a canine after marsupialization of an infected dentigerous cyst," *American Journal of Orthodontics & Dentofacial Orthopedics*, vol. 137, no. 5, pp. 690–693, 2010.

[10] M. Hyomoto, M. Kawakami, M. Inoue, and T. Kirita, "Clinical conditions for eruption of maxillary canines and mandibular premolars associated with dentigerous cysts," *American Journal of Orthodontics and Dentofacial Orthopedics*, vol. 124, no. 5, pp. 515–520, 2003.

[11] R. Fujii, M. Kawakami, M. Hyomoto, J. Ishida, and T. Kirita, "Panoramic findings for predicting eruption of mandibular premolars associated with dentigerous cyst after marsupialization," *Journal of Oral and Maxillofacial Surgery*, vol. 66, no. 2, pp. 272–276, 2008.

[12] Y. Yahara, Y. Kubota, T. Yamashiro, and K. Shirasuna, "Eruption prediction of mandibular premolars associated with dentigerous cysts," *Oral Surgery, Oral Medicine, Oral Pathology, Oral Radiology and Endodontology*, vol. 108, no. 1, pp. 28–31, 2009.

32

Artefacts in Cone Beam CT Mimicking an Extrapalatal Canal of Root-Filled Maxillary Molar

Carla Cristina Camilo,[1] Manoel Brito-Júnior,[1] André Luis Faria-e-Silva,[2] Alex Carvalho Quintino,[1] Adrianne Freire de Paula,[1] Antônio Miranda Cruz-Filho,[3] and Manoel Damião Sousa-Neto[3]

[1] *Department of Dentistry, State University of Montes Claros, Avenue Rui Braga s/n, 39401-089 Montes Claros, MG, Brazil*
[2] *Department of Dentistry, School of Dentistry, Federal University of Sergipe, Rua Cláudio Batista s/n, 49060-100 Aracaju, SE, Brazil*
[3] *Department of Restorative Dentistry, Faculty of Dentistry, University of São Paulo, Avenue Bandeirantes 3900, 14040-900 Ribeirão Preto, SP, Brazil*

Correspondence should be addressed to Manoel Brito-Júnior; manoelbritojr@gmail.com

Academic Editors: C. Evans and M. Manfredi

Despite the advantages of cone-beam computed tomography (CBCT), the images provided by this diagnostic tool can produce artifacts and compromise accurate diagnostic assessment. This paper describes an endodontic treatment of a maxillary molar where CBCT images suggested the presence of a nonexistent third root canal in the palatal root. An endodontic treatment was performed in a first maxillary molar with palatal canals, and the tooth was restored with a cast metal crown. The patient returned four years later presenting with a discomfort in chewing, which was reduced after occlusal adjustment. CBCT was prescribed to verify additional diagnostic information. Axial scans on coronal, middle, and apical palatal root sections showed images similar to a third root canal. However, sagittal scans demonstrated that these images were artifacts caused by root canal fillings. A careful interpretation of CBCT images in root-filled teeth must be done to avoid mistakes in treatment.

1. Introduction

Knowledge about the anatomy of the root canal system is essential for successful endodontic therapy and permits a correct diagnosis followed by thorough cleaning and shaping of root canals [1, 2]. An accurate observation of internal anatomy is important mainly in teeth presenting complex and variable configurations related to root canals, such as maxillary molars. Unfortunately, these teeth present important variations in number of roots and root canals. The presence of three roots (two buccal and one palatal) and three root canals is a frequent condition for this tooth. It is not uncommon for there to be a second root canal in the mesiobuccal root, increasing the total of root canals to four [2]; however, the presence of an additional root canal has been reported for mesiobuccal, distobuccal, and palatal roots [3–6]. These anatomical variations can compromise the endodontic therapy when not observed.

Traditionally, radiographs are used to assess the anatomic aspect of root canals, enabling verification of the number and location of root canals and the presence of curvatures that could hinder the instrumentation [7]. However, the correct visualization of the root canal system can be jeopardized by the two-dimensional view of radiographs, while the object evaluated presents three dimensions. Recently, the use of three-dimensional (3D) imaging techniques such as cone beam computed tomography (CBTC) has gained popularity in endodontic therapy [8].

The 3D images provided by CBCT permit the view of greater details of the root canal anatomy than radiographic images [9]. The improved evaluation of the internal anatomy of root canal systems is an important diagnostic tool for

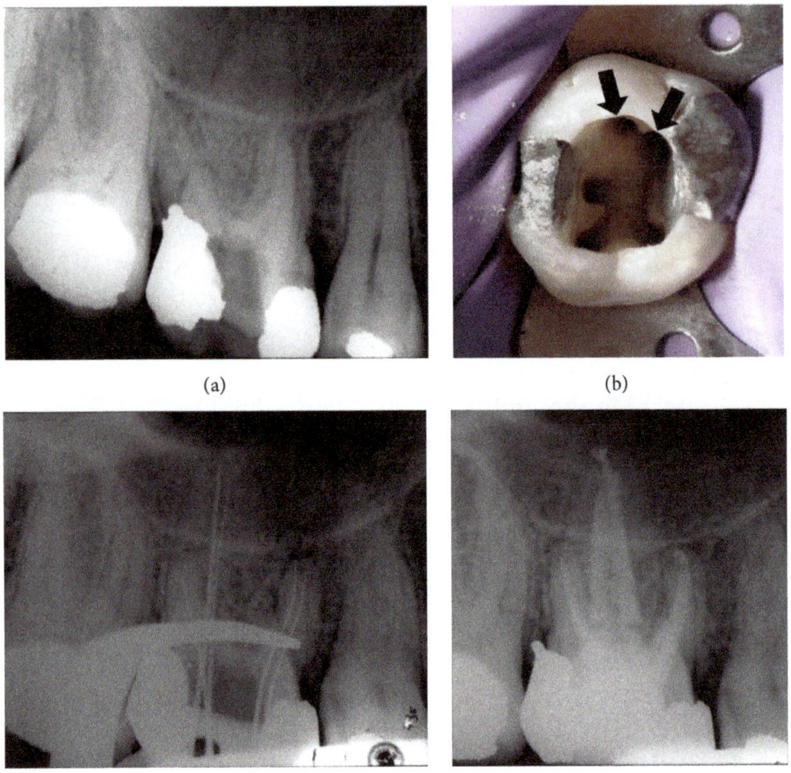

FIGURE 1: (a) Initial radiographic aspect of tooth number 3. (b) Endodontic access showing the presence of five root canal entrances. (c) Radiograph for working length determination. (d) Radiographic aspect after root canal fillings.

the proper therapy of all root canals in morphologically complex teeth [10, 11]. Despite these advantageous, however, artifacts can be produced in the CBCT images that may lead to a misdiagnosis related to the number and localization of root canals [12]. In this situation, an accurate clinical diagnosis assumes crucial importance to the prevention of unwanted procedure errors.

This paper describes the endodontic management of a first maxillary molar for which artifacts in a CBCT follow-up exam mimicked an extra palatal canal.

2. Case Presentation

A 27-year-old man was referred for endodontic treatment of tooth number 3. The patient related episodes of spontaneous pain in the previous week, while an emergency procedure was performed. Clinical examination revealed that the pulp chamber was exposed, and no response to thermal pulp testing (Endo-Ice, Maquira Indústria de Produtos Odontológicos Ltda, Maringá, PR, Brazil) was observed. Slight responses to palpation and percussion were verified. A periapical radiograph showed normality of the periapical region (Figure 1(a)). The diagnosis of pulp necrosis was established and the endodontic treatment initiated.

Under local anesthesia and rubber dam, the coronal access was performed and the root canals' entrance was explored using an endodontic explorer. Identified were the two mesiobuccal canals, the distobuccal canal, and, unexpectedly, two orifices in the palatal root, corresponding to mesio- and distopalatine canals (Figure 1(b)). After the root canals instrumentation, the radiograph taken for working length determination confirmed the presence of five root canals (Figure 1(c)). Chemomechanical preparation was performed by using ProTaper NiTi rotatory instruments (Dentsply-Maillefer, Ballaigues, Switzerland) and irrigation with 2.5% sodium hypochlorite. A calcium-hydroxide-based paste (Calen, SS White, Rio de Janeiro, RJ, Brazil) was used as intracanal dressing and the provisional restoration was performed with a zinc oxide and eugenol restorative material (IRM, Dentsply, Petrópolis, RJ, Brazil).

The patient returned for a second appointment after eight days. The temporary restoration was removed under local anesthesia and rubber dam. The intracanal dressing was removed, and the root canals were dried and filled with gutta-percha cones (Konne, Belo Horizonte, MG, Brazil) and sealer (Endofill, Dentsply, Petropolis, RJ, Brazil) by lateral condensation technique. Afterwards, the tooth was restored with composite resin.

Four years later, the patient returned to the clinic complaining of discomfort when chewing on tooth number 3, which had received a cast metal restoration approximately six months earlier. Clinical examination showed that the tooth had no tenderness on palpation and no mobility. The mean probing pocket depth was within normal limits. Slight pain

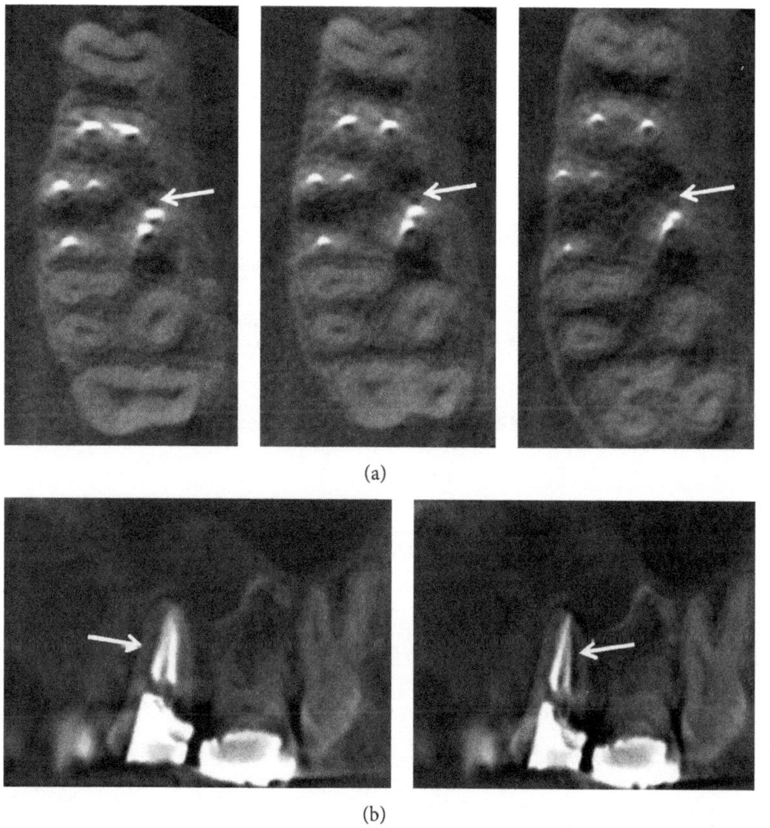

FIGURE 2: (a) From left to right, axial scans of coronal, middle, and apical root sections suggesting the presence of a third root canal in the palatal root (arrows). (b) Sagittal scans demonstrating that the third canal observed at previous images was an artifact (arrows). Note the presence of hypodense periapical areas on the palatal root.

to percussion was observed and the radiograph showed absence of periapical lesion. Upon checking the occlusion, a premature contact was detected on the metal restoration of tooth number 3. Occlusal adjustment was performed, resulting in a gradual resolution of the symptoms.

Despite this, the patient was advised that CBCT examination could be useful in providing additional information on the case. Thus, a small-volume CBCT scan (Kodak 9000 3D, Carestream Health, Inc., Rochester, NY, USA) of tooth number 3 with exposure parameters of 70 kV, 5.0 mA, and 0.076 mm (isotropic voxel) was obtained after informed consent from the patient. An image suggesting the presence of a third root canal in the palatal root was observed in the axial scans (Figure 2(a)); however, sagittal scans demonstrated that the previous images were artifacts caused by root canal fillings (Figure 2(b)). Small hypodense periapical areas also were observed in the sagittal views (Figure 2(b)). These images were possibly related to the occlusal trauma or to a healing process of a preoperative lesion not detected radiographically at the initiation of treatment. Thus, it was decided to monitor the case without any additional treatment.

3. Discussion

Additional anatomical information in maxillary molars is provided by CBCT images when compared with limited two-dimensional techniques [13–15]. Despite CBCT not being available during initial treatment in the present case, all root canals were identified and treated based on the operator's knowledge and skills [16]. Careful clinical inspection and suitable access to the cavity were performed, permitting the identification of two-canal orifices on the palatal root, which represents an unusual root canal configuration [3, 4]. CBCT was recommended at the follow-up period, considering the clinical findings and the importance of 3D images to identify untreated root canals [11]. At first, a diagnostic dilemma was established owing to the possible presence of an extra canal in the palatal root observed on CBCT images. However, these images were characterized as artifacts produced by root canal fillings after a detailed CBCT data assessment.

An understanding of CBCT technology, including its properties and limitations, is essential to prevent misleading findings. CBCT was introduced into dentistry in the late 1990s, and it is characterized as an imaging modality under constant improvement [8]. High-quality bony definition, low radiation dose, and compact design are advantages of CBCT scans over conventional computed tomography [8, 17]. In addition, CBCT allows a faster image reconstruction in the axial, sagittal, and coronal planes, providing 3D views for diagnosing and managing endodontic complications [9].

One disadvantage of CBCT is the scattered radiation that produces streaking image artifacts, which can prevent diagnostic accuracy. This problem generally occurs during data acquisition after lower jaw movement (motion artifacts) or when a metal object or a dense filling material exists on the tooth structure (metal artifacts) [18]. Untrue CBCT images were observed near metallic intracanal posts, jeopardizing the diagnosis of root perforations [19] and root fractures [20]. Metal artifacts apparently degrade the quality of CBCT images by increasing background noise with a simultaneous decrease in contrast [18]. These artifacts are caused by the beam-hardening effect (i.e., lower energy photons are absorbed in preference to higher-energy photons).

Scanning and reconstructed parameters similar to those used in this paper resulted in suitable image quality for root canal anatomy assessment [21]. The CBCT device used (Kodak 9000 3D) is categorized as small-volume CBCT, based on its scan field of view (FoV), which covers only few teeth or one jaw [8, 22]. Usually, small FoV provides better image quality with lower effective radiation and fewer artifacts when compared with medium and large FoV devices [22]. However, artifacts still occur using a small FoV, reducing the accuracy, sensitivity, and specificity of the CBCT technique, particularly in root-filled teeth [23. 24].

A careful interpretation of CBCT data adjusted to the diagnostic task is necessary to attain the examination goals [23]. Krithikadatta et al. [12] reported contradictory findings between CBCT images and clinical aspects evaluating the root canal anatomy of a mandibular first molar. They found clinically the existence of a single root canal within the mesial root, while CBCT artifacts mimicked an additional untreated canal. This challenging case showed the importance of recognizing imaging artifacts for differential diagnosis of anatomical root canal morphology [12]. In the present case, CBCT scans also suggested an extra canal, but the analysis of the images in different reconstructed planes provided sufficient information to correct diagnosis.

One major reason to interpret CBCT images with caution in the present case was the uncommon occurrence of three palatal canals in the maxillary molars, something only documented in few reports [24, 25]. On the other hand, the presence of an additional canal could justify the hypodense periapical areas, which would be representative of an apical periodontitis. In this scenario, a nonsurgical endodontic retreatment could be indicated; however, the final diagnosis was made in conjunction with the clinical findings, and the monitoring of the case was chosen. In summary, this case indicates that CBCT images should be interpreted carefully in root-filled teeth, taking into account the possibility of artifacts that mimic the presence of additional canals.

References

[1] F. J. Vertucci, "Root canal morphology and its relationship to endodontic procedures," *Endodontic Topics*, vol. 10, no. 1, pp. 3–29, 2005.

[2] M. Torabinejad and R. Walton, *Endodontics: Principles and Practiceedition*, Saunders/Elsevier, St. Louis, Mo, USA, 4th edition, 2009.

[3] F. J. Vertucci, "Root canal anatomy of the human permanent teeth," *Oral Surgery, Oral Medicine, Oral Pathology, Oral Radiology and Endodontology*, vol. 58, no. 5, pp. 589–599, 1984.

[4] Q. D. de Deus and B. Horizonte, "Frequency, location, and direction of the lateral, secondary, and accessory canals," *Journal of Endodontics*, vol. 1, no. 11, pp. 361–366, 1975.

[5] K. Gulabivala, T. H. Aung, A. Alavi, and Y. L. Ng, "Root and canal morphology of Burmese mandibular molars," *International Endodontic Journal*, vol. 34, no. 5, pp. 359–370, 2001.

[6] S. Sert, V. Aslanalp, and J. Tanalp, "Investigation of the root canal configurations of mandibular permanent teeth in the Turkish population," *International Endodontic Journal*, vol. 37, no. 7, pp. 494–499, 2004.

[7] G. Plotino, N. M. Grande, R. Pecci, R. Bedini, C. H. Pameijer, and F. Somma, "Three-dimensional imaging using microcomputed tomography for studying tooth macromorphology," *Journal of the American Dental Association*, vol. 137, no. 11, pp. 1555–1561, 2006.

[8] C. Durack and S. Patel, "Cone beam computed tomography in endodontics," *Brazilian Dental Journal*, vol. 23, no. 3, pp. 179–191, 2012.

[9] P. S. D'Addazio, C. N. Campos, M. Özcan, H. G. C. Teixeira, R. M. Passoni, and A. C. P. Carvalho, "A comparative study between cone-beam computed tomography and periapical radiographs in the diagnosis of simulated endodontic complications," *International Endodontic Journal*, vol. 44, no. 3, pp. 218–224, 2011.

[10] K. M. de Toubes, M. I. Côrtes, M. A. Valadares, L. C. Fonseca, E. Nunes, and F. F. Silveira, "Comparative analysis of accessory mesial canal identification in mandibular first molars by using four different diagnostic methods," *Journal of Endodontics*, vol. 38, no. 4, pp. 436–441, 2012.

[11] S. H. La, D. H. Jung, E. C. Kim, and K. S. Min, "Identification of independent middle mesial canal in mandibular first molar using cone-beam computed tomography imaging," *Journal of Endodontics*, vol. 36, no. 3, pp. 542–545, 2010.

[12] J. Krithikadatta, J. Kottoor, C. S. Karumaran, and G. Rajan, "Mandibular first molar having an unusual mesial root canal morphology with contradictory cone-beam computed tomography findings: a case report," *Journal of Endodontics*, vol. 36, no. 10, pp. 1712–1716, 2010.

[13] T. C. Blattner, N. George, C. C. Lee, V. Kumar, and C. D. J. Yelton, "Efficacy of cone-beam computed tomography as a modality to accurately identify the presence of second mesiobuccal canals in maxillary first and second molars: a pilot study," *Journal of Endodontics*, vol. 36, no. 5, pp. 867–870, 2010.

[14] F. Baratto Filho, S. Zaitter, G. A. Haragushiku, E. A. de Campos, A. Abuabara, and G. M. Correr, "Analysis of the internal anatomy of maxillary first molars by using different methods," *Journal of Endodontics*, vol. 35, no. 3, pp. 337–342, 2009.

[15] R. Bauman, W. Scarfe, S. J. Clark, J. Morelli, J. Scheetz, and A. Farman, "Ex vivo detection of mesiobuccal canals in maxillary molars using CBCT at four different isotropic voxel dimensions," *International Endodontic Journal*, vol. 44, no. 8, pp. 752–758, 2011.

[16] J. Corcoran, M. J. Apicella, and P. Mines, "The effect of operator experience in locating additional canals in maxillary molars," *Journal of Endodontics*, vol. 33, no. 1, pp. 15–17, 2007.

[17] J. B. Ludlow and M. Ivanovic, "Comparative dosimetry of dental CBCT devices and 64-slice CT for oral and maxillofacial radiology," *Oral Surgery, Oral Medicine, Oral Pathology, Oral Radiology and Endodontology*, vol. 106, no. 1, pp. 106–114, 2008.

[18] J. F. Barrett and N. Keat, "Artifacts in CT: recognition and avoidance," *Radiographics*, vol. 24, no. 6, pp. 1679–1691, 2004.

[19] M. R. Bueno, C. Estrela, J. A. P. de Figueiredo, and B. C. Azevedo, "Map-reading strategy to diagnose root perforations near metallic intracanal posts by using cone beam computed tomography," *Journal of Endodontics*, vol. 37, no. 1, pp. 85–90, 2011.

[20] F. F. Costa, B. F. Gaia, O. S. Umetsubo, and M. G. Cavalcanti, "Detection of horizontal root fracture with small-volume cone-beam computed tomography in the presence and absence of intracanal metallic post," *Journal of Endodontics*, vol. 37, no. 10, pp. 1456–1459, 2011.

[21] J. Michetti, D. Maret, J. P. Mallet, and F. Diemer, "Validation of cone beam computed tomography as a tool to explore root canal anatomy," *Journal of Endodontics*, vol. 36, no. 7, pp. 1187–1190, 2010.

[22] Z. D. Kajan and M. Taromsari, "Value of cone beam CT in detection of dental root fractures," *Dentomaxillofacial Radiology*, vol. 41, no. 1, pp. 3–10, 2012.

[23] S. Lofthag-Hansen, A. Thilander-Klang, and K. Gröndahl, "Evaluation of subjective image quality in relation to diagnostic task for cone beam computed tomography with different fields of view," *European Journal of Radiology*, vol. 80, no. 2, pp. 483–488, 2011

[24] M. Wong, "Maxillary first molar with three palatal canals," *Journal of Endodontics*, vol. 17, no. 6, pp. 298–299, 1991.

[25] F. Maggiore, Y. T. Jou, and S. Kim, "A six-canal maxillary first molar: case report," *International Endodontic Journal*, vol. 35, no. 5, pp. 486–491, 2002.

33

Gingival Anaplastic Large-Cell Lymphoma Mimicking Hyperplastic Benignancy as the First Clinical Manifestation of AIDS: A Case Report and Review of the Literature

Rafaela Elvira Rozza-de-Menezes,[1] Stefânia Jeronimo Ferreira,[1] Diogo Lenzi Capella,[1] Stephan Schwartz,[1] Ana Helena Willrich,[2] Lúcia de Noronha,[3] Aline Cristina Batista Rodrigues Johann,[4] and Paulo Henrique Couto Souza[1]

[1] *Department of Stomatology, Faculty of Dentistry, School of Health and Biosciences, Pontifical Catholic University of Paraná, Imaculada Conceição, 1155 Prado Velho, 80-215-901 Curitiba, PR, Brazil*
[2] *Departament of Pathology, Erasto Gaertner Hospital, Dr. Ovande do Amaral, 201-Jardim América, 81-520-060 Curitiba, PR, Brazil*
[3] *Department of Pathology, School of Medicine, Pontfical Catholic University of Paraná, Imaculada Conceição, 1155 Prado Velho, 80-215-901 Curitiba, PR, Brazil*
[4] *Department of Oral Pathology, Faculty of Dentistry, School of Health and Biosciences, Pontifical Catholic University of Paraná, Curitiba, Imaculada Conceição, 1155 Prado Velho, 80-215-901 Curitiba, PR, Brazil*

Correspondence should be addressed to Aline Cristina Batista Rodrigues Johann; aline.johann@pucpr.br

Academic Editors: M. Ashkenazi, M. A. Polack, and A. Scribante

This paper presents an unusual case of gingival ALCL, which mimicked a benign hyperplastic lesion that occurred in a 57-year-old white man representing the first clinical manifestation of acquired immunodeficiency syndrome (AIDS). The patient was referred to the Dental Clinic of PUCPR complaining of a lobulated nodule on the gingiva of his upper central incisors. The presence of advanced chronic periodontitis and dental plaque raised suspicion for a benignancy. An excisional biopsy was performed, and large pleomorphic cells with an abundant cytoplasm, sometimes containing prominent nucleoli and "Hallmark" cells, were observed through hematoxylin and eosin staining. The tumor cells showed strong CD30 expression, EMA, Ki-67, and LCA, and negative stain for $p80^{NPM/ALK}$, CKAE1/AE3, CD20, CD3, CD56, and CD15. The final diagnosis was ALCL (ALK-negative). Further laboratory tests revealed positivity for human immunodeficiency virus (HIV). The patient was submitted to chemotherapy, but four months after diagnosis, the patient died due to pneumonia and respiratory failure. Oral anaplastic large-cell lymphoma (ALCL) is a rare disorder. Only 5 cases involving the gingiva have been reported, and to our knowledge, this is the first case reported of the ALCL, which mimicked a hyperplastic benignancy as the first clinical manifestation of AIDS.

1. Introduction

Malignant lymphomas (MLs) are a large group of neoplasms affecting the lymphoid system and are subdivided into two main groups: Hodgkin's and non-Hodgkin's lymphomas (NHLs) [1]. ML is considered an opportunistic neoplasm because it frequently affects immunocompromised patients. The prevalence of ML has increased considerably with improved acquired immune deficiency syndrome (AIDS) survivorship [2, 3]. NHLs appear in 3% of HIV-seropositive patients [4]. The NHLs may be present outside the lymphoid system, in which case they are called extranodal [5]. This type of lymphoma is located at an extranodal site in 40% of cases [5] and its extranodal presentation occurs in almost 75% of human-immunodeficiency-virus- (HIV-) seropositive patients [2]. Furthermore, only 2% to 3% of these extranodal cases occur in the oral cavity [6].

In the group of NHLs, mature T cell and natural killer (NK) cell neoplasms make up only 12% of NHL cases worldwide [1]. Within this heterogeneous category, anaplastic large-cell lymphoma (ALCL) is found [7, 8] and is listed in the Revised European-American Classification of Lymphoid Neoplasms (REAL) as an independent entity [9]. A couple of ALCL cases have been reported, although some were the B-cell phenotype now classified as an anaplastic type of diffuse large B-cell lymphoma [10]; therefore, these cases were excluded from the present review. ALCL is characterized by proliferation of the anaplastic large lymphoid cells with abundant cytoplasm and strong expression of CD30 antigen; however, its final diagnosis is a challenge for oral pathologists [8, 11–17]. Two distinct clinical entities of ALCL are recognized by the World Health Organization (WHO) lymphoma classification: cutaneous and systemic lymphomas [1, 5]. The cutaneous ALCLs are characterized by indolent growth and may show spontaneous remission and good prognosis [18, 19]. The systemic ALCLs can be ALK-positive or -negative [18]. The ALK-positive ALCLs usually occur in male pediatric patients and show a good prognosis taking into account their affective response to chemotherapy, whereas the ALK-negative ALCLs occur in elderly patients and present a poor prognosis [18, 20].

ALCL especially affects the skin of the body [6]. This T-type lymphoma in the oral cavity is an extremely rare disorder characterizing 1% of lymphomas overall [19]. From the scientific literature, we found around 15 cases of ALCL in the oral cavity [2, 6, 8, 11–17, 21, 22]. Only 5 cases of ALCL located in gingiva have been reported in the literature [12, 17, 22], and our case is the fourth reported occurrence of ALCL in the oral cavity of a HIV-seropositive patient [2, 11]. Besides, this paper is the first to present an unusual case of oral ALK-negative ALCL that mimicked a benign hyperplastic lesion as a first clinical manifestation of AIDS.

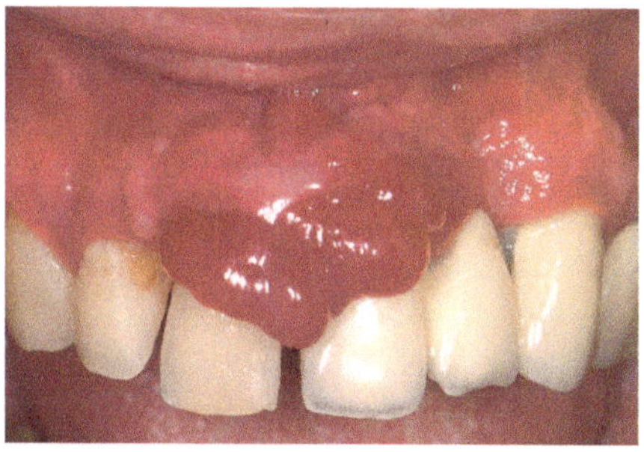

FIGURE 1: Clinical presentation: a 2,5 cm red nodule, pedunculated, located on the gingival between upper central incisors.

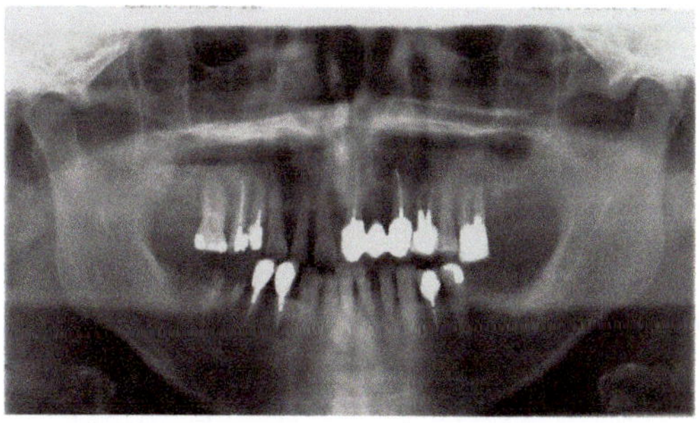

FIGURE 2: Radiographic image: panoramic radiography showing the extensive bone resorption in the anterior area of the maxilla compatible with advanced periodontal disease.

2. Case Report

A 57-year-old white man was referred to the Dental Clinic of PUCPR complaining of an asymptomatic hyperplastic lesion on the gingiva of his upper central incisors, which had grown significantly in the last two months. The patient was a nonsmoker and his medical history did not reveal other relevant information. The extraoral examination showed a small swelling of the upper lip and absence of cervical lymphadenopathy. The intraoral examination showed advanced chronic periodontitis and the presence of a lobulated reddish nodule, pedunculated, measuring around 2.5 cm on the gingival area between both upper central incisors which had mobility and accumulation of dental plaque (Figure 1). The lesion did not have an ulcerated surface, and palpation revealed a soft consistency with bleeding on the surface. Panoramic radiography showed a significant resorption of bone mainly in the anterior area of the maxillary, compatible with advanced chronic periodontitis (Figure 2).

Taking into account that the first impression of the lesion revealed clinical characteristics of a benignancy, as the pedunculated nodule, circumscribed, freely moveable, the presence of dental plaque, and advanced chronic periodontitis, we initially suspected that it could be related to a reactive hyperplastic lesion. These lesions include pyogenic granuloma, focal fibrous hyperplasia, peripheral giant cell granuloma, and peripheral ossifying fibroma. Therefore, considering these main hypotheses, an excisional biopsy of the nodule was performed under local anesthesia. Furthermore, the patient was referred for periodontal treatment.

Hematoxylin and eosin-stained sections showed a lesion characterized by a diffuse proliferation of lymphoid tumor cells underneath an epithelium (Figure 3(a)). The slices also showed large pleomorphic cells with an abundant cytoplasm, sometimes containing prominent nucleoli. "Hallmark" cells with eccentric, horse-shoe, or kidney-shaped nuclei were also observed (Figure 3(b)). The tumor cells frequently demonstrated mitotic figures. Immunohistochemical analysis using a streptavidin-biotin protocol [14] was performed with the antibodies: CKAE1/AE3, CD20, CD3, CD30, Ki-67, epithelial membrane antigen (EMA), CD56, leukocyte common antigen (LCA), $p80^{NPM/ALK}$, and CD15. The tumor cells showed strong CD30 expression with a membrane and Golgi distribution in the majority of tumor cells (Figure 3(c)). Ki-67 positive stain was observed in 90% of tumor cells (Figure 3(d)). Positive stain in tumor cells was also identified for EMA and LCA. Negative stain was identified for $p80^{NPM/ALK}$, CKAE1/AE3, CD56, and CD15. The tumor was a null-cell type (negatively stained for CD20 and CD3). Based on clinical, histological, and immunohistochemical findings, the final diagnosis was extranodal ALK-negative ALCL.

The patient was referred to a specialized oncology hospital where further laboratory and imaging tests showed positivity for HIV, negativity for both hepatitis B and C, normal full blood count proportions of white and red blood

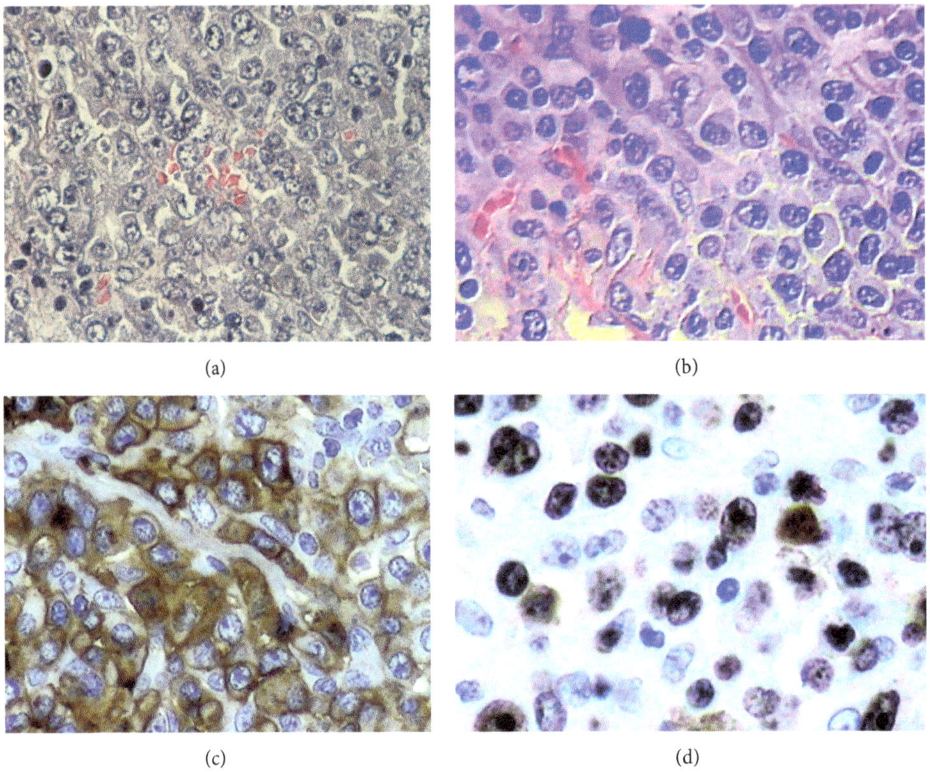

FIGURE 3: Histologic features: (a) diffuse proliferation of lymphoid tumor cells (hematoxylin-eosin stain (HE), magnification ×200) was observed. (b) Large pleomorphic cells with an abundant cytoplasm, sometimes containing prominent nucleoli, were verified. "Hallmark" cells with eccentric, horse-shoe, or kidney-shaped nuclei were also identified (HE, magnification ×400). Immunohistochemical findings: sections showing tumor cells are positive for (c) CD30 with a membrane and Golgi distribution (streptavidin-biotin, ×400 magnification) and (d) Ki-67 (streptavidin-biotin, ×400 magnification).

cells and platelets, and absence of lymphadenopathies and metastasis. The following chemotherapy protocol consisted of six cycles of CHOP (cyclophosphamide 750 mg/m^2, doxorubicin 50 mg/m^2, vincristine 2 mg, and oral prednisone 100 mg) for five days [23]. However, four months after diagnosis, the patient died due to pneumonia and respiratory failure.

3. Discussion

This case report presents a rare case of ALCL in an extranodal site of a Brazilian male HIV-seropositive patient. Since ALCL was first described as a clinical entity by Stein et al. (1985) [20], this lesion was classified as Ki-1+ ALCL and currently as Ki-1 (CD30) [17], which corresponds to a cohesive proliferation of large pleomorphic cells that express CD30. The ALCL is subdivided according to the immunohistochemical features in precursor T cells or null cells, in 60% and 25% of the cases, respectively [2]. Therefore, immunohistochemistry is imperative for the correct diagnosis of ALCL considering that the cells are positive for CD30 antigen and several other markers such as EMA that is present in slightly more than 50% of cases [2]. LCA is usually positive but may be used negative in 30% to 40% of cases [2]. In most cases, other markers such as Ki-67, CD3, and CD45RO (T-cell phenotype), TIA-1 (T-cell intracytoplasmic antigen-1), perforin, granzyme B, and p80$^{NPM/ALK}$ will be positive [6, 17].

The clinicopathologic features of ALK-carrying ALCLs were first investigated by Shiota and Mori [24]. The authors found that ALK-positive is a distinctive entity clinically and pathogenetically and should be differentiated from ALK-negative. Indeed, based on the most recent findings, the WHO classification currently considers two ALCL types, negative and ALK-positive [25, 26]. The tumors that show a positive reaction for ALK have greater cell proliferation and can show a relatively better prognosis [19]. Recently, studies have proposed that proteins such as aberrant fusion protein (NPM-ALK), JAK-STAT, and PI3K/STAT may be a potential target in ALK-positive lymphomas [26–28]. The findings about specific antigens also suggest that ALK represents an ideal tumor antigen for vaccination-based therapies of ALCL and other ALK-positive tumors [29]. On the other hand, the cases of ALK-negative ALCL show an inaccurate behavior with a relatively unfavorable prognosis [18]. To make the diagnosis of ALK-negative ALCL, there must be a large cell predominant population with abundant cytoplasm and pleomorphic, embryo or hallmark nuclei or wreath-like giant cells, and strong CD30 expression with a membrane and Golgi distribution in virtually every cell with a highly anaplastic T-cell phenotype [17, 19]. As the current case did not express ALK, it was classified as an ALK-negative ALCL. In addition, the tumor did not show expression of NK or T-cell markers; therefore, it was classified as a null cell lymphoma. ALK-negative ALCL normally occurs in adults

Table 1: Clinical, radiological, and ALK-profile features of oral anaplastic large-cell lymphomas.

Age	Gender	Oral area	Clinical findings	Radiographic findings	HIV	Diagnostic hypothesis	ALK	References
ND	ND	ND	ND	ND	ND	ND	ND	Takahashi et al. [8]
36	M	Retromolar trigone	Mass with ulcerated surface	Diffuse radiolucency with poorly margins	+	Nonspecific infection	ND	Hicks et al. [2]
42	M	Retromolar trigone	Enlargement surrounding a crateriform ulcer	Not relevant	+	Pericoronitis or nonspecific infection	ND	Hicks et al. [2]
12	F	Gingiva	Scaly, swollen, and bleeding gingival surface	Bone resorption causing teeth displacement	+	Gingivitis	ND	Willard et al. [11]
12	M	Hard palate	Mass involving the nasal cartilage and floor of the orbit	ND	ND	ND	ND	Papadimitriou et al. [21]
75	F	Upper gingiva	Periodontitis (deep pockets) and redness of the gingiva	Bone resorption adjacent to teeth 11, 12, and 13	ND	Periodontitis	ND	Rosenberg et al. [12]
61	M	Lower gingiva	Well-delimited ulceration	ND	ND	Eosinophilic granuloma	ND	Rosenberg et al. [12]
48	M	Upper lip	Nonfluctuant, firm, and swelling lesion	ND	ND	Nonspecific infection	ND	Chandu et al. [13]
76	F	Upper lip	Well-delimited ulceration	ND	ND	ND	ND	Chim et al. [14]
65	F	Hard palate, buccal mucosa, and floor of the mouth	Well-delimited ulceration	ND	–	ALCL	ND	Born et al. [15]
77	M	Left side of soft palate	Mass with ulcerated surface	ND	–	Lymphoma, salivary gland neoplasm, or necrotizing sialometaplasia	ND	Savarrio et al. [6]
77	M	Tongue	Nodule with ulcerated surface	A low density mass	ND	Nonspecific infection	+	Notani et al. [16]
76	F	Upper and lower gingiva	Swollen gingival	Bone resorption	ND	Chronic marginal periodontitis	–	Matsumoto et al. [17]
34	F	Upper gingiva	White/gray ulcerated mass with erythematous border	ND	ND	Lymphomatoid papulosis, fungal infection, or traumatic ulcer	–	Grandhi et al. [22]
53	M	Tongue	Mass with ulcerated surface	ND	ND	ND	–	Grandhi et al. [22]
57	M	Gingiva in maxillary incisor area	A lobulated reddish nodule, bleedin,g and pedunculated	Bone resorption	+	Reactive hyperplasic lesion[a]	–	Present case

ND: not described, F: female; M: male; +: positive; –: negative; [a]includes pyogenic granuloma, focal fibrous hyperplasia, peripheral giant cell granuloma, and peripheral ossifying fibroma.

(40–65 years) with a modest male prevalence [3], as seen in our patient, a 57-year-old man.

Based on cases found in the review of the literature (Table 1), there is a slight male prediction (female : male, 1 : 1.5), and the patients presented at a mean age of 53.4 years old (standard deviation, 22.4). Most of the tumors were located in the gingiva (5 cases), followed by the palate (3 cases), tongue (2 cases), retromolar trigone (2 cases), lip (2 cases), floor of the mouth (1 case), and buccal mucosa (1 case). The main radiographic findings were bone resorption [11, 12, 17], and the main diagnostic hypothesis more frequent is nonspecific infection (4 cases) [2, 13, 16]. To the best of our knowledge, the present case reports the first gingival ALCL, which mimicked a benign hyperplastic lesion as the first clinical manifestation of AIDS. Positivity to HIV was reported in 3 cases [2, 11]. About 14% of the ALCL cases were ALK-negative [17]; our case is the fourth case reported [17, 22]. This highlights that studies about ALK protein were developed in the 1990s. Only in 2002 [16], $p80^{NPM/ALK}$ was first included in the immunohistochemical studies involving oral ALCLs. Currently, there is only one case reported that showed ALK expression in ALCL involving oral cavity [16].

Interestingly, cases of ALCL present in the gingiva also suggested that the majority of clinical aspects mimicked gingivitis or advanced chronic periodontitis with ulcers, bleeding, and swelling. All clinical aspects of ALCLs in oral cavity were associated with extensive bone resorption, which made the clinical diagnosis of ALCL more difficult. Clinical cases have reported other entities of oral lymphomas that mimicked a benignancy in HIV-seropositive patients [30]. We found only 15 cases of oral ALCL reported in the English literature (Table 1). The current case showed an unusual appearance of a reactive hyperplastic lesion associated with advanced chronic periodontitis. Indeed, this fact emphasizes the need for a thorough clinical history, HIV investigation, and also high index suspicion in both dentists and pathologists.

Oral lymphomas also occur more frequently in patients with HIV infection [31] as well as those iatrogenically immunosuppressed [31, 32]. Mechanisms other than the loss of immune surveillance appear to be involved with HIV-associated malignances [11]. In our case, the oral lymphoma with distinctive clinical appearance and associated with periodontitis occurred in an HIV-seropositive patient and was the first manifestation of AIDS. Some studies have also suggested that HIV is a risk factor for the development of ALCL, but this hypothesis is not clear yet. Similarly, the relative risk for the development of an NHL in HIV patients is approximately 3%, making the prognosis worse [2, 4]. A few cases of oral ALCL in patients with HIV infection have been reported in the literature [2, 11]. It is important to point out that ALCL prognosis is usually associated with immune status, and the death of the patient in this case due to the presence of pneumonia and respiratory failure was directly related to his poor immune systemic condition [20].

ALCL is normally treated by intensive chemotherapy with CHOP (cyclophosphamide 750 mg/m^2, doxorubicin 50 mg/m^2, vincristine 2 mg, and oral prednisone 100 mg from the first to the fifth day of chemotherapy) [23]. This CHOP regimen was administered every 3 weeks for a total of six cycles. Several studies demonstrate the high rate of complete remission (70%–95%) and 70%–85% long-term overall survival [23]. However, unfortunately, in the current case, the patient died.

4. Summary

In our case, it is important to highlight that the rapid growth of the lesion in the last two months reported by the patient and the presence of dental plaque and advanced chronic periodontitis indicated a reactive process in the gingiva. For this reason, the first decision to make an excisional biopsy of the lesion was kept. It is also important to stress that, if it was known that the patient was HIV-positive, our conduct would be completely different. Unfortunately, the final diagnosis was a malignant lesion.

We presented an unusual case of ALK-negative ALCL on the gingiva associated with advanced chronic periodontitis that mimicked some clinical features of a hyperplastic gingival benignancy, which manifested in a 57-year-old HIV-seropositive man. ALCL is a systemic malignant disease characterized by the extranodal type which rarely occurs in the oral cavity as the first manifestation of acquired immunodeficiency syndrome. Thus, we emphasize the importance of an accurate clinical, including HIV investigation, histological, and immunohistochemical analysis of oral lesions to establish the correct diagnosis of those lesions which in daily practice are considered benign.

Disclosure

The authors declare no conflict of interests concerning this paper. The authors have full control of all primary data of their paper. This paper is not supported by any institutional or corporate affiliation.

Acknowledgments

The authors thank Ana Paula Camargo Martins and Marina Viola Azevedo for their most valuable laboratory technical assistance.

References

[1] S. A. Rosenerg, C. W. Berand, and B. W. Brown Jr., "National Cancer Institute sponsored study of classifications of non-Hodgkin's lymphomas. Summary and description of a working formulation for clinical usage," *Cancer*, vol. 49, no. 10, pp. 2112–2135, 1982.

[2] M. J. Hicks, C. M. Flaitz, C. M. Nichols, M. A. Luna, and M. V. Gresik, "Intraoral presentation of anaplastic large-cell Ki-1 lymphoma in association with HIV infection," *Oral Surgery Oral Medicine and Oral Pathology*, vol. 76, no. 1, pp. 73–81, 1993.

[3] E. S. Jaffe, N. L. Harris, H. Stein, and J. V. Vardiman, "World Health Organization: classification of tumors. Pathology and genetics: tumours of haematopoietic and lymphoid tissues,"

in *Pathology and Genetics of Tumours of Haematopoietic and Lymphoid Tissues*, pp. 119–205, IARC, Lyon, France, 2001.

[4] V. Beral, T. Peterman, R. Berkelman, and H. Jaffe, "AIDS-associated non-Hodgkin lymphoma," *The Lancet*, vol. 337, no. 8745, pp. 805–809, 1991.

[5] S. Kemp, G. Gallagher, S. Kabani, V. Noonan, and C. O'Hara, "Oral non-Hodgkin's lymphoma: review of the literature and World Health Organization classification with reference to 40 cases," *Oral Surgery, Oral Medicine, Oral Pathology, Oral Radiology and Endodontology*, vol. 105, no. 2, pp. 194–201, 2008.

[6] L. Savarrio, J. Gibson, D. J. Dunlop, N. O'Rourke, and E. J. Fitzsimons, "Spontaneous regression of an anaplastic large cell lymphoma in the oral cavity: first reported case and review of the literature," *Oral Oncology*, vol. 35, no. 6, pp. 609–613, 1999.

[7] O. Merkel, L. Kenner, and S. D. Turner, "Anaplastic large cell lymphoma: the current state of play from a European prospective as presented at the second annual meeting of the European Research Initiative on ALCL, 27-28 June 2011," *Leukemia*, vol. 25, no. 12, pp. 1795–1796, 2011.

[8] H. Takahashi, S. Fujita, H. Okabe, N. Tsuda, and F. Tezuka, "Immunophenotypic analysis of extranodal Non-Hodgkin's lymphomas in the oral cavity," *Pathology Research and Practice*, vol. 189, no. 3, pp. 300–311, 1993.

[9] N. L. Harris, E. S. Jaffe, H. Stein et al., "A revised European-American classification of lymphoid neoplasms: a proposal from the International Lymphoma Study Group," *Blood*, vol. 84, no. 5, pp. 1361–1392, 1994.

[10] M. Piris, D. C. Brown, K. C. Gatter, and D. Y. Mason, "CD30 expression in non-Hodgkin's lymphoma," *Histopathology*, vol. 17, no. 3, pp. 211–218, 1990.

[11] C. C. Willard, R. D. Foss, T. J. Hobbs, and P. L. Auclair, "Primary anaplastic large cell (KI-1 positive) lymphoma of the mandible as the initial manifestation of acquired immunodeficiency syndrome in a pediatric patient," *Oral Surgery, Oral Medicine, Oral Pathology, Oral Radiology and*, vol. 80, no. 1, pp. 67–70, 1995.

[12] A. Rosenberg, D. H. Biesma, D. M. D. S. Sie-Go, and P. J. Slootweg, "Primary extranodal CD30-positive T-cell non-Hodgkin's lymphoma of the oral mucosa: report of two cases," *International Journal of Oral and Maxillofacial Surgery*, vol. 25, no. 1, pp. 57–59, 1996.

[13] A. Chandu, D. A. Mitchell, and A. M. Corrigan, "Cutaneous CD30 positive large T cell lymphoma of the upper lip: a rare presentation," *British Journal of Oral and Maxillofacial Surgery*, vol. 35, no. 3, pp. 193–195, 1997.

[14] C. S. Chim, A. C. L. Chan, and L. Raymond, "Primary CD30-positive anaplastic large cell lymphoma of the lip," *Oral Oncology*, vol. 34, no. 4, pp. 313–315, 1998.

[15] S. Born, G. Gaber, K. Willgeroth, U. Wagner, E. Haneke, and W. C. Marsch, "Metastasising malignant lymphoma mimicking necrotising and hyperplastic gingivostomatitis," *European Journal of Dermatology*, vol. 9, no. 7, pp. 569–573, 1999.

[16] K. Notani, M. Shindoh, T. Takami, Y. Yamazaki, T. Kohgo, and H. Fukuda, "Anaplastic large cell lymphoma (ALCL) in the oral mucosa with repeating recurrence and spontaneous regression of ulceration: report of a case.," *Oral Medicine & Pathology*, vol. 7, no. 2, pp. 79–82, 2002.

[17] N. Matsumoto, H. Ohki, S. Mukae et al., "Anaplastic large cell lymphoma in gingiva: case report and literature review," *Oral Surgery, Oral Medicine, Oral Pathology, Oral Radiology and Endodontology*, vol. 106, no. 4, pp. e29–e34, 2008.

[18] R. L. ten Berge, J. J. Oudejans, G. J. Ossenkoppele, and C. J. L. M. Meijer, "ALK-negative systemic anaplastic large cell lymphoma: differential diagnostic and prognostic aspects—a review," *Journal of Pathology*, vol. 200, no. 1, pp. 4–15, 2003.

[19] E. Campo, A. Chott, M. C. Kinney et al., "Update on extranodal lymphomas. Conclusions of the Workshop held by the EAHP and the SH in Thessaloniki, Greece," *Histopathology*, vol. 48, no. 5, pp. 481–504, 2006.

[20] H. Stein, D. Y. Mason, and J. Gerdes, "The expression of the Hodgkin's disease associated antigen Ki-1 in reactive and neoplastic lymphoid tissue: evidence that Reed-Sternberg cells and histiocytic malignancies are derived from activated lymphoid cells," *Blood*, vol. 66, no. 4, pp. 848–858, 1985.

[21] J. C. Papadimitriou, L. V. Abruzzo, P. M. Bourquin, and C. B. Drachenberg, "Correlation of light microscopic, immunocytochemical and ultrastructural cytomorphology of anaplastic large cell Ki-1 lymphoma, an activated lymphocyte phenotype: a case report," *Acta Cytologica*, vol. 40, no. 6, pp. 1283–1288, 1996.

[22] A. Grandhi, A. L. Boros, N. Berardo, R. F. Reich, and P. D. Freedman, "Two cases of CD30+, anaplastic lymphoma kinase (ALK)-negative anaplastic large cell lymphoma with oral manifestations," *Oral Surgery, Oral Medicine, Oral Pathology, Oral Radiology*, vol. 115, no. 2, pp. e41–e47, 2013.

[23] P. Porcu and C. R. Nichols, "Evaluation and management of the "new" lymphoma entities: mantle cell lymphoma, lymphoma of mucosa-associated lymphoid tissue, anaplastic large-cell lymphoma, and primary mediastinal B-cell lymphoma," *Current Problems in Cancer*, vol. 22, no. 5, pp. 283–368, 1998.

[24] M. Shiota and S. Mori, "Anaplastic large cell lymphomas expressing the novel chimeric protein p80npm/alk: a distinct clinicopathologic entity," *Leukemia*, vol. 11, supplement 3, pp. 538–540, 1997.

[25] G. Inghirami and S. A. Pileri, "Anaplastic large-cell lymphoma," *Seminars in Diagnostic Pathology*, vol. 28, no. 3, pp. 190–201, 2011.

[26] P. P. Piccaluga, A. Gazzola, C. Mannu et al., "Pathobiology of anaplastic large cell lymphoma," *Advances in Hematology*, vol. 2010, Article ID 345053, 10 pages, 2010.

[27] H. M. Amin, T. J. McDonnell, Y. Ma et al., "Selective inhibition of STAT3 induces apoptosis and G1 cell cycle arrest in ALK-positive anaplastic large cell lymphoma," *Oncogene*, vol. 23, no. 32, pp. 5426–5434, 2004.

[28] H. M. Amin, L. J. Medeiros, Y. Ma et al., "Inhibition of JAK3 induces apoptosis and decreases anaplastic lymphoma kinase activity in anaplastic large cell lymphoma," *Oncogene*, vol. 22, no. 35, pp. 5399–5407, 2003.

[29] R. Chiarle, C. Martinengo, C. Mastini et al., "The anaplastic lymphoma kinase is an effective oncoantigen for lymphoma vaccination," *Nature Medicine*, vol. 14, no. 6, pp. 676–680, 2008.

[30] N. Bagul, G. S. Mamatha, and A. Mahalle, "Plasmablastic lymphoma of gingiva mimicking a reactive lesion: a case report," *Case Reports in Dentistry*, vol. 2012, Article ID 259307, 4 pages, 2012.

[31] E. Zapater, J. V. Bagán, F. Carbonell, and J. Basterra, "Malignant lymphoma of the head and neck," *Oral Diseases*, vol. 16, no. 2, pp. 119–128, 2010.

[32] B. Safai, B. Diaz, and J. Schwartz, "Malignant neoplasms associated with human immunodeficiency virus infection," *Ca-A Cancer Journal for Clinicians*, vol. 42, no. 2, pp. 74–95, 1992.

Splinting of Longitudinal Fracture: An Innovative Approach

Rashmi Bansal, Priyanka Chowdhary, Anuraag Gurtu, Nakul Mehrotra, and Abhinav Kishore

Department of Conservative Dentistry & Endodontics, Institute of Dental Sciences, Bareilly 243006, India

Correspondence should be addressed to Rashmi Bansal; drrashmirajeshbansal@gmail.com

Academic Editor: Jiiang H. Jeng

Trauma may result in craze lines on the enamel surface, one or more fractured cusps of posterior teeth, cracked tooth syndrome, splitting of posterior teeth, and vertical fracture of root. Out of these, management of some fractures is of great challenge and such teeth are generally recommended for extraction. Literature search reveals attempts to manage such fractures by full cast crown, orthodontic wires, and so forth, in which consideration was given to extracoronal splinting only. However, due to advancement in materials and technologies, intracoronal splinting can be achieved as well. In this case report, longitudinal fractures in tooth #27, tooth #37, and tooth #46 had occurred. In #27, fracture line was running mesiodistally involving the pulpal floor resulting in a split tooth. In teeth 37 and 46, fractures of the mesiobuccal cusp and mesiolingual cusp were observed, respectively. They were restored with cast gold inlay and full cast crown, respectively. Longitudinal fracture of 27 was treated with an innovative approach using intracanal reinforced composite with Ribbond, external reinforcement with an orthodontic band, and full cast metal crown to splint the split tooth.

1. Introduction

Conservation is becoming the basis of dentistry due to advancements in adhesive materials and technologies [1]. Longitudinal tooth fractures, which were once considered irreparable, can now be preserved [2]. The success of such teeth depends on its early identification and management. Based on location, direction, extent, prognosis, and treatment modalities, they can be classified as craze lines on the enamel surface, one or more fractured cusps of posterior teeth, cracked tooth syndrome, splitting of posterior tooth, and vertical fracture of root [3].

Craze lines are the least complicated type of fractures, extending on any surface buccally or lingually running through the marginal ridges. Fractured cusp initiating from the crown may extend subgingivally, through the buccal or lingual groove. Split tooth type of fractures has subgingival extension involving both the marginal ridges. The more centered the split occlusally, the greater the tendency to extend apically [2].

Posterior tooth fractures occur mainly due to masticatory forces, large restoration, or endodontically treated teeth and rarely due to acute trauma [4, 5]. Management of different longitudinal fractures depends upon the extent of fracture line and vitality of the tooth (Figure 1). Amongst various types of longitudinal fractures, the most devastating and controversial to treat is the split tooth involving the pulp chamber. A literature search for the management of split tooth reveals that if the fracture extends to a root surface, the mobile segment can be removed followed by surgical crown lengthening and orthodontic extrusion of the retained segment [2]. The rationale behind such treatment is that when fracture line extends below the attachment it becomes a site for infection, subsequently leading to bony defect. If the fractured segment of the split tooth is immobile, in such situation the cusp removal is not required; instead a full coverage restoration can be placed to hold the segments. For reinforcement-ligature wires [6], composite resin [7], adhesives [8], full coverage crowns, intentional reimplantation [9], and lasers like CO_2 and Nd-YAG, used to fuse the fracture segments [10, 11], have been successfully tried. In all these cases, the fracture line involving the pulpal floor was sealed with adhesive restorations, which is not a bioactive material and cannot promote cementogenesis at fracture site in the furcation area.

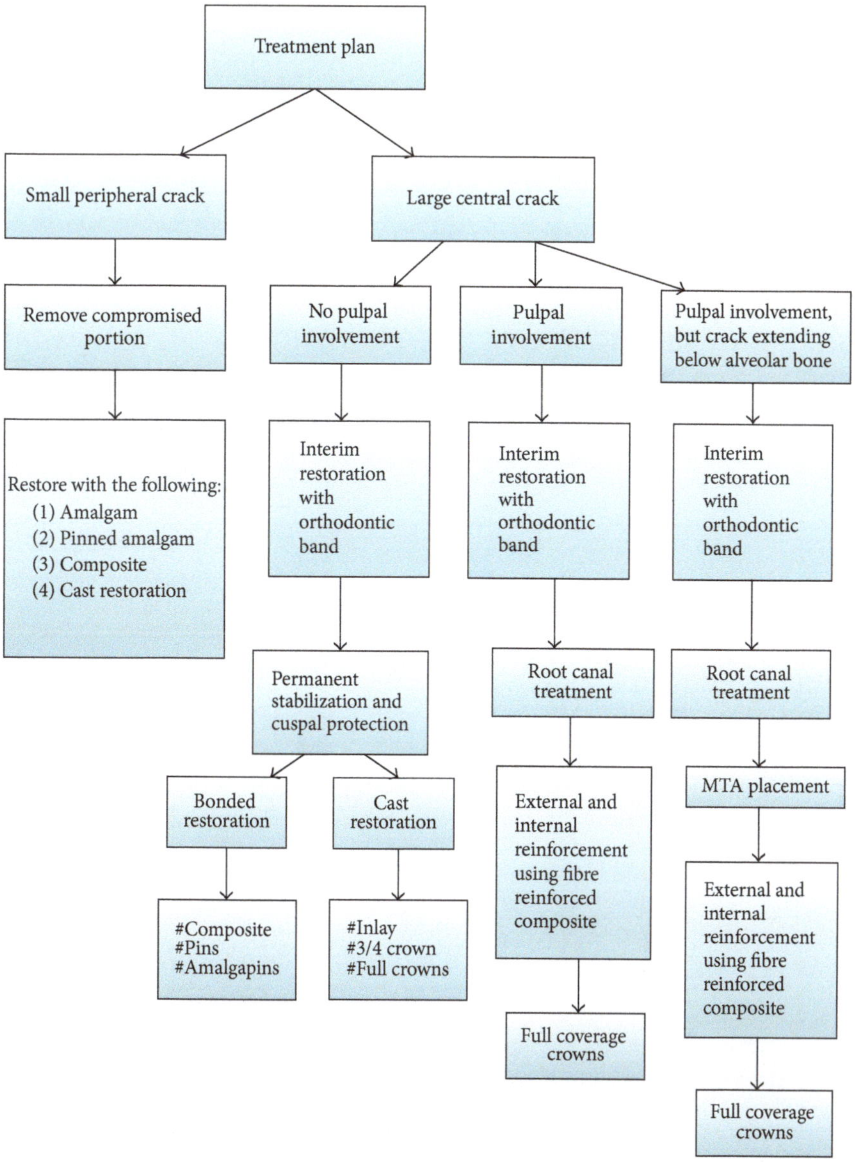

FIGURE 1: Treatment protocol for longitudinal fracture of teeth.

This paper presents an innovative approach to the management of split tooth (tooth #27) due to trauma by internal and external reinforcement. Cementogenesis was promoted at the fracture site in the furcation area by using MTA as a bioactive material. Further, in the same patient, fractured cusps of teeth 37 and 46 were also successfully managed by cast gold inlay and full cast crown, respectively.

2. Case Presentation

A male patient, 19 years of age, came to the Department of Conservative Dentistry and Endodontics with chief complaint of multiple fractured teeth in both upper and lower jaws causing pain and discomfort for the last two weeks. The patient gave a history of trauma two weeks ago due to injury by hand pump handle. Extraoral examination revealed no significant findings. Intraoral examination of all quadrants revealed longitudinal fractures involving 27, 37, and 46 (Figures 2–9).

On visual inspection of 27, the fracture line was running mesiodistally involving both the marginal ridges (Figures 2 and 7). The fracture segments cannot be displaced, but they can be visualized by wedging with a probe (Figure 2). There was no dentine between the fractured segments on the pulpal floor. The fracture line had extended subgingivally through the pulp chamber into the furcation area. Exploration of periodontium along the fracture line indicates no sign of periodontal attachment loss, although tooth was tender on percussion and nonvital on pulp testing. An intraoral periapical radiograph revealed that lamina dura of mesiobuccal

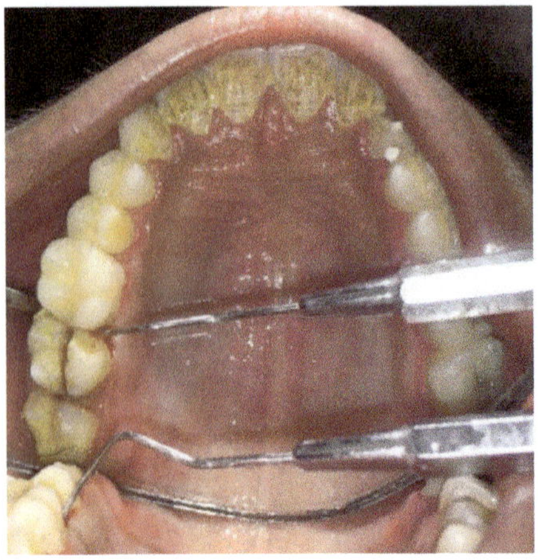

FIGURE 2: Preoperative photograph showing split tooth of 27.

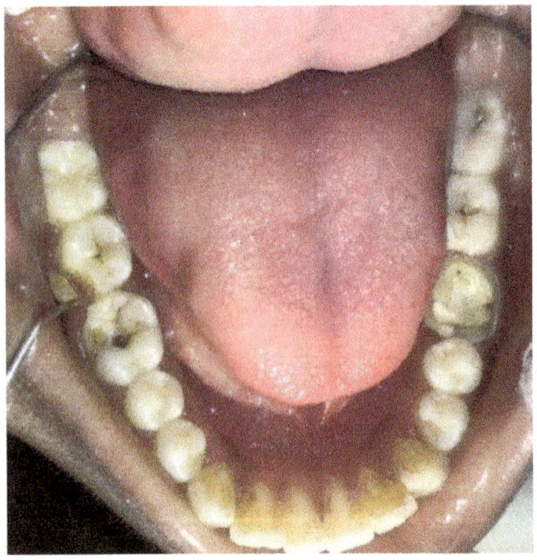

FIGURE 3: Preoperative photograph showing fractured cusps in 37 and 46.

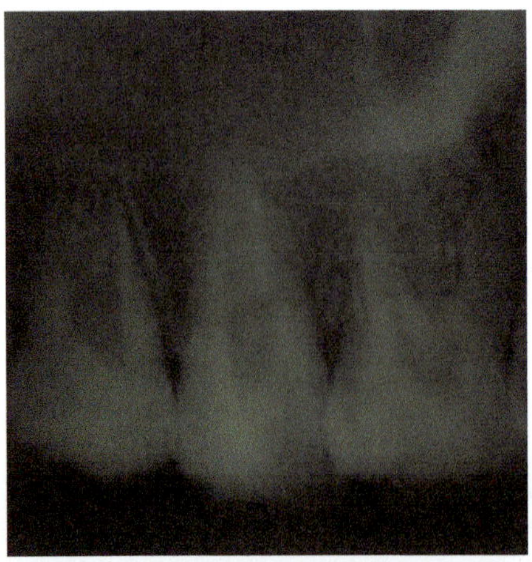

FIGURE 4: Preoperative radiograph of 27.

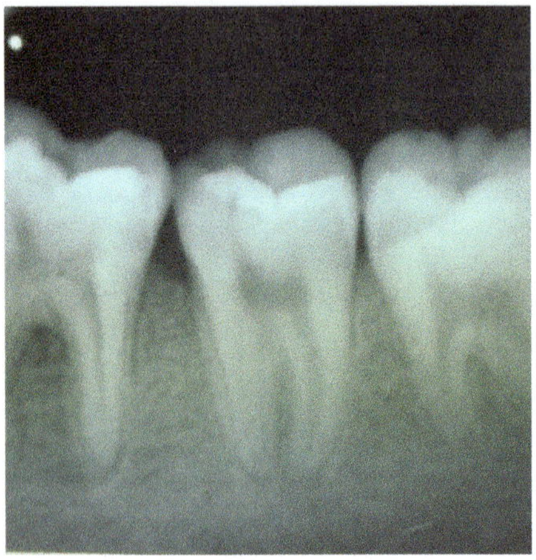

FIGURE 5: Preoperative radiograph of 37.

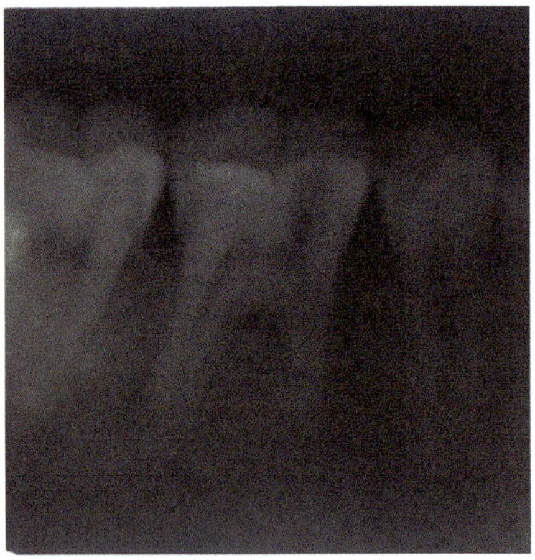

FIGURE 6: Preoperative radiograph of 46.

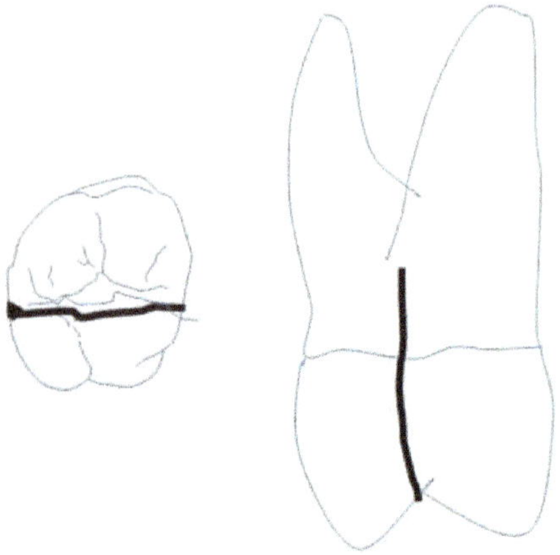

FIGURE 7: Extent of fracture line in 27.

and distobuccal root was involved. Fracture line was not appreciable on the radiograph (Figure 4). It was diagnosed as a split tooth of 27 involving the pulpal floor.

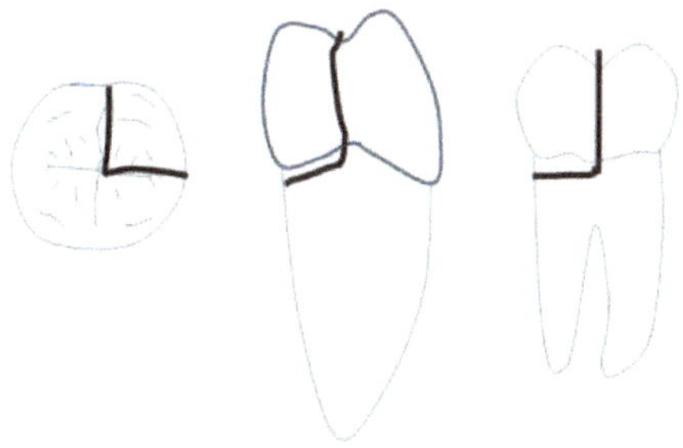

FIGURE 8: Extent of fracture line in 37.

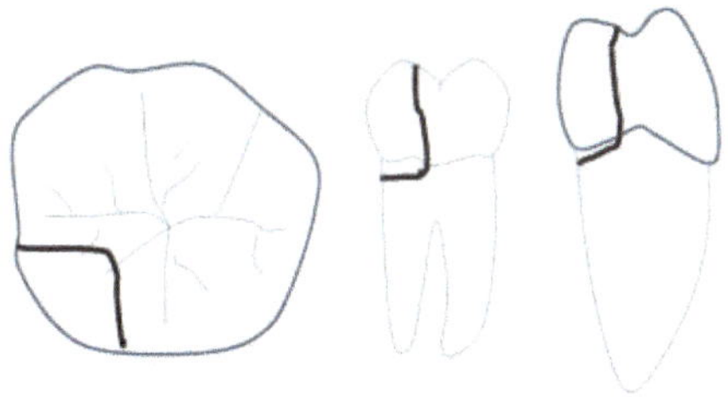

FIGURE 9: Extent of fracture line in 46.

On examination of the lower left quadrant, there was a fracture of a mesiobuccal cusp with respect to 37. The fracture line had both mesiodistal and buccolingual components. It was running cervically from buccal groove towards the centre of occlusal surface and then extending mesially involving the mesial marginal ridge (Figure 8). Both fractured segments were in position but can be visualized by exploring with a probe (Figure 3). Further, the subgingival extent of fracture line was 1 mm below the cementoenamel junction (CEJ), and it was not involving the pulp chamber. Periodontium was intact along the fracture line. An intraoral periapical radiograph revealed intact lamina dura (Figure 5). The tooth was not mobile and not tender on percussion. Vitality test was positive. It was diagnosed as fractured mesiobuccal cusp with respect to 37, not involving the pulp.

On examination of the lower right quadrant, there was a fracture of mesiolingual cusp with respect to 46. The fractured segments were not displaced but could be separated by exploration with the probe. Further, the fracture line was extending up to the coronal third of the root surface, without involving the pulpal floor (Figure 9). Periodontium was not compromised along the fracture line and percussion test was negative. Vitality test was positive. Intraoral periapical radiograph revealed fracture line (Figure 6). It was diagnosed as fractured mesiolingual cusp with respect to 46.

Comprehensive treatment was planned for each tooth depending on the vitality and extent of fracture line mesiodistally, buccolingually, and gingivally. Before initiation of the treatment, diagnosis, treatment, and prognosis were discussed with the patient.

Immediately after the diagnosis, the tooth was stabilized using orthodontic band (RMO 0.180 × 0.005 mm) (Figure 10). In the same appointment, endodontic treatment was initiated. Fracture line was cleaned of any debris with

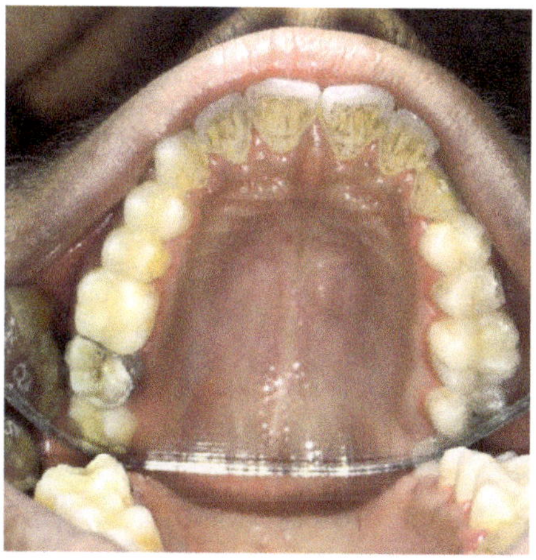

FIGURE 10: Photograph showing stabilization of split tooth with respect to 27 using orthodontic band.

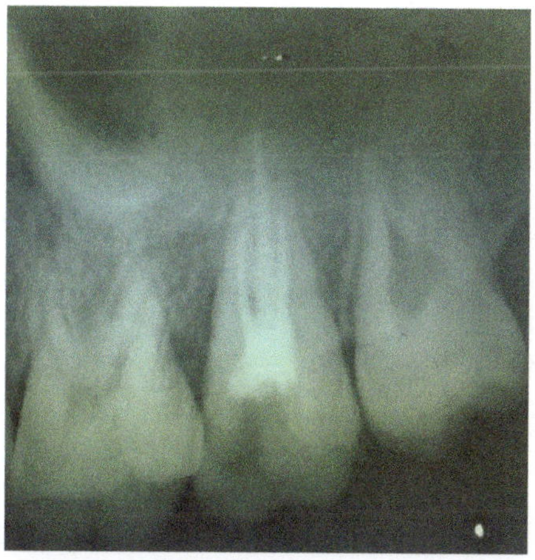

FIGURE 11: Postobturation radiograph with respect to 27.

30% H_2O_2 (Shree Sai Chemicals, Ghaziabad, Uttar Pradesh, India). The biomechanical preparation was done using Rotary V-Taper (30/0.04%) (SS White) (Figure 11). Single cone gutta-percha obturation using MTA Fillapex, as the root canal sealer, was completed. Mineral Trioxide Aggregate (ProRoot MTA, Dentsply, DeTrey, Germany) was placed on the pulpal floor at the fracture site where dentine was missing. A wet cotton pellet was placed in the pulp chamber followed by temporary restoration. The patient was recalled after 3 days. In the next appointment, temporary restoration was removed and access cavity was thoroughly debrided with saline and dried. From each canal, 3 mm of gutta-percha was removed with Peeso Reamer size-3 (Dentsply Maillefer, Ballaigues, Switzerland), and preparation was checked radiographically (Figure 12). Three pieces of 1 cm Ribbond (Ribbond Inc., USA) fibre were taken. The root canal orifices were etched and rinsed and bonding agent was applied. Into each of the three canals, 3 mm of Ribbond fibres was inserted and was stabilized in the root canal with the help of flowable composite (G-aenial Universal Flo, GC Corporation, Tokyo,

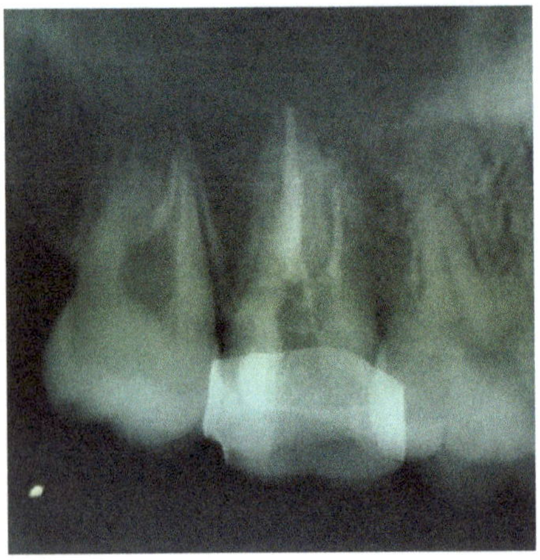

Figure 12: Radiograph showing 3 mm of intracanal space preparation with respect to 27.

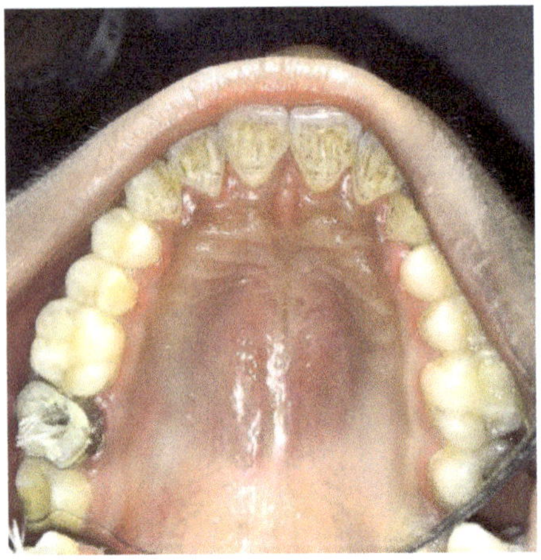

Figure 13: Photograph showing 3 mm placement of Ribbond in the canal.

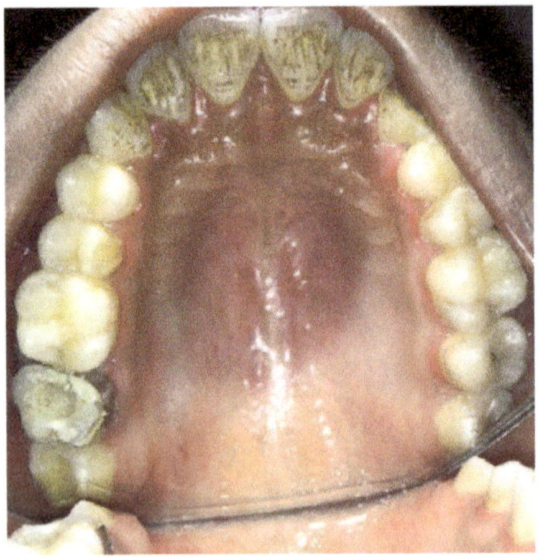

Figure 14: Photograph showing meshwork of fibre in the pulp chamber.

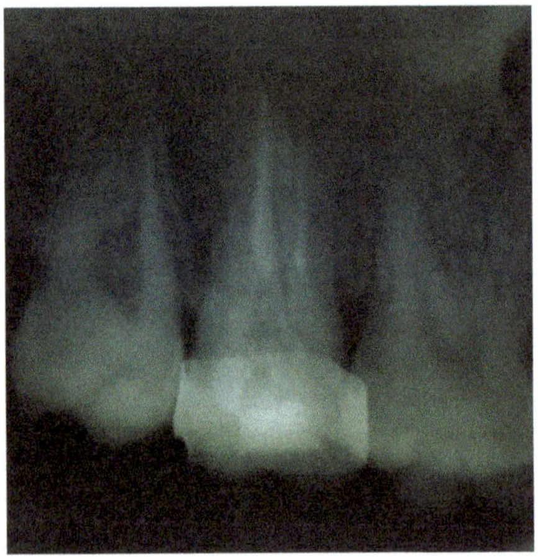

Figure 15: Radiograph showing internal reinforcement with Ribbond in 27.

Japan) and cured (Figure 13). After curing, around 7 mm of remaining fibres was kept outside the canal orifice. Then, these fibres were spread on the floor of the pulp chamber and intermingled to create a meshwork for the internal reinforcement (Figure 14). A flowable composite was placed over this fibrous meshwork and manipulated slightly with the help of plastic instrument (API) along the buccolingual and mesiodistal directions so as to form a unique composite Ribbond meshwork along the floor of the pulp chamber which was later cured. Subsequently, core buildup composite (Tetric Ceram Ivoclar Vivadent, Germany) was done. After 15 days, the orthodontic band was removed and crown preparation was done. Temporary crown was cemented which was later replaced by metal ceramic crown (Figures 15 and 16).

Fractured mesiobuccal cusp in 37 was removed carefully (Figure 17) and tooth preparation was done for class II cast metal inlay with cusp capping. Tooth preparation was extended more apically, and an indirect pattern was fabricated (Figures 18 and 19). Cast gold inlay was fabricated, luted

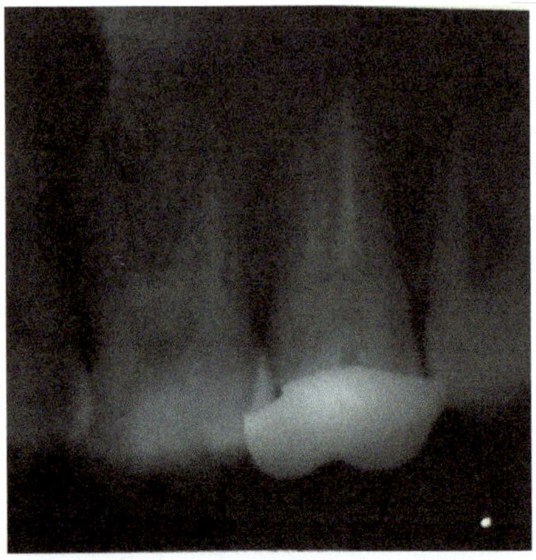

Figure 16: Radiograph showing external reinforcement with metal crown in tooth 27.

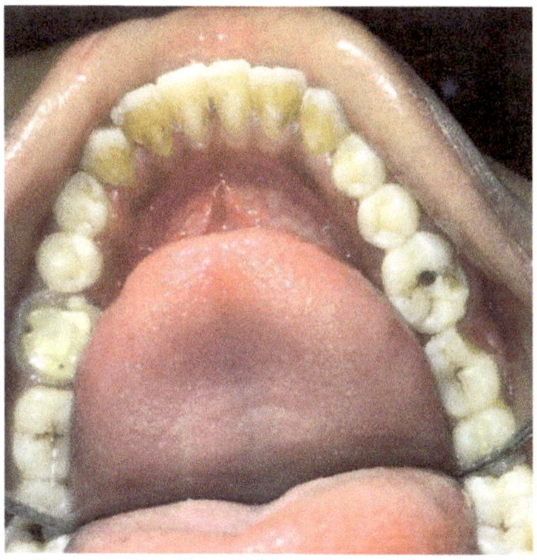

FIGURE 17: Mesiobuccal cusp in tooth 37 removed.

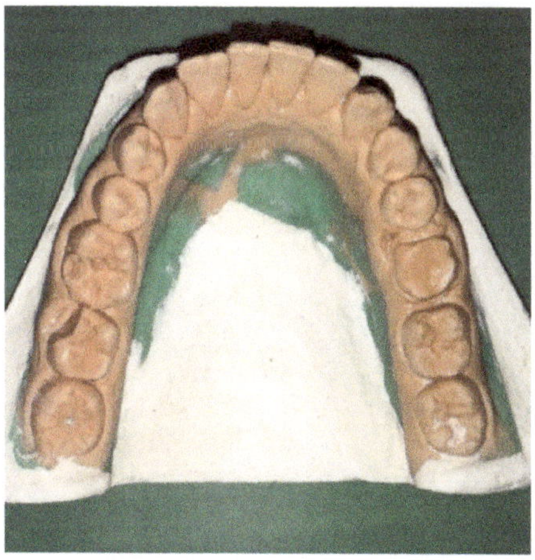

FIGURE 18: Preoperative cast of tooth 37.

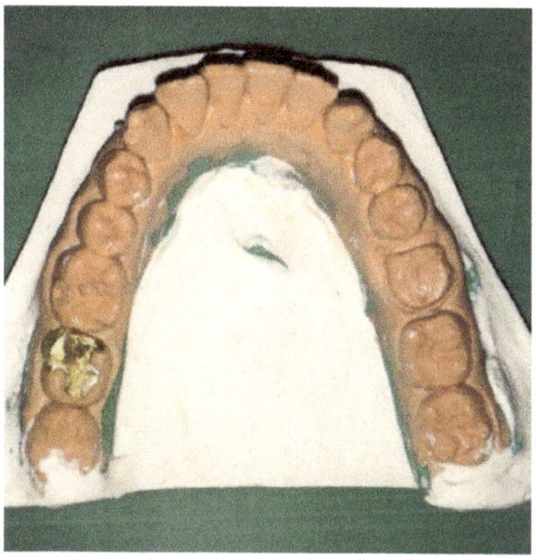

FIGURE 19: Inlay casting try-in on the cast with respect to 37.

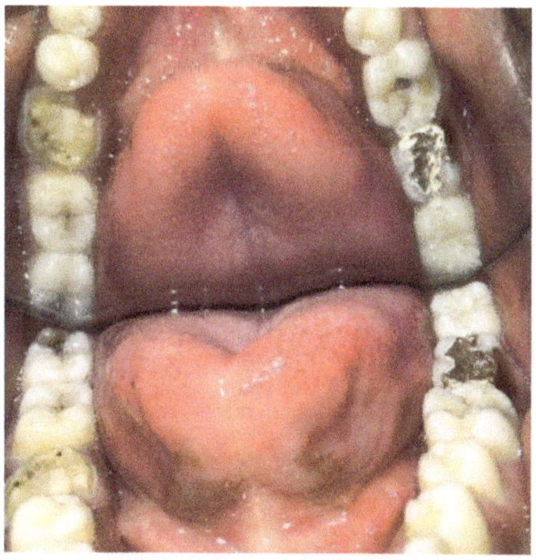

FIGURE 20: Photograph showing inlay luted with respect to 37 (occlusal view).

using glass ionomer cement type I (GC Corporation, Tokyo, Japan) (Figures 20, 21, and 22), and checked radiographically (Figure 23).

As the fracture line was not involving the pulp chamber in 46 but was extending subgingivally, and tooth was vital initially, the fractured cusp was not removed; instead it was bonded with the help of composite resin and stabilized with orthodontic band (Figure 24). On subsequent appointment, the tooth had become nonvital and a sinus tract had also appeared in its relation. Hence, endodontic treatment was completed (Figure 25). Internal and external reinforcement were achieved in the same manner as mentioned for tooth 27.

3. Discussion

Two classic patterns of longitudinal fracture were seen in this case report. In one (#27), the fracture was located centrally, extending to the pulp, and, in others (#37 and #46), the fracture was more peripherally directed and resulting in a cuspal fracture.

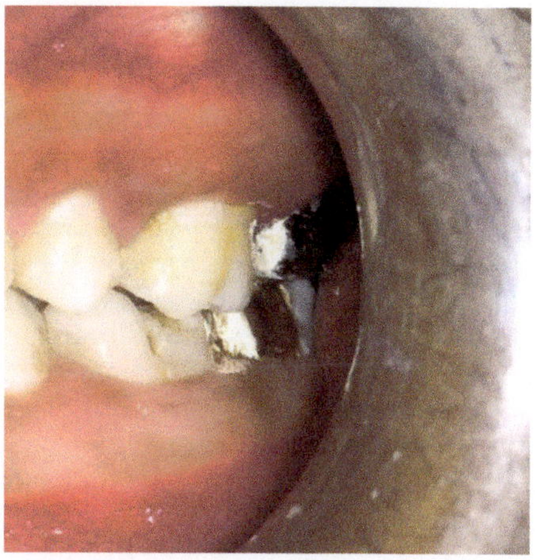

FIGURE 21: Photograph showing inlay luted with respect to 37 (buccal view).

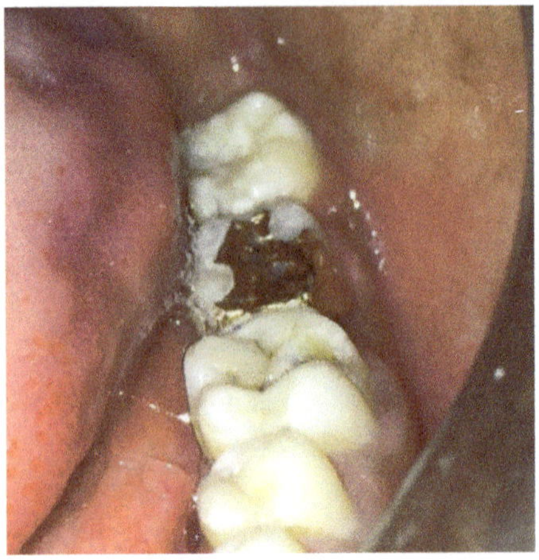

FIGURE 22: Photograph showing inlay luted with respect to 37 (occlusal view).

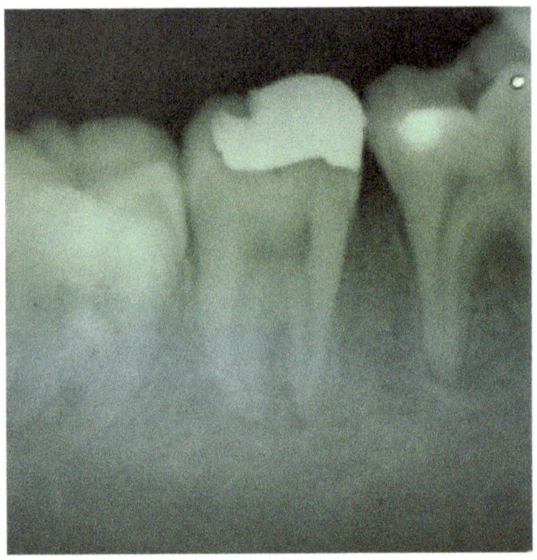

FIGURE 23: Radiograph showing luted inlay with respect to 37.

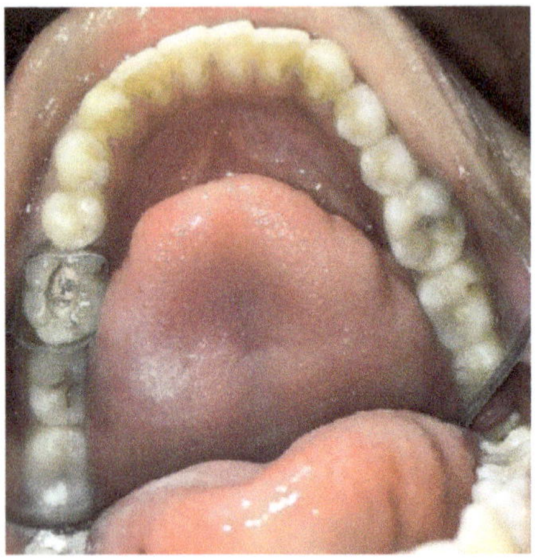

FIGURE 24: Photograph showing stabilization of fractured cusp with respect to 46.

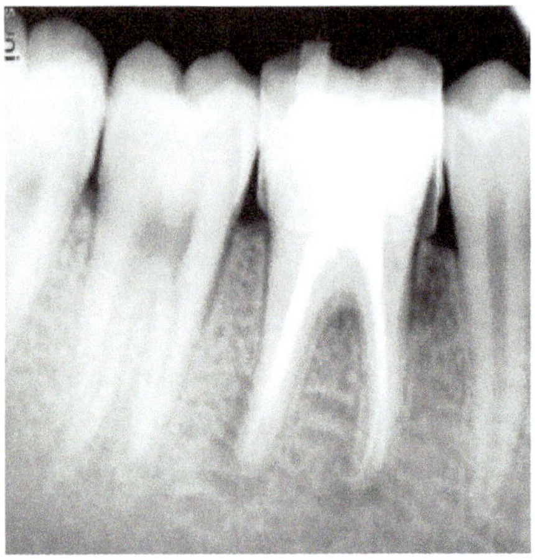

FIGURE 25: Postobturation radiograph of 46.

In tooth #27, the fracture was crossing both the marginal ridges involving the pulpal floor and there was no dentine connection between the two segments. Such teeth are usually difficult to restore and generally advised for extraction, as granulation tissue grows in the furcation area which results in loss of periodontal attachment. Further, bonding of two fragments together is difficult as the cuspal flexure during occlusion may result in failure of the bond [12]. However, with advancements in biomaterials and adhesive materials both aspects were successfully managed in tooth #27. MTA being bioactive, biocompatible, and having biomineralizing properties allows cementum to grow at the furcation area and aids in the regeneration of periodontal ligament [13]. Hence, MTA was used to seal the pulpal floor at the fracture site. Perfect approximation of split section was achieved with orthodontic banding. As MTA sets in the presence of moisture [14, 15], matrix was not required to contain the MTA. Since MTA is weak in compressive strength, it was reinforced by flowable composite to bear the occlusal forces.

The tooth was further reinforced internally and externally using orthodontic band and fibre Ribbond. The orthodontic band provided a good interim stabilization of fracture segment. Recent studies have proved that orthodontic band reduces cuspal flexure by one-half compared to teeth without bands [16]. Internal reinforcement was achieved using Ribbond, possessing high strength fibres with cross-link weave. Ribbond also has enhanced bond ability, thereby resisting crack opening and creating a strong bond between the fractured segments. Stresses can be redistributed along the direction of the fibre to intact portions of the teeth and away from the bonded surface [17].

To reduce the polymerization shrinkage, incremental placement of composite using pulse curing technique was used. This reduced the stress development at the cavosurface margin and reinforced the remaining tooth structure [18]. Full coverage metal crown was fabricated and cemented over the treated tooth, which gave external reinforcement of fractured segments. Literature search reveals case reports on managing such fracture by intentional reimplantation procedure. 4-META adhesive was used to bond split tooth after extraction. With such technique, resorption of root after reimplantation remains a concern. Further intentional reimplantation is an invasive procedure [10]. CO_2 and Nd-YAG lasers were found ineffective in fusing the segments [11].

In tooth #37, the fracture line was not extending below the cervical line and was not involving the pulp. Cast gold inlay with cusp capping of mesiobuccal cusp was planned instead of composite restoration, as resin shows polymerization shrinkage, which can further displace and weaken the fractured segments, rendering them more susceptible to masticatory forces [19]. During tooth preparation, the preparation margins were extended more apically and bevelling the fractured segment to minimize the displacement [12].

Tooth 46 was vital and fracture line was not involving the pulp. Hence, initially, fracture segment was reattached with composite and stabilized with orthodontic bands. The tooth was examined periodically. After two weeks, tooth became nonresponsive to vitality test and an intraoral sinus also developed in its relation. So root canal treatment was initiated and completed. The tooth was restored and permanently stabilized by internal and external reinforcement as done for tooth #27.

During the endodontic procedure in tooth #27 and tooth #46 to avoid excessive wedging forces during lateral condensation which may cause the split to spread, single cone obturation (30/4%) was done after biomechanical preparation with Rotary V-Taper file (SS White, Lakewood, NJ). For irrigation, metronidazole (JB Chemicals, Bharuch, Gujarat) was used. As the fracture line was involving the palatal canal in tooth #27, MTA based sealer (MTA Fillapex, Angelus, Brazil) was used. The post was also avoided for anchorage as they may exert wedging forces, and, instead, Ribbond fibre reinforced resin was used in its place.

4. Conclusion

With recent advancements in adhesives, split tooth resulting in longitudinal fractures that were once considered irreparable and recommended for extraction can now be successfully restored and reinforced both internally and externally. Further, with the introduction of biomaterials fracture lines involving the pulpal floor can be managed by the apposition of new cement at the fracture site. In addition, vital teeth with the longitudinal fracture of the cusp, not involving the pulp, can be conservatively managed by cast gold inlay or full cast crown.

Competing Interests

The authors declare that they have no competing interests.

References

[1] K. Loomba, A. Loomba, R. Bains, and V. K. Bains, "A proposal for classification of tooth fractures based on treatment need," *Journal of Oral Science*, vol. 52, no. 4, pp. 517–529, 2010.

[2] E. M. Rivera and R. E. Walton, "Longitudinal tooth fractures: findings that contribute to complex endodontic diagnoses," *Endodontic Topics*, vol. 16, no. 1, pp. 82–111, 2007.

[3] M. Abou-Rass, "Crack lines: the precursors of tooth fractures—their diagnosis and treatment," *Quintessence International*, vol. 14, no. 4, pp. 437–447, 1983.

[4] S. G. S. Ellis, "Incomplete tooth fracture—proposal for a new definition," *British Dental Journal*, vol. 190, no. 8, pp. 424–428, 2001.

[5] J. D. Bader, D. A. Shugars, and J. A. Martin, "Risk indicators for posterior tooth fracture," *Journal of the American Dental Association*, vol. 135, no. 7, pp. 883–892, 2004.

[6] A. Gurtu, A. Singhal, C. Guha, and S. M. Sharma, "Management of vertical fracture—a case report," *Journal of Dental Sciences & Oral Rehabilitation*, pp. 34–35, 2011.

[7] K. N. Jyoti, "Management of vertically fractured maxillary second molar," *Journal of Dental Sciences and Research*, vol. 2, pp. 45–50, 2010.

[8] I. B. Bender and J. B. Freedland, "Adult root fracture," *The Journal of the American Dental Association*, vol. 107, no. 3, pp. 413–419, 1983.

[9] N. Masaka, "Long-term observation of fractured tooth roots preserved by adhesion," *Adhesive Dentistry. Japanese*, vol. 13, pp. 156–170, 1995.

[10] G. Aesert, "Management of vertical tooth fractures," *Endocrine Practice*, vol. 4, pp. 32–38, 2001.

[11] S. Arakawa, C. M. Cobb, J. W. Rapley, W. J. Killoy, and P. Spencer, "Treatment of root fracture by CO_2 and Nd:YAG lasers: an in vitro study," *Journal of Endodontics*, vol. 22, no. 12, pp. 662–667, 1996.

[12] B. J. Casciari, "Altered preparation design for cracked teeth," *Journal of the American Dental Association*, vol. 130, no. 4, pp. 571–572, 1999.

[13] M. Parirokh and M. Torabinejad, "Mineral trioxide aggregate: a comprehensive literature review—part III: clinical applications, drawbacks, and mechanism of action," *Journal of Endodontics*, vol. 36, no. 3, pp. 400–413, 2010.

[14] L. L. Hench and J. Wilson, "Surface-active biomaterials," *Science*, vol. 226, no. 4675, pp. 630–636, 1984.

[15] H. W. Roberts, J. M. Toth, D. W. Berzins, and D. G. Charlton, "Mineral trioxide aggregate material use in endodontic treatment: a review of the literature," *Dental Materials*, vol. 24, no. 2, pp. 149–164, 2008.

[16] E. S. Pane, J. E. A. Palamara, and H. H. Messer, "Stainless steel bands in endodontics: effects on cuspal flexure and fracture resistance," *International Endodontic Journal*, vol. 35, no. 5, pp. 467–471, 2002.

[17] S. Belli, F. K. Cobankara, O. Eraslan, G. Eskitascioglu, and V. Karbhari, "The effect of fiber insertion on fracture resistance of endodontically treated molars with MOD cavity and reattached fractured lingual cusps," *Journal of Biomedical Materials Research—Part B Applied Biomaterials*, vol. 79, no. 1, pp. 35–41, 2006.

[18] S. Deliperi, D. N. Bardwell, and A. Papathanasiou, "In vitro evaluation of composite microleakage using different methods of polymerization," *American Journal of Dentistry*, vol. 16, pp. 73–76, 2003.

[19] F. W. Allara Jr., K. E. Diefenderfer, and J. D. Molinaro, "Effect of three direct restorative materials on molar cuspal fracture resistance," *American Journal of Dentistry*, vol. 17, no. 4, pp. 228–232, 2004.

35

Nasopalatine Duct Cyst

Pratik Dedhia,[1] Shely Dedhia,[2] Amol Dhokar,[1] and Ankit Desai[3]

[1] *Department of Oral Medicine and Radiology, Terna Dental College, Nerul, Navi Mumbai 400706, India*
[2] *Department of Pediatric and Preventive Dentistry, Nair Hospital Dental College, Mumbai Central, Mumbai 400008, India*
[3] *Department of Periodontics, Terna Dental College, Nerul, Navi Mumbai 400706, India*

Correspondence should be addressed to Shely Dedhia; drshelyjain@gmail.com

Academic Editors: R. S. Brown, C. Evans, E. Hochuli-Vieira, K. Nakamori, and K. Seymour

The nasopalatine cyst is the most common epithelial and nonodontogenic cyst of the maxilla. The cyst originates from epithelial remnants from the nasopalatine duct. The cells may be activated spontaneously during life or are eventually stimulated by the irritating action of various agents (infection, etc.). It is different from a radicular cyst. The definite diagnosis should be based on clinical, radiological, and histopathological findings. The treatment is enucleation of the cystic tissue, and only in rare cases a marsupialisation needs to be performed. A case of a nasopalatine duct cyst in a 35-year-old male is reviewed. The typical radiologic and histological findings are presented.

1. Introduction

The nasopalatine duct cyst (NPDC) was first ever described by Meyer in 1914 [1, 2]. Nasopalatine duct cyst, also termed as incisive canal cyst, arises from embryogenic remnants of nasopalatine duct, the communication between the nasal cavity and anterior maxilla in the developing fetus. Most of these cysts develop in the midline of anterior maxilla near the incisive foramen [3]. It is one of the most common nonodontogenic cysts of the oral cavity occurring in about 1% of the population [4].

NPDCs affect a wide age range; however, most present in the fourth through sixth decades of life, and most studies show a significantly higher frequency in men than woman, with the ratio being 2.5 : 1 [5–11]. Patients may be asymptomatic, with the lesion being detected on routine radiographs; however, many will present with one or more symptoms. Complaints are often found to be associated with an infection of a previously asymptomatic nasopalatine duct cysts and consist primarily of swelling, drainage, and pain [10, 12]. The vitality of nearby teeth should not be affected; however, it is not uncommon to see evidence of endodontic therapy because the nasopalatine duct cyst was previously clinically misdiagnosed as a periapical cyst or granuloma.

The present case of NPDC is one such typical pathology with the classical presentation which could have been easily misdiagnosed as a periapical lesion.

2. Case Report

2.1. History. A 35-year-old male reported to the dental clinic with the chief complaint of painless swelling over the palate and anterior maxilla. The swelling was gradually increasing in size for the past 3 months with associated displacement of maxillary central incisors. There was no associated history of trauma.

On examination, a well defined firm nontender swelling was seen on the left side of anterior hard palate and crossing over the midline to the right side. The crown of left central incisor was displaced labially and mesially, overlapping the crown of right central incisor (Figure 1). A provisional diagnosis of periapical cyst was given but the vitality tests of the central incisors were negative. The differential diagnosis was established with other conditions such as an nasopalatine duct cyst, enlarged nasopalatine duct, central giant cell granuloma, a root cyst associated to the upper central incisors, a supernumerary tooth follicular cyst, primordial

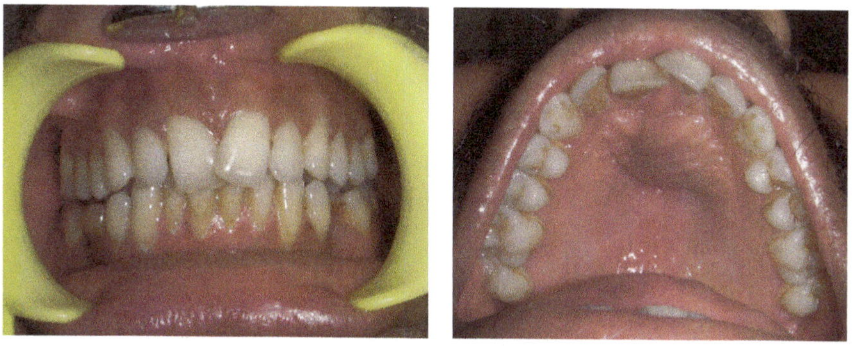

(a) (b)

FIGURE 1: Preoperative intraoral swelling.

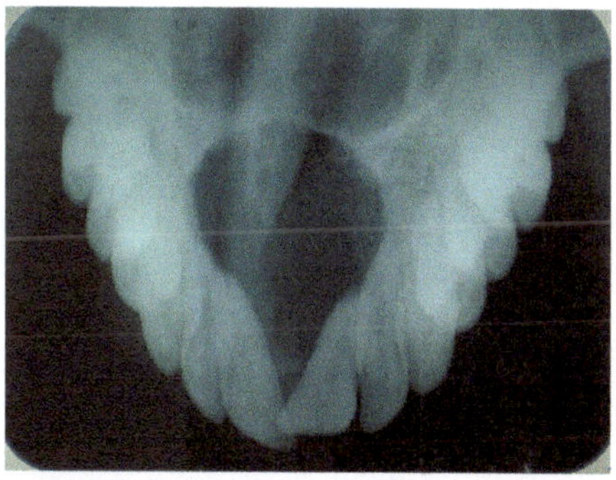

FIGURE 2: Maxillary occlusal view showing well defined radiolucency in the anterior maxilla.

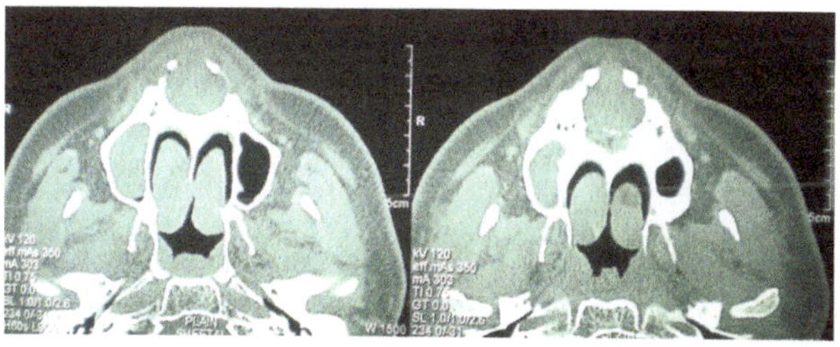

FIGURE 3: Axial sections of CT scan showing the well-defined round radiolucency.

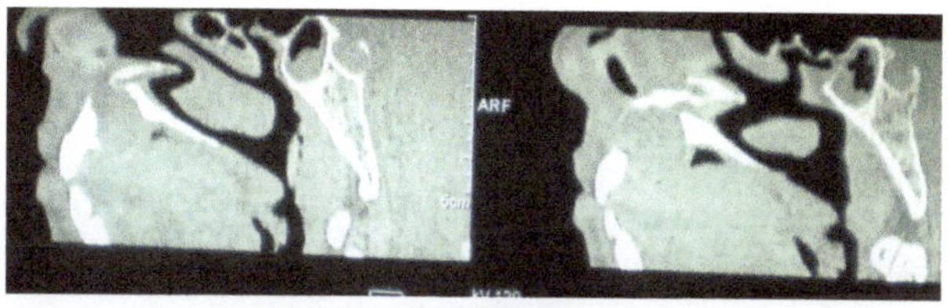

FIGURE 4: Sagittal sections of CT scan.

cyst, and nasoalveolar cyst. Radiological investigations were subsequently advised.

2.2. Radiographic Features. Maxillary occlusal radiograph showed a well-defined round radiolucency approximately 2.5 cm in size with corticated margins in the midline and between the central incisors which was the typical radiographic feature of NPDC (Figure 2). The lesion was causing displacement of the roots of the incisors. Superiorly it was extending till the floor of nasal fossa. Also there was deviation of the nasal septum to the right side.

CT scan also showed a well-defined radiolucency in anterior maxilla in the region of incisive canal, 2.6 cm × 2.8 cm in size. Mesiodistally the radiolucency was causing displacement of the roots of both maxillary central incisors and it was not extending laterally beyond the roots of incisors. Inferiorly it was extending till the crest of interdental bone. Loss of cortication was seen along the buccal and palatal aspects of the lesion in the sagittal sections. The lesion was causing mild elevation of the floor of nasal fossa in the anterior region with deviation of the nasal septum to the right side (Figures 3, 4, and 5). Mucosal polyp was seen associated with the floor of left maxillary sinus. A radiographic diagnosis of NPDC was established and surgical enucleation was planned.

2.3. Treatment. A surgical enucleation was done with intact removal of the cyst (Figure 6) and the specimen was sent for histopathological examination which showed cystic lining composed of stratified squamous epithelium about 2-3 cell layer thick. Lining was flattened and showed pseudostratification at places (Figure 7). This was conclusive for NPDC.

3. Discussion

NPDCs are usually central or unilateral with no prevalence of side occurrence. Radiographically, they are seen as well-defined round or oval radiolucencies in the midline, although some lesions may appear heart-shaped [6], either because they become notched by the nasal septum during their expansion or because the nasal spine is superimposed on the radiolucent area.

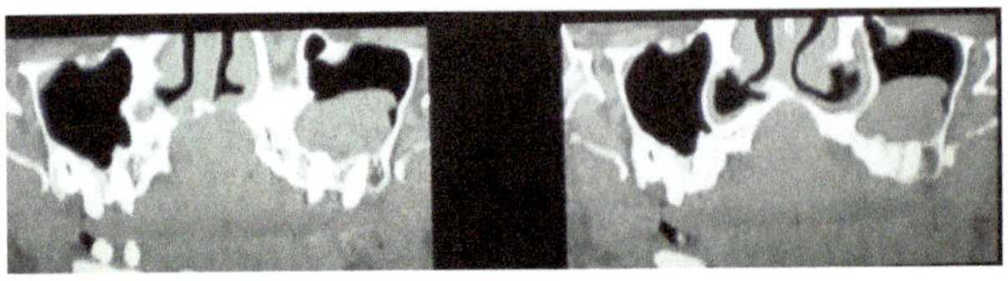

FIGURE 5: Panoramic reconstruction of CT scan.

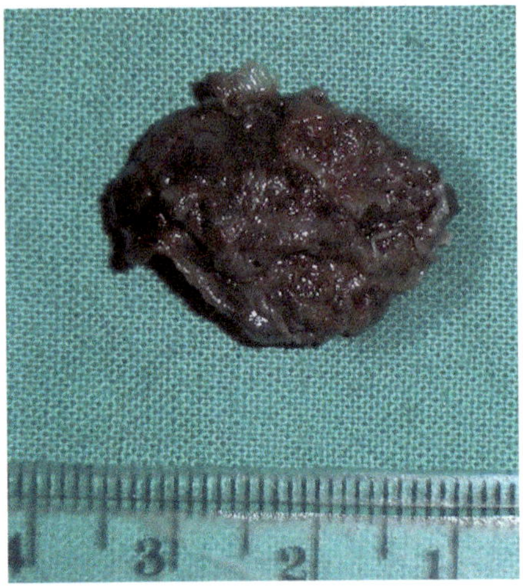

FIGURE 6: Gross specimen of the enucleated cyst.

Due to similar signs and symptoms, the NPDC may be easily misdiagnosed by the clinicians as a periapical lesion. This is why many authors believe that its prevalence is actually higher than presented in the literature [13]. Although a large NPDC might show the adjacent incisors roots to be within the cystic cavity, the lamina dura will be usually intact and the pulp usually vital, whereas a radicular cyst is associated with a pulpless tooth and involves a portion of the root, usually with loss of continuity of the lamina dura. In the reported case, the lesions were close to the apexes of the maxillary anterior teeth which were vital.

A reported 71.8% of NPDCs have squamous, columnar, cuboidal, or some combination of these epithelial types; respiratory epithelium is seen in only 9.8% [12, 14, 15]. In this case the squamous epithelium was present with stratification.

The present case had typical clinical, radiographic, and histopathological features of a nasopalatine duct cyst. The importance of this case is in the diagnosis of such lesions which can easily be misinterpreted as periapical cyst and inadvertent root canal therapy of surrounding vital teeth can be avoided.

4. Conclusion

Nasopalatine duct cysts are the most common nonodontogenic cyst of the oral cavity seen in the general population. NPDCs must be distinguished from other maxillary anterior radiolucencies. Vitality testing of teeth adjacent to or involved with a cyst-like lesion is mandatory and the final diagnosis could only be performed after histological analysis. It is important that practitioners are aware of the features of the NPDC.

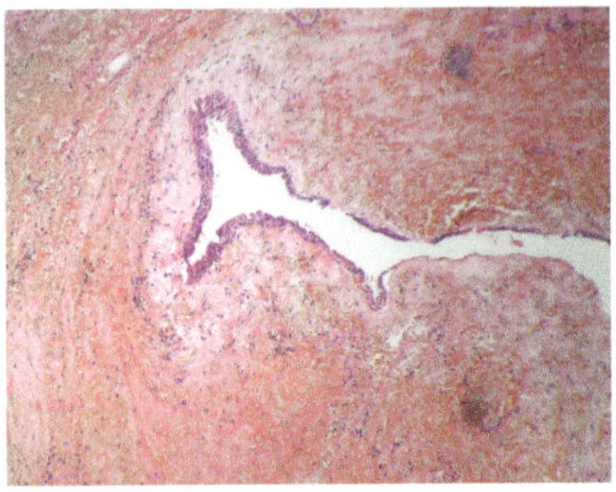

FIGURE 7: Photomicrograph of nasopalatine duct cyst showing stratified squamous epithelium.

References

[1] A. W. Meyer, "A unique supernumerary Paranasal sinus directly above the superior incisors," *Journal of Anatomy*, vol. 48, pp. 118–129, 1914.

[2] K. A. Elliott, C. B. Franzese, and K. T. Pitman, "Diagnosis and surgical management of nasopalatine duct cysts," *Laryngoscope*, vol. 114, no. 8 I, pp. 1336–1340, 2004.

[3] S. P. Lewis, *Wysocki. Contemporary Oral and Maxillofacial Pathology*, pp. 62-63, Mosby, St. Louis, Mo, USA, 2nd edition.

[4] B. Neville, "Developmental defects of the oral and maxillofacial region," in *Textbook of Oral Pathology*, p. 25, Saunders, Philadelphia, Pa, USA, 1st edition.

[5] H. C. Killey and L. W. Kay, "An analysis of 471 benign cystic lesions of the jaws," *International Surgery*, vol. 46, no. 6, pp. 540–545, 1966.

[6] M. Shear and P. M. Speight, *Cysts of the Oral and Maxillofacial Regions*, Blackwell Munksgaard, Oxford, UK, 4th edition, 2007.

[7] M. Hedin, A. Klamfeldt, and G. Persson, "Surgical treatment of nasopalatine duct cysts. A follow-up study," *International Journal of Oral Surgery*, vol. 7, no. 5, pp. 427–433, 1978.

[8] I. Bodin, G. Isacsson, and P. Julin, "Cysts of the nasopalatine duct," *International Journal of Oral and Maxillofacial Surgery*, vol. 15, no. 6, pp. 696–706, 1986.

[9] N. Ely, E. C. Sheehy, and F. Mcdonald, "Nasopalatine duct cyst: a case report," *International Journal of Paediatric Dentistry*, vol. 11, no. 2, pp. 135–137, 2001.

[10] K. S. Swanson, G. E. Kaugars, and J. C. Gunsolley, "Nasopalatine duct cyst: an analysis of 334 cases," *Journal of Oral and Maxillofacial Surgery*, vol. 49, no. 3, pp. 268–271, 1991.

[11] R. H. B. Allard, W. A. M. van der Kwast, and I. van der Waal, "Nasopalatine duct cyst. Review of the literature and report of 22 cases," *International Journal of Oral Surgery*, vol. 10, no. 6, pp. 447–461, 1981.

[12] R. Vasconcelos, M. F. de Aguiar, W. Castro, V. C. de Araujo, and R. Mesquita, "Retrospective analysis of 31 cases of nasopalatine duct cyst," *Oral Diseases*, vol. 5, no. 4, pp. 325–328, 1999.

[13] E. Santora Jr., A. J. Ballantyne, and E. C. Hinds, "Nasoalveolar cyst: report of case," *Journal of Oral Surgery*, vol. 28, no. 2, pp. 117–120, 1970.

[14] J. D. Gnanasekhar, S. V. Walvekar, A. M. Al-Kandari, and Y. Al-Duwairi, "Misdiagnosis and mismanagement of a nasoplatine duct cyst and its corrective therapy. A case report," *Oral Surgery, Oral Medicine, Oral Pathology, Oral Radiology, and Endodontology*, vol. 80, no. 4, pp. 465–470, 1995.

[15] A. M. Abrams, F. V. Howell, and W. K. Bullock, "Nasopalatine cysts," *Oral Surgery, Oral Medicine, Oral Pathology*, vol. 16, no. 3, pp. 306–332, 1963.

36

Description of a Rare Case of Nodular Fasciitis of the Apical Aspect of the Upper Buccal Sulcus

Ana Amélia Souza,[1] Eldon Guttenberg Cariri Neto,[1] Vera Cavalcanti de Araújo,[1] Fabricio Passador-Santos,[1] Maria Teresa de Seixas Alves,[2] and Andresa Borges Soares[1]

[1] *Department of Oral Pathology, Sao Leopoldo Mandic Institute and Research Center, Rua José Rocha Junqueira13, Ponte Preta, 13045-755 Campinas, SP, Brazil*

[2] *Department of Pathology, Escola Paulista de Medicina, Rua Botucatu 740, Vila Clementino, 04023-900 Sao Paulo, SP, Brazil*

Correspondence should be addressed to Andresa Borges Soares; andresabs@hotmail.com

Academic Editor: Evanthia Chrysomali

This report describes a rare case of nodular fasciitis (NF) of the oral cavity, discussing the clinical, histological, and immunohistochemical characteristics. Histopathologic diagnosis of this type of lesion can be challenging due to its differential diagnosis, which principally includes sarcoma. The patient presented with a painless, well-defined nodule, reported as increasing in size, located at the apical aspect of the upper left buccal sulcus. Histologically, the lesion revealed spindle cell proliferation arranged in fascicles, while immunohistochemistry demonstrated positivity for smooth muscle actin. Eight months after complete surgical excision, no signs of local recurrence have been observed.

1. Introduction

Nodular fasciitis (NF) is a benign reactive soft tissue lesion, frequently found in the subcutaneous tissues and muscle fascia, which shows proliferation of myofibroblasts and fibroblasts. While NF has been frequently reported at many anatomical sites, namely, the upper extremities, the trunk, head and neck, and, lastly, the lower extremities, it is extremely rare in the oral cavity [1, 2].

NF was first described by Konwaler et al. as a subcutaneous pseudosarcomatous fibromatosis and has subsequently been nominated as infiltrative fasciitis and pseudosarcomatous fasciitis [3–5]. Several authors believe that the lesion represents a reactive or inflammatory condition triggered by local injury or infection [6]. However, the presence of a reciprocal translocation involving chromosome 15 has been recently described, which may categorize this lesion as a true neoplasm [7–9]. Erickson-Johnson et al. [10] confirmed the presence of the translocation in 44 cases of NF. The authors also identified a new translocation-induced fusion gene, *MYH9-USP6*, and postulated that NF could be the first example of a self-limiting human lesion that can be characterized by a recurrent somatic gene fusion event.

The histopathological diagnosis of NF can be challenging, as its differential diagnosis includes other significant soft tissue lesions, such as sarcoma. NF is characterized by myofibroblast and fibroblast proliferation. Immunohistochemical panels are often needed to aid in diagnosis, with NF showing positivity for vimentin, smooth muscle actin, and muscle specific actin [11–15].

The present report describes the clinical and histopathologic features of a rare case of nodular fasciitis of the oral cavity.

2. Case Report

A 17-year-old white female presented to a private dental clinic complaining of a painless swelling to the apical aspect of the upper left buccal sulcus, which had increased in size over the preceding seven weeks. The medical history was otherwise unremarkable.

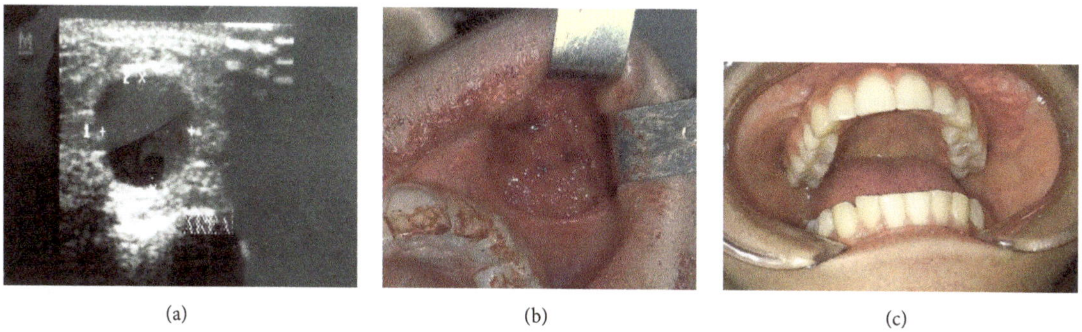

FIGURE 1: (a) Ultrasound examination showing the presence of a hypoechoic tumoral mass. (b) Transoperative view. (c) Follow-up at 8 months.

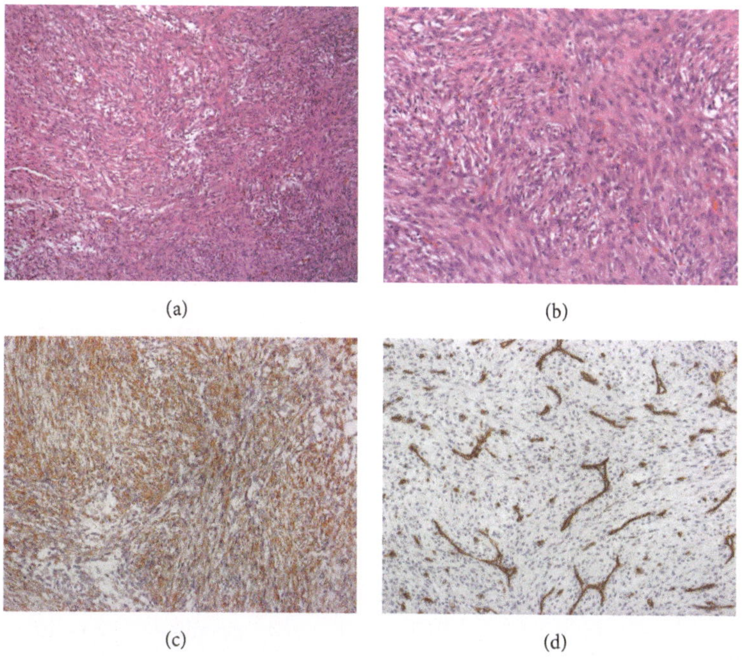

FIGURE 2: (a) Proliferation of spindle cells arranged in fascicles (Hematoxylin and Eosin stain, original magnification 10x). (b) Cells of nodular fasciitis with elongated shape, oval nuclei, and eosinophilic cytoplasm (Hematoxylin and Eosin stain, original magnification 40x). (c) Immunohistochemical stain showing strong positivity for smooth muscle actin (smooth muscle actin stain, original magnification 20x). (d) Immunohistochemistry stain showing negativity for CD34 (CD34 stain, original magnification 20x).

Initial inspection revealed a gross asymmetry of the face, with no palpable lymph nodes. Intraoral examination demonstrated a well-defined, rubbery, painless, nonulcerated mass at the apical aspect of the upper left buccal sulcus. Ultrasound examination showed a rounded hypoechoic mass (Figure 1(a)). An excisional biopsy of the soft tissue mass was performed, and a clinical diagnosis of a benign tumor was suggested. The lesion was completely excised during biopsy (Figure 1(b)). The surgical specimen consisted of an irregular, fibrous, yellow soft tissue mass.

The specimen was fixed in 10% buffered formalin, with paraffin sections being prepared for light microscopy following standard procedures. Microscopic examination of the Hematoxylin and Eosin (H&E) stained sections revealed spindle cell proliferation arranged in fascicles. In general, the cells were elongated, with oval nuclei and eosinophilic cytoplasm. Rare mitotic figures were observed, yet no atypical mitoses were present. Scarce discrete cell pleomorphism was observed, with myxoid areas also present. A chronic inflammatory process scattered throughout the lesion was observed (Figures 2(a) and 2(b)).

Immunohistochemistry revealed spindle cell positivity to the smooth muscle actin (clone 1A4) (Figure 2(c)) antibody, while an absence of reactivity was seen for CD34 (clone M 7165) (Figure 2(d)), AE1/AE3 (clone M3515), and S-100 (clone Z0311).

No sign of local recurrence has been observed after eight months of follow-up (Figure 1(c)).

3. Discussion

The case reported, herein, fulfills the clinical, histological, and immunohistochemical criteria for the diagnosis of NF, a rare benign tumor of the oral cavity. The challenge in diagnosis of oral NF comes from the fact that the lesion is rare in the oral cavity, as well as the fact that it has a significant histopathologic differential diagnosis [11].

According to the literature, NF is typically diagnosed in young adults between the ages of 20 and 40 years [12–15]. Lima et al. [16] published a literature review of oral cavity NF over the past 10 years, which revealed an average age of 34 years, with a maximum age of 50 and minimum of 8 years. In the present case, the lesion arose in a 17-year-old female, which is considered younger age than that previously described for patients with NF.

The clinical features of NF are rather nonspecific, with it usually being described as a well circumscribed nonencapsulated mass, soft and elastic in consistency, which firmly adheres to the underlying tissues [13, 14]. Oral NF lesions are most common in the buccal and labial mucosa, as well as tongue, with the parotid gland and floor of the mouth also being affected [2, 12–18]. NF can present as multiple nodules in a single area, with multiple anatomic sites rarely affected concurrently [13]. In the present case, the lesion was a well-defined, rubbery, painless, nonulcerated mass located at the apical aspect of the upper left buccal sulcus. Ultrasound of the lesion revealed a round, hypoechoic mass.

NF is characterized by rapid growth, which often leads to tissue distortion, mimicking its malignant counterpart [11, 12]. In the present case, the lesion was reported as having increased in size over the course of seven weeks, which corroborates the literature [11–14, 16, 18, 19].

Histologically, NF is classified into three subtypes, according to the tissue plane involved: subcutaneous, intramuscular, and fascial. The lesion is usually attached to the fascia from which it arises and extends into the subcutaneous fat in an irregular fashion. Occasionally, it may also arise from the fibrous septa of the subcutaneous fat, only secondarily extending to the fascia [12, 16]. NF is usually a well circumscribed yet nonencapsulated mass composed of fibroblastic and myofibroblastic proliferation arranged in short fascicles and untidy bundles. Typical histologic findings include a myxoid and, in some cases, highly cellular stroma, exhibiting abundant mitotic activity, with the absence of cellular atypia. Myxoid degeneration may also be observed, while other areas are more fibrotic and hyalinized, displaying evidence of adjacent microhemorrhage with granulation tissue. Moreover, some lesions may display multinucleated giant cells [11–14]. The histological features of the present case are similar to those previously described. The lesion consisted of spindle cells arranged in fascicles, exhibiting oval nuclei and eosinophilic cytoplasm. While rare mitotic figures were observed, there were no atypical mitoses. Scarce discrete cellular pleomorphism was also observed. Myxoid areas were present, with a chronic inflammatory process and erythrocytes found scattered throughout the histological sections.

Despite the histopathological characteristics of the present case being similar to those of other NF cases, immunohistochemistry was an essential aid for the final diagnosis. In the literature, the immunohistochemical profile of NF includes positivity for vimentin, α-smooth muscle actin, and muscle specific actin, demonstrating the myofibroblastic differentiation of the spindle cells [11, 12, 16]. NF has also been described as being negative for CD34, cytokeratins, desmin, and the S-100 protein [5, 11, 12, 16]. In the present case, the spindle-like cells were positive for smooth muscle actin and negative for cytokeratin, CD34, and S100.

NF is a challenging diagnosis owing to its unusual clinical features, as well as its histological features, which are similar to other lesions [13, 14, 16]. Due to its rapid growth and the presence of mitoses and spindle cells and its rich cellularity, the differential diagnoses of sarcoma, including sarcomatoid carcinoma, fibrosarcoma, and leiomyosarcoma, are important [20]. It is important to highlight, however, that sarcoma is characterized by its prominent nuclear atypia, long, sweeping bundles, herringbone or storiform arrangement, atypical mitoses, and necrotic background, none of which are found in NF, as corroborated by the present report [21].

NF should also be distinguished from highly cellular lesions, such as fibrous histiocytoma, which displays dense fascicles of fibroblastic cells, chronic inflammation, lipophages, and giant cells. The myxoid appearance of NF can lead to a misdiagnosis of myxoma, myofibroma, fibrous histiocytoma, and fibromatosis or malignant peripheral nerve sheath tumor [22]. Myxoma, myofibroma, fibrous histiocytoma, and fibromatosis can, however, be distinguished from nodular fasciitis by their growth pattern and cytological features [13, 23].

While the treatment of choice for NF is surgical excision [12, 13, 16, 17], Yanagisawa and Okada [24] and de Carli et al. [20] have described total and partial spontaneous regression, respectively. Following surgical excision, recurrence is extremely rare, even when the excision is incomplete. In the current case report, surgical excision was performed and, after eight months of follow-up, no sign of recurrence has been observed.

In conclusion, NF is a benign lesion that can occur at any anatomical site, yet it is rare in the oral cavity. Despite its rarity, the dental surgeon and oral pathologist must have an adequate understanding of the lesion in order to establish an accurate diagnosis and offer appropriate treatment.

Competing Interests

The authors declare no potential competing interests with respect to the research, authorship, and/or publication of this paper.

References

[1] E. J. Jang, T. I. Park, S. C. Nam, and J. Y. Park, "Nodular fasciitis in the submandibular gland," *Diagnostic Cytopathology*, vol. 36, no. 11, pp. 805–808, 2008.

[2] D. Dayan, V. Nasrallah, and M. Vered, "Clinico-pathologic correlations of myofibroblastic tumors of the oral cavity: I.

Nodular fasciitis," *Journal of Oral Pathology and Medicine*, vol. 34, no. 7, pp. 426–435, 2005.

[3] B. E. Konwaler, L. Keasbey, and L. Kaplan, "Subcutaneous pseudosarcomatous fibromatosis (fasciitis)," *American Journal of Clinical Pathology*, vol. 25, no. 3, pp. 241–252, 1955.

[4] R. V. Hutter, F. W. Stewart, and F. W. Foote Jr., "Fasciitis. A report of 70 cases with follow-up proving the benignity of the lesion," *Cancer*, vol. 15, pp. 992–1003, 1962.

[5] M. Martínez-Blanco, J. V. Bagán, J. R. Alba, and J. Basterra, "Maxillofacial nodular fasciitis: a report of 3 cases," *Journal of Oral and Maxillofacial Surgery*, vol. 60, no. 10, pp. 1211–1214, 2002.

[6] M. Leventis, E. Vardas, A. Gkouzioti, E. Chrysomali, and I. Chatzistamou, "Oral nodular fasciitis: report of a case of the buccal mucosa," *Journal of Cranio-Maxillofacial Surgery*, vol. 39, no. 5, pp. 340–342, 2011.

[7] S. H. Birdsall, J. M. Shipley, B. M. Summersgill et al., "Cytogenetic findings in a case of nodular fasciitis of the breast," *Cancer Genetics and Cytogenetics*, vol. 81, no. 2, pp. 166–168, 1995.

[8] L. R. Donner, T. Silva, and S. M. Dobin, "Clonal rearrangement of 15p11.2, 16p11.2, and 16p13.3 in a case of nodular fasciitis: additional evidence favoring nodular fasciitis as a benign neoplasm and not a reactive tumefaction," *Cancer Genetics and Cytogenetics*, vol. 139, no. 2, pp. 138–140, 2002.

[9] G. V. N. Velagaleti, J. K. Tapper, N. E. Panova, M. Miettinen, and Z. Gatalica, "Cytogenetic findings in a case of nodular fasciitis of subclavicular region," *Cancer Genetics and Cytogenetics*, vol. 141, no. 2, pp. 160–163, 2003.

[10] M. R. Erickson-Johnson, M. M. Chou, B. R. Evers et al., "Nodular fasciitis: a novel model of transient neoplasia induced by MYH9-USP6 gene fusion," *Laboratory Investigation*, vol. 91, no. 10, pp. 1427–1433, 2011.

[11] P. Nair, W. A. Barrett, and T. Theodossy, "Oral nodular fasciitis: case report," *British Journal of Oral and Maxillofacial Surgery*, vol. 42, no. 4, pp. 360–362, 2004.

[12] W. Han, Q. Hu, X. Yang, Z. Wang, and X. Huang, "Nodular fasciitis in the orofacial region," *International Journal of Oral and Maxillofacial Surgery*, vol. 35, no. 10, pp. 924–927, 2006.

[13] A. Naidu and M. A. Lerman, "Clinical pathologic conference case 3: nodular fasciitis," *Head and Neck Pathology*, vol. 5, no. 3, pp. 276–280, 2011.

[14] V. Reiser, M. Alterman, B. Shlomi et al., "Oral intravascular fasciitis: a rare maxillofacial lesion," *Oral Surgery, Oral Medicine, Oral Pathology and Oral Radiology*, vol. 114, no. 2, pp. e40–e44, 2012.

[15] N. Chaithanyaa, P. Somannavar, and N. A. Annajal, "Nodular fasciitis over the anterior wall of the maxillary sinus: a case report and review of the literature," *Oral Surgery, Oral Medicine, Oral Pathology and Oral Radiology*, vol. 115, no. 1, pp. e10–e15, 2013.

[16] F. J. Lima, M. L. Diniz De Sousa Lopes, F. José De Oliveira Nóbrega, and É. J. Dantas Da Silveira, "A rare case of intraoral nodular fasciitis: diagnosis and immunohistochemical profile," *Journal of Oral and Maxillofacial Surgery*, vol. 72, no. 3, pp. 529–536, 2014.

[17] A. C. Chi, W. S. Dunlap, M. S. Richardson, and B. W. Neville, "Intravascular fasciitis: report of an intraoral case and review of the literature," *Head and Neck Pathology*, vol. 6, no. 1, pp. 140–145, 2012.

[18] X. Y. Lin, L. Wang, Y. Zhang et al., "Variable Ki67 proliferative index in 65 cases of nodular fasciitis, compared with fibrosarcoma and fibromatosis," *Diagnostic Pathology*, vol. 8, article 50, 2013.

[19] A. K. Sharma, G. Scott, and P. L. Westesson, "MRI sign of nodular fasciitis: a case report," *Oral Surgery, Oral Medicine, Oral Pathology, Oral Radiology, and Endodontology*, vol. 105, pp. e53–e56, 2008.

[20] M. L. de Carli, K. Sá Fernandes, D. dos Santos Pinto Jr., A. L. Witzel, and M. T. Martins, "Nodular fasciitis of the oral cavity with partial spontaneous regression (nodular fasciitis)," *Head and Neck Pathology*, vol. 7, no. 1, pp. 69–72, 2013.

[21] W.-X. Peng, M. Kudo, T. Yamamoto et al., "Nodular fasciitis in the parotid gland: a case report and review of the literature," *Diagnostic Cytopathology*, vol. 41, no. 9, pp. 829–833, 2013.

[22] T. Imai, M. Michizawa, and M. Nakazawa, "Nodular fasciitis in the buccal region with rapid growth after incisional biopsy mimicking sarcoma," *Journal of Craniofacial Surgery*, vol. 24, no. 6, pp. e615–e617, 2013.

[23] B. Bhattacharya, H. P. Dilworth, C. Iacobuzio-Donahue et al., "Nuclear β-catenin expression distinguishes deep fibromatosis from other benign and malignant fibroblastic and myofibroblastic lesions," *The American Journal of Surgical Pathology*, vol. 29, no. 5, pp. 653–659, 2005.

[24] A. Yanagisawa and H. Okada, "Nodular fasciitis with degeneration and regression," *Journal of Craniofacial Surgery*, vol. 19, no. 4, pp. 1167–1170, 2008.

37

Long-Term Follow-Up of a Revascularized Immature Necrotic Tooth Evaluated by CBCT

C. M. L. She, G. S. P. Cheung, and C. F. Zhang

Comprehensive Dental Care, Endodontics, Faculty of Dentistry, The University of Hong Kong, Hong Kong

Correspondence should be addressed to C. F. Zhang; zhangcf@hku.hk

Academic Editor: Ali I. Abdalla

This case study reports the successful treatment of an immature upper premolar with periapical pathosis and sinus tract using revascularization technique. Clinical and radiographic examination demonstrated the recovery of vitality, continued root development, and periapical healing at the 7-month follow-up. In addition, severe calcification of the canal was noted at the 36-month follow-up. At the 66-month follow-up, cone-beam computed tomography (CBCT) revealed complete periapical healing, apical closure, increase in root length and thickness of dentin, and severe calcification of the root canal. Even though the nature of tissue within the root canal is unknown, revascularization appears to give good clinical and radiographic success. This case report highlights that severe calcification of the canal is one of the long-term outcomes of revascularized root canals.

1. Introduction

It is often challenging to treat cases of pulpal necrosis involving immature teeth with open apices, as the root canal walls are often thin and prone to fracture. This makes it difficult for root canal instrumentation and obturation [1]. Historically, immature teeth with open apices have been treated by apexification, with placement of intracanal calcium hydroxide medicament to induce the formation of a calcific barrier at the root apex [2]. However, the strong alkalinity of calcium hydroxide may result in the denaturing of the carboxylate and phosphate groups, initiating a collapse of the bonding between the collagen network and hydroxyapatite crystals of the root dentin, thereby increasing the risk of root fracture [3]. Nowadays, apexification is no longer practiced routinely [4].

To overcome the shortcomings of apexification, mineral trioxide aggregate (MTA) has been advocated as the apical root filling to create a barrier [4]. The advantages include shorter treatment time and favorable healing of the periapical tissues due to the good sealing ability and biocompatibility of MTA [2, 5]. However, these teeth are still prone to fracture due to the short root length and insufficient dentin thickness [3, 6].

More recently, revascularization/regenerative procedures have been favored as they allow for the continued growth of immature root. The concept of revascularization is such that it focuses on gaining of blood supply into the disinfected root canal space, triggering a process similar to wound healing in surgical procedures [7]. The primary goal of regenerative endodontic procedures would be to achieve resolution of periapical lesion with absence of any clinical signs or symptoms. The secondary goal would be to achieve an increase in root length and thickness of dentinal walls, along with eventual apical closure. Finally, the tertiary goal would be to obtain positive responses to pulp sensibility testing [8]. There has been a scarcity of long-term case reports in the literature on revascularization of immature teeth with induction of blood clot formation. Most of the published studies have rather short follow-up periods, with the longest reported as 5 years for those involving induction of blood clot formation and 13 years for those without induction of blood clot [9–11]. It is essential to have long-term evaluation of such cases to find out the treatment outcomes, which may include canal calcification.

2. Case Report

A 12-year-old male patient with noncontributory medical history was referred to Prince Phillip Dental Hospital, a dental teaching hospital in Hong Kong, for root canal treatment of tooth 15. The patient complained of swelling on the upper right region for the past 3 months. Clinical examination revealed a fractured tubercle (dens evaginatus) of tooth 15. A draining sinus tract was observed on the buccal attached gingiva between tooth 14 and tooth 15. Tooth 15 was tender to percussion and palpation and had negative responses to cold and electric pulp testing. Radiographic examination revealed immature root formation of tooth 15, with a periapical radiolucency measuring approximately 5 mm in diameter. A diagnosis of an open apex with necrotic pulp and chronic apical abscess was made based on the clinical and radiographic findings.

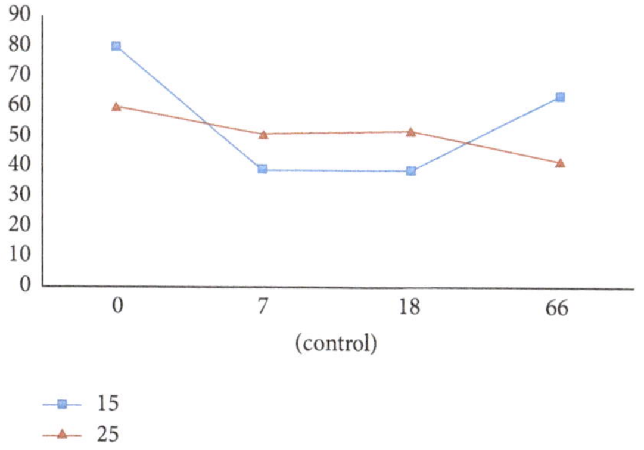

FIGURE 1: Graph showing the electric pulp testing (EPT) readings of tooth 15 and tooth 25 (control).

3. Treatment

After informed consent was taken, local anesthesia was given using 2% Xylestesin with 1 : 80 000 epinephrine (3M ESPE, Neuss, Germany), and tooth 15 was isolated with a rubber dam. An access cavity was prepared using a high-speed handpiece with copious water spray. The necrotic pulpal remnants were removed under copious irrigation with 3% sodium hypochlorite (15 mL) and sterile saline, along with gentle debridement of the canal walls. Working length was determined by estimating the radiographic working length. The canal was dressed with calcium hydroxide medicament (Calasept, Nordiska Dental, Ängelholm, Sweden) by injecting it directly into the canal and a temporary filling consisting of Cavit (3M ESPE AG, Seefeld, Germany) and Intermediate Restorative Material (IRM) (Dentsply Caulk, Milford, USA) was placed.

At the second visit 3 weeks later, the buccal sinus tract was noted to have healed and the tooth was asymptomatic. The tooth was reopened to replace the calcium hydroxide dressing. At the third visit another 2 weeks later, local anesthesia was given using 3% Mepivastesin (3M ESPE, Neuss, Germany). The root canal was irrigated copiously with sterile saline and dried with sterile paper points (Dentsply Maillefer, Ballaigues, Switzerland). Bleeding was induced by overinstrumentation of the canal length with a size #40 K-file, and a blood clot was formed at the middle third of the root. Grey MTA (ProRoot, Dentsply Tulsa Dental, Johnson City, TN, USA) was placed over the blood clot, followed by a moist cotton pellet above. The access cavity was then restored with IRM (Dentsply Caulk, Milford, USA). The patient was seen 1 week later and the temporary restoration was removed under rubber dam isolation. After confirming that the MTA has set, the tooth was restored with glass-ionomer cement (GC Corporation, Tokyo, Japan) and universal composite resin (3M ESPE, St. Paul, MN, USA).

4. Follow-Up Examinations

In follow-up visits (at 4, 7, 18, 36, and 66 months postoperatively), no clinical signs or symptoms were detected. Healing of the periapical lesion was observed at the 4-month follow-up. After 7 months, continued root growth was noted, and the tooth gave positive responses to both cold and electric pulp tests (Figure 1). Apical closure was observed at the 18-month follow-up. At the 36-month and 66-month follow-up, periapical radiograph revealed severe calcification of the canal (Figure 2). A CBCT examination of the tooth was done at the 66-month follow-up, which demonstrated a narrowed canal lumen (Figure 3). Clinical examination revealed greyish discoloration at the cervical region of the crown (Figure 4).

5. Discussion

Regenerative endodontics has been described as procedures to replace the original structure and histology of damaged or lost dentin, root structures, and cells of the pulp-dentin complex [12]. However, animal histological studies demonstrated the ingrowth of periodontal-like, cementum-like, and bone-like tissues into the pulpal space, rather than true pulpal regeneration [12]. Furthermore, continued root growth after revascularization of immature permanent necrotic teeth depends on the ability of Hertwig's epithelial root sheath (HERS) to survive after apical periodontitis or abscess [13].

Published case reports have shown that successful treatment outcome can be obtained when there is (i) eradication of bacteria from the root canal system, (ii) construction of a scaffold for the ingrowth of new tissue, and (iii) prevention of reinfection by creating a bacteria-tight seal [14]. The choice of irrigants and medicaments has to be made based on their antimicrobial effectiveness, with the minimum destruction to stem cells and growth factors. Both calcium hydroxide and triple antibiotic paste are effective in disinfection of canals [15]. Triple antibiotic paste was used by Banchs and Trope [16], and it has proven to be a very effective antimicrobial agent both in vitro and in vivo [17]. However, it has the disadvantage of causing discoloration of teeth and may be cytotoxic to stem cells at high concentrations. An in vitro study has shown that antibiotic paste with concentrations higher than 1 mg/mL would affect the survival of stem cells in the apical papilla, whereas calcium hydroxide promoted stem cell survival [15]. Hence, recently there seems to be a trend

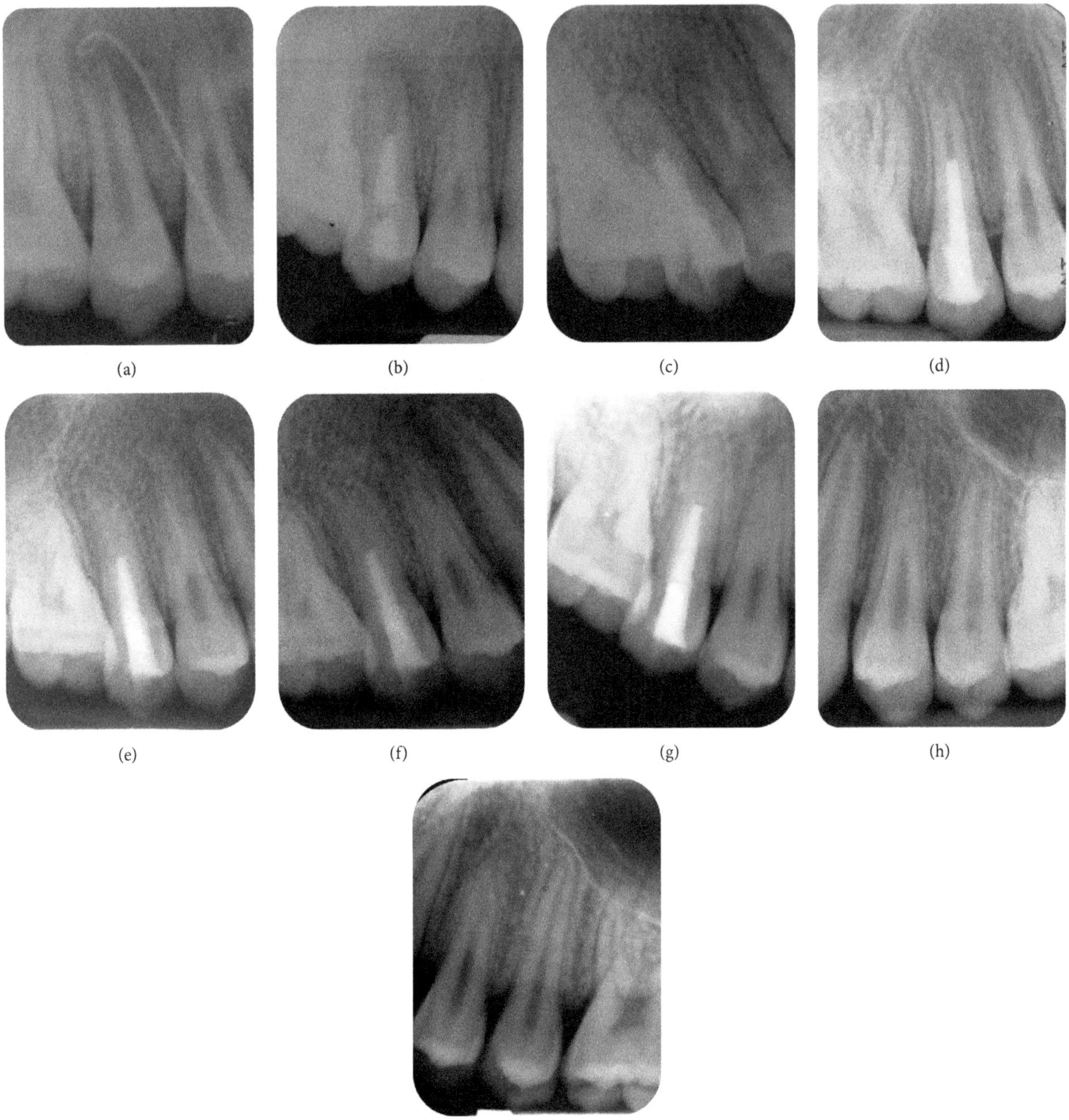

FIGURE 2: Periapical radiographs. (a) Preoperative, sinus tracing with gutta-percha. (b) After placement of MTA into the root canal. (c) 4-month follow-up showing healing of periapical lesion. (d) 7-month follow-up showing increase in root length. (e) 18-month follow-up showing apical closure. (f) 36-month follow-up showing a narrowed canal lumen. (g) 66-month follow-up showing absence of canal lumen. (h) Tooth 25 (control) at 7-month follow-up. (i) Tooth 25 (control) at 66-month follow-up.

of reverting back to the use of calcium hydroxide intracanal medicament, instead of the triple antibiotic paste.

A limited field-of-view CBCT was used to assess the treatment outcome of this tooth 15 at the 66-month follow-up. It is effective in assessing radiographic changes that may occur in the medullary bone, with the advantage of viewing at various (sagittal, coronal, and transverse) directions [18]. The advantages of CBCT can be clearly seen by comparing the periapical radiograph of tooth 15 with its corresponding CBCT image (Figures 2 and 3), where the former displayed absence of a canal space, while the latter was able to pick up a narrowed canal lumen.

In this case report, severe calcification of canal space was noted, similar to findings reported by other authors [13]. It

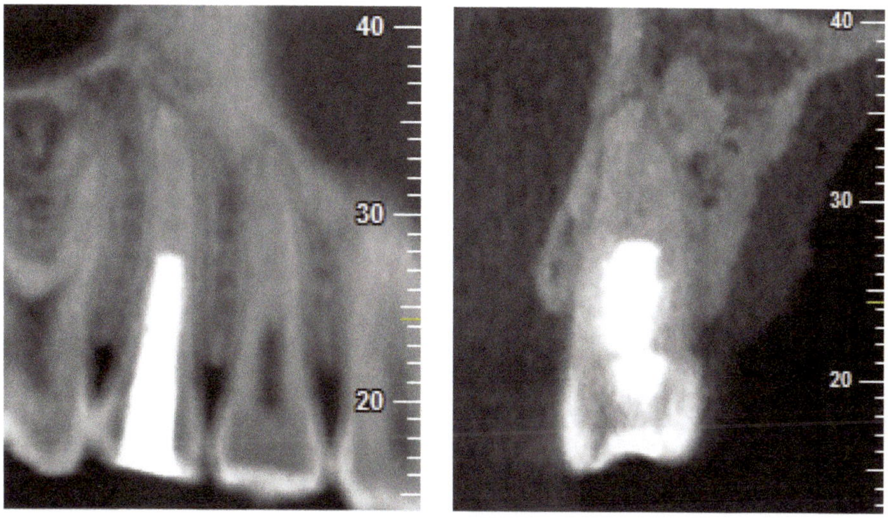

(a) (b)

FIGURE 3: CBCT images at 66 months showing the presence of a narrowed canal lumen due to severe calcifications. (a) CBCT (sagittal view). (b) CBCT (coronal view).

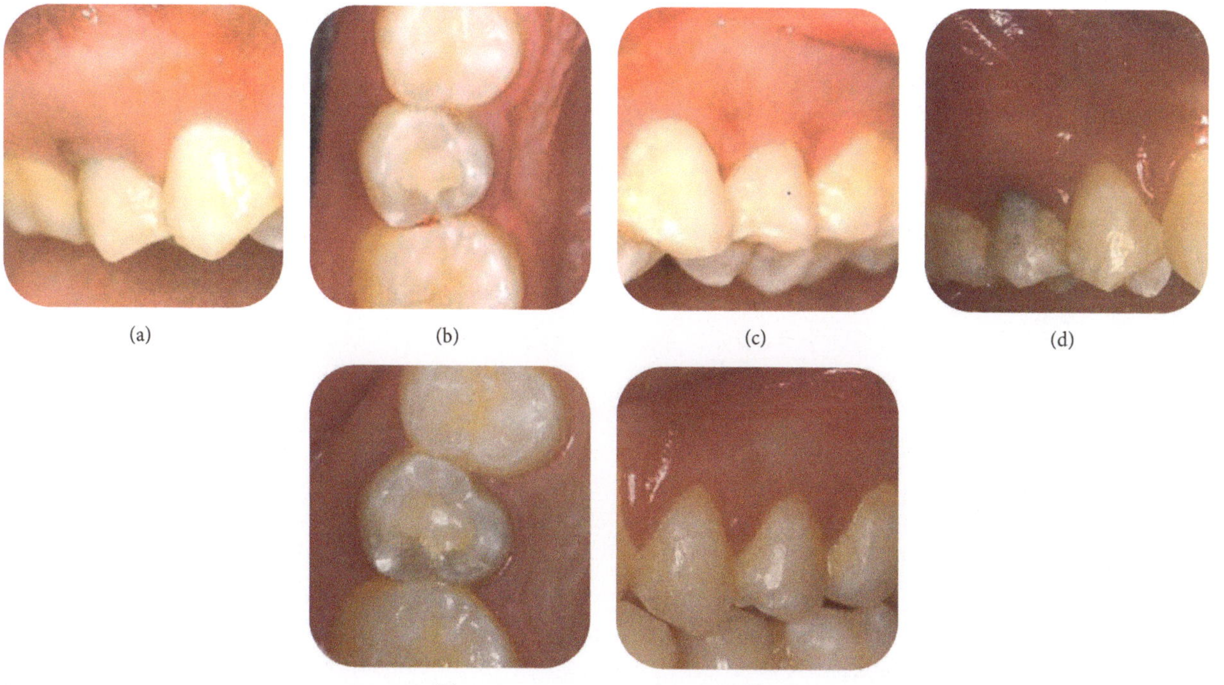

(a) (b) (c) (d) (e) (f)

FIGURE 4: Intraoral photos (1st row: 7-month follow-up, 2nd row: 66-month follow-up). (a) Tooth 15, buccal view. (b) Tooth 15, occlusal view. (c) Tooth 25 (control), buccal view. (d) Tooth 15, buccal view, showing greyish discoloration on the cervical crown of tooth. (e) Tooth 15, occlusal view. (f) Tooth 25, buccal view.

is one of the five types of treatment outcomes associated with regenerative endodontic procedure reported by Chen et al. [13]. Pulp canal obliteration is a known consequence of traumatic injuries to teeth, tooth replantation, and periodontal disease. However, it is not known if the mechanism is similar in the revascularization of immature permanent teeth with pulp necrosis. The possibility of internal replacement resorption or unification of intracanal solid tissue to apical alveolar bone cannot be ruled out [13]. It is also unknown if there would be any complications associated with pulp canal obliteration, such as pulpal necrosis with apical periodontitis, that has been shown in some teeth affected by traumatic injury [19].

In conclusion, this case report showed good clinical and radiographic outcomes for a revascularization procedure involving an immature tooth with pulpal necrosis and chronic apical abscess. However, clinical success may not equate to histological success. Long-term root canal calcification may be one of the treatment outcomes of revascularized teeth.

Conflict of Interests

The authors deny any conflict of interests related to this study.

References

[1] M. A. D. Al Ansary, P. F. Day, M. S. Duggal, and P. A. Brunton, "Interventions for treating traumatized necrotic immature permanent anterior teeth: inducing a calcific barrier & root strengthening," *Dental Traumatology*, vol. 25, no. 4, pp. 367–379, 2009.

[2] M. Trope, "Treatment of the immature tooth with a non-vital pulp and apical periodontitis," *Dental Clinics of North America*, vol. 54, no. 2, pp. 313–324, 2010.

[3] J. O. Andreasen, B. Farik, and E. C. Munksgaard, "Long-term calcium hydroxide as a root canal dressing may increase risk of root fracture," *Dental Traumatology*, vol. 18, no. 3, pp. 134–137, 2002.

[4] G. T.-J. Huang, "Apexification: the beginning of its end," *International Endodontic Journal*, vol. 42, no. 10, pp. 855–866, 2009.

[5] S. Simon, F. Rilliard, A. Berdal, and P. Machtou, "The use of mineral trioxide aggregate in one-visit apexification treatment: a prospective study," *International Endodontic Journal*, vol. 40, no. 3, pp. 186–197, 2007.

[6] M. Rafter, "Apexification: a review," *Dental Traumatology*, vol. 21, no. 1, pp. 1–8, 2005.

[7] B. Nygaard-Ostby and O. Hjortdal, "Tissue formation in the root canal following pulp removal," *Scandinavian Journal of Dental Research*, vol. 79, no. 5, pp. 333–349, 1971.

[8] G. T.-J. Huang, "A paradigm shift in endodontic management of immature teeth: conservation of stem cells for regeneration," *Journal of Dentistry*, vol. 36, no. 6, pp. 379–386, 2008.

[9] E. G. Kontakiotis, C. G. Filippatos, and A. Agrafioti, "Levels of evidence for the outcome of regenerative endodontic therapy," *Journal of Endodontics*, vol. 40, no. 8, pp. 1045–1053, 2014.

[10] J. Kottoor and N. Velmurugan, "Revascularization for a necrotic immature permanent lateral incisor: a case report and literature review," *International Journal of Paediatric Dentistry*, vol. 23, no. 4, pp. 310–316, 2013.

[11] S. I. Iwaya, M. Ikawa, and M. Kubota, "Revascularization of an immature permanent tooth with periradicular abscess after luxation," *Dental Traumatology*, vol. 27, no. 1, pp. 55–58, 2011.

[12] X. Zhu, Y. Wang, Y. Liu, G. T.-J. Huang, and C. Zhang, "Immunohistochemical and histochemical analysis of newly formed tissues in root canal space transplanted with dental pulp stem cells plus platelet-rich plasma," *Journal of Endodontics*, vol. 40, no. 10, pp. 1573–1578, 2014.

[13] M. Y.-H. Chen, K.-L. Chen, C.-A. Chen, F. Tayebaty, P. A. Rosenberg, and L. M. Lin, "Responses of immature permanent teeth with infected necrotic pulp tissue and apical periodontitis/abscess to revascularization procedures," *International Endodontic Journal*, vol. 45, no. 3, pp. 294–305, 2012.

[14] A. S. Law, "Considerations for regeneration procedures," *Journal of Endodontics*, vol. 39, supplement 3, pp. S44–S56, 2013.

[15] N. B. Ruparel, F. B. Teixeira, C. C. R. Ferraz, and A. Diogenes, "Direct effect of intracanal medicaments on survival of stem cells of the apical papilla," *Journal of Endodontics*, vol. 38, no. 10, pp. 1372–1375, 2012.

[16] F. Banchs and M. Trope, "Revascularization of immature permanent teeth with apical periodontitis: new treatment protocol?" *Journal of Endodontics*, vol. 30, no. 4, pp. 196–200, 2004.

[17] E. Hoshino, N. Kurihara-Ando, I. Sato et al., "In-vitro antibacterial susceptibility of bacteria taken from infected root dentine to a mixture of ciprofloxacin, metronidazole and minocycline," *International Endodontic Journal*, vol. 29, no. 2, pp. 125–130, 1996.

[18] R. Lenzi and M. Trope, "Revitalization procedures in two traumatized incisors with different biological outcomes," *Journal of Endodontics*, vol. 38, no. 3, pp. 411–414, 2012.

[19] A. Robertson, F. M. Andreasen, G. Bergenholtz, J. O. Andreasen, and J. G. Norén, "Incidence of pulp necrosis subsequent to pulp canal obliteration from trauma of permanent incisors," *Journal of Endodontics*, vol. 22, no. 10, pp. 557–560, 1996.

38

Nonsyndromic Bilateral Multiple Impacted Supernumerary Mandibular Third Molars: A Rare and Unusual Case Report

G. Siva Prasad Reddy, G. V. Reddy, I. Venkata Krishna, and Shravan Kumar Regonda

Department of Oral and Maxillofacial Surgery, Panineeya Institute of Dental Sciences, Road No. 5, Kamala Nagar, Dilsukhnagar, Hyderabad, Andhra Pradesh 500060, India

Correspondence should be addressed to G. Siva Prasad Reddy; gspreddy@yahoo.com

Academic Editors: A. Epivatianos, C. Evans, and M. W. Roberts

A supernumerary tooth is that which is present additionally to the normal series and can be found in any region of the dental arch. An impacted tooth is defined as the one which is embedded in the alveolus, so that its eruption is prevented, or the tooth is locked in position by bone or the adjacent teeth. The occurrence of multiple supernumerary teeth in only one patient in the absence of an associated systemic condition or syndrome is considered as a rare phenomenon. The occurrence of supernumerary teeth in the lower molar region is rare. A prevalence of less than 2% of cases occurring in this region has been estimated. Their occurrence presents a clinical problem for orthodontists and oral surgeons. The cause, frequency, complications, and surgical operation of impacted teeth are always interesting subjects for study and research. An impacted tooth can result in caries, pulp disease, periapical and periodontal disease, temporomandibular joint disorder, infection of the fascial space, root resorption of the adjacent tooth, and even oral and maxillofacial tumours. The management of impacted wisdom teeth has changed over the past 20 years from removal of nonsymptomatic third molars to simple observation. The aim of this paper is to present a rare case of bilateral multiple impacted supernumerary mandibular third molars.

1. Introduction

Supernumerary teeth may be defined as any teeth or tooth substance in excess of the usual configuration of 20 deciduous and 32 permanent teeth. Supernumerary teeth may occur in single, multiple, unilateral, or bilateral and in one or both the jaws.

The occurrence of multiple supernumerary teeth is a rare phenomenon and is often found in association with syndromes such as cleidocranial dysplasia, Gardners syndrome, or cleft lip and palate [1, 2]. Only a few examples of nonsyndromic multiple supernumerary teeth have been reported in the literature [3].

The most common supernumerary teeth, listed in order of frequency, are the maxillary midline supernumeraries, maxillary fourth molars, maxillary paramolars, mandibular premolars, maxillary lateral incisors, mandibular fourth molars, and maxillary premolars. Supernumerary teeth occur in the upper jaw ten times more frequently than in the lower jaw [4]. Multiple impacted teeth may be related to metabolic disorders. In some cases, however, impaction of multiple teeth is not accompanied by a fixed complex of symptoms. Although multiple supernumerary teeth without associated syndromes are rare, their occurrence can create a variety of clinical problems such as crowding, delayed eruption, diastema, rotations, cystic lesions, and resorption of the adjacent teeth. Hence, suitable treatment after proper clinical and radiographic evaluation is essential.

The aim of this case report is to document a rare and an unusual case of multiple impacted supernumerary mandibular third molars in an adult patient which is a unique presentation in the absence of any syndrome and to discuss our proposed clinical approach.

2. Case Report

A 22-year-old man was referred by a private dental practitioner to our unit with a chief complaint of pain in the lower right back tooth. The medical history, family history, and extraoral examination were not suggestive of any syndrome

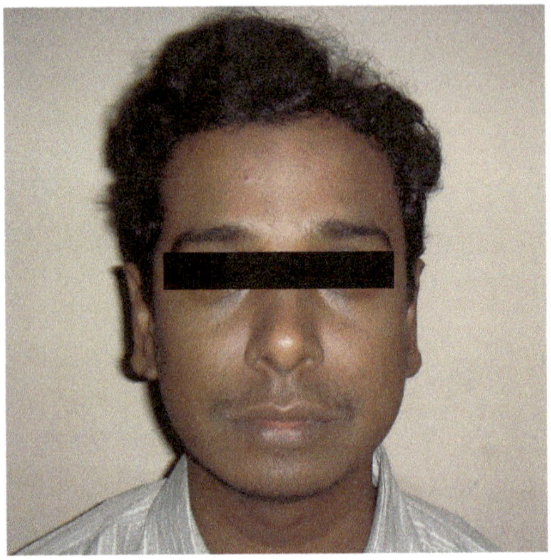

FIGURE 1: Frontal view of the patient.

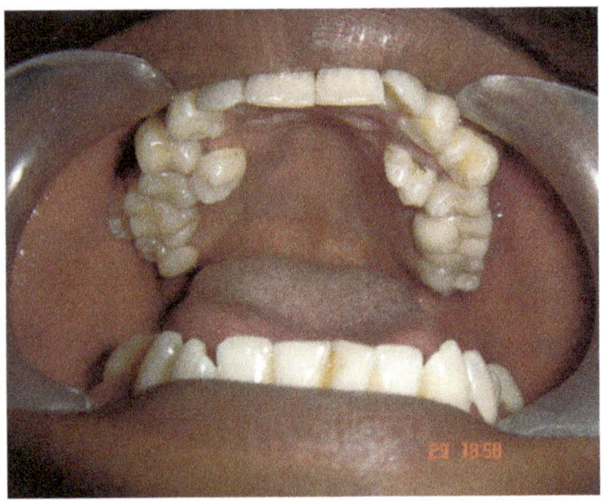

FIGURE 2: Intraoral photograph showing supernumerary teeth in the maxillary arch.

or metabolic disorder. General physical examination did not show any abnormality (Figure 1).

On local examination the patient had an impacted mandibular third molar which was grossly decayed. Other clinical findings included a total of six supernumerary teeth, four in the maxilla, and two in the mandible (Figures 2 and 3).

3. Radiographic Examination

In addition to the clinically noticed supernumerary teeth, the panoramic radiograph revealed the presence of impacted multiple supernumerary third molars in the mandible bilaterally (Figure 4). In total, the patient had ten supernumerary teeth. There are six impacted mandibular third molars: three on each side and of which two are supernumerary.

It was stated that unerupted supernumerary teeth that are asymptomatic do not appear to affect the dentition in any way, and those that are found by chance are sometimes best left in place and kept under observation. In this case,

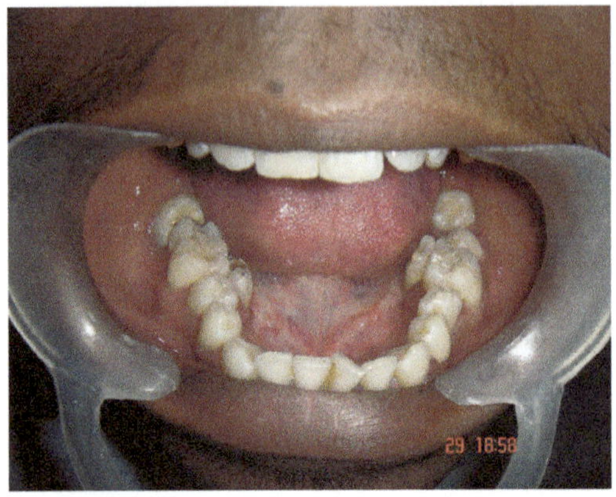

FIGURE 3: Intraoral photograph showing supernumerary teeth in the mandibular arch.

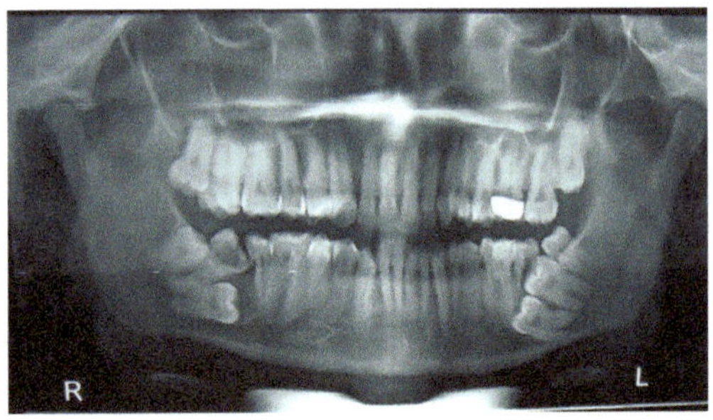

FIGURE 4: Orthopantomograph showing multiple supernumerary impacted teeth.

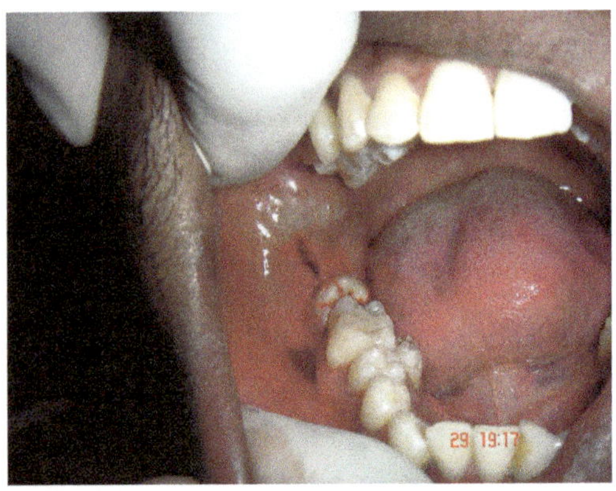

FIGURE 5: Incision and flap design for removal of mandibular third molar.

as the chief complaint of the patient was pain on the right side, two impacted third molars were surgically removed on that side under local anesthesia, the third one is left intact as it was asymptomatic, and its removal could cause serious complications like bleeding from the inferior dental canal (IDC) and fracture of the mandible (Figures 5, 6, 7, and 8).

The patient was explained about the surgical removal of the remaining impacted teeth under general anesthesia. He

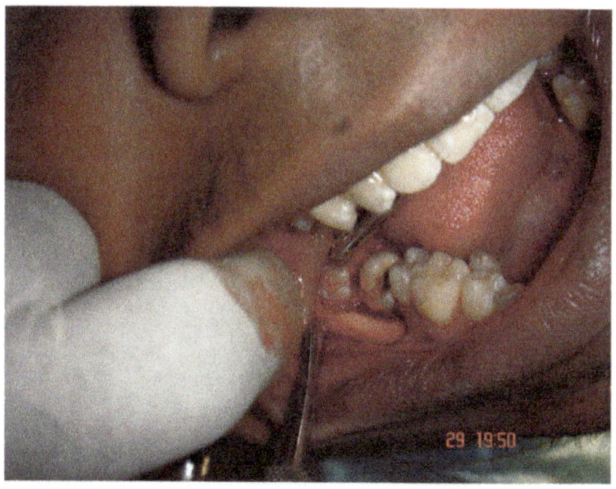

FIGURE 6: Exposed mandibular impated third molar and supernumerary teeth.

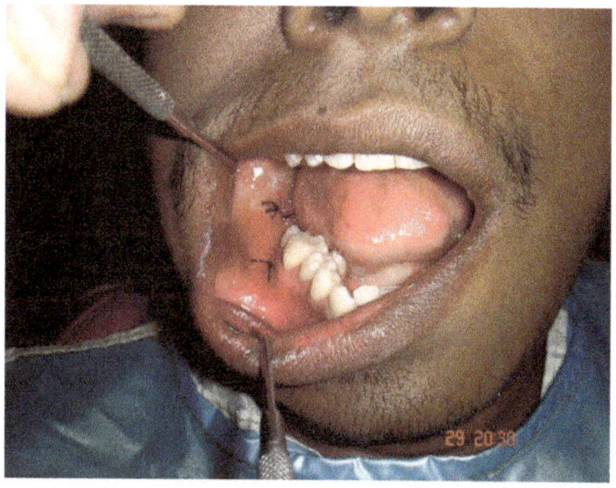

FIGURE 8: Closure of the surgical wound with mersilk suture.

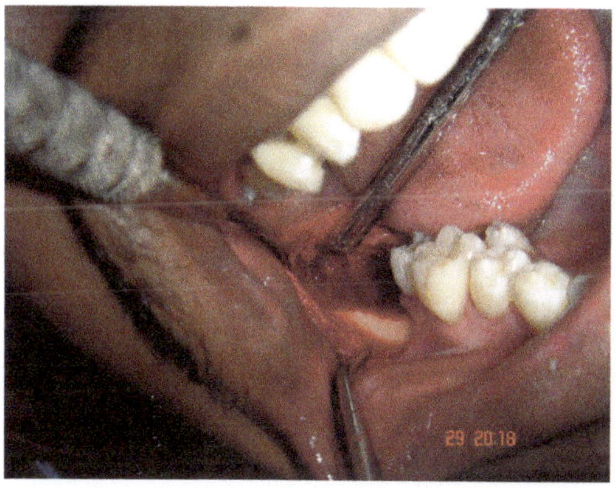

FIGURE 7: Sockets of extracted mandibular third molar and supernumerary teeth.

was also explained about the possible complications and their management. The patient did not come for further followup.

4. Discussion

The etiology of hyperdontia still remains unclear. Various theories have been proposed to explain the etiology of supernumerary teeth. They are (A) atavism or reversion, (B) heredity, (C) aberrations during embryologic formation, (D) progress zone, and (E) unified etiologic explanation [5]. Hyperactivity of the dental lamina is the most commonly accepted cause. Lack of space or crowding of dental arches, the premature loss of the primary teeth with subsequent partial closure of the area, and rotation of tooth buds are some of the most common causes contributing to impaction.

Supernumerary teeth can be classified according to the following:

(A) morphology: rudimentary or supplemental;

(B) number: single or multiple;

(C) location: mesiodens, paramolars, or distomolars.

The supernumerary teeth present in various different forms. If they are similar to a natural tooth, they are called by the same name, for instance, supernumerary canine, and otherwise, when its morphology is abnormal, it is just indicated as a supernumerary tooth located in a certain area. The occurrence of supernumerary teeth in the region of mandibular molars is less frequent than in the region of maxillary molars. Currently, more than 20 syndromes and developmental anomalies have been associated with supernumerary teeth [6]. The apparently morphologically normal finding of multiple supernumerary teeth in the absence of an associated systemic condition or syndrome is an uncommon phenomenon.

Supernumerary teeth may erupt normally or remain impacted, but in either case their presence may lead to clinical problems. Most problems associated with supernumeraries are because of their potential to interfere with normal occlusal development or with orthodontic mechanics such as crowding, separation, impaction, or delayed eruption of permanent teeth, malocclusion, rotations, retained deciduous teeth, palatally displaced permanent canines, abnormal eruption sequence, and compromised space closure. In addition to these, supernumerary teeth can also cause cyst formation. Hirose et al. [7] reported a case of multiple impacted teeth in upper jaw associated with large follicular cyst in the right maxillary sinus.

Radiographic examination is required to diagnose impacted supernumerary teeth, their position, their relation to the adjacent tooth, and the distance of the impacted permanent tooth to the occlusal plane. Whenever supernumerary teeth are diagnosed, single or multiple, a decision regarding the appropriate management should be made carefully. Surgical removal of the teeth may cause damage to adjacent structures. Cozza et al. [8] emphasized the importance of removing supernumerary teeth to eliminate the cause of a possible delayed eruption of the permanent dentition. Jones et al. stated that the removal of mandibular third molar by sagittal splitting of the mandible allows adequate access, controlled removal of bone, and enables the inferior alveolar nerve to be directly identified and protected [9].

In our opinion, the clinical management of multiple supernumerary teeth poses a great challenge to clinicians. Therefore, it is important to initiate appropriate consultation and an interdisciplinary approach for the treatment.

Acknowledgment

The authors sincerely thank Dr. Guruprasad Reddy (Dental Surgeon, Nizampet, Hyderabad) for referring this patient to their unit.

References

[1] A. I. Orhan, L. Özer, and K. Orhan, "Familial occurrence of non-syndromal multiple supernumerary teeth: a rare condition," *Angle Orthodontist*, vol. 76, no. 5, pp. 891–897, 2006.

[2] D. Yildirim, H. H. Yilmaz, and U. Aydin, "Case report: multiple impacted permanent and deciduous teeth," *Dentomaxillofacial Radiology*, vol. 33, no. 2, pp. 133–135, 2004.

[3] G. R. Bayar, K. Ortakoglu, and M. Sencimen, "Multiple impacted teeth : report of three cases," *European Journal of Dentistry*, vol. 2, pp. 73–78, 2008.

[4] A. Parihar, R. Ram Kishore, N. Vilas, and R. Madhu, "Multiple impacted permanent and supernumerary teeth: a case report," *Journal of Clinical and Diagnostic Research*, vol. 4, no. 5, pp. 3287–3288, 2010.

[5] V. K. Bharadwaj, J. R. Kaundal, A. Chug, S. Vaid, A. Soni, and M. Chandel:, "Rare occurrence of bilaterally impacted mandibular supernumerary teeth," *Dental Hypothesis*, vol. 3, no. 2, pp. 83–85, 2012.

[6] F. M. Rosa, A. Stankiewicz, and I. M. Faraco, "Impaction of mandibular molar by supernumerary tooth: case report," *Journal of Dentistry for Children*, vol. 75, no. 2, pp. 181–184, 2008.

[7] K. Hirose, S. Suzuki, and T. A. Kuroda, "Long-term follow- up case of multiple impacted teeth assosiated with large follicular cyst in maxilla," *Journal of the Stomatological Society*, vol. 67, no. 2, pp. 213–220, 2000.

[8] P. Cozza, M. Mucedero, F. Ballanti, and L. Toffol, "Supernumerary teeth and mental retardation: the importance of early surgical intervention," *European Journal of Paediatric Dentistry*, vol. 7, no. 1, pp. 45–49, 2006.

[9] T. A. Jones, T. Garg, and A. Monaghan, "Removal of a deeply impacted mandibular third molar through a sagittal split ramous osteotomy approach," *British Journal of Oral and Maxillofacial Surgery*, vol. 42, no. 4, pp. 365–368, 2004.

Hypophosphatemic Rickets in Siblings: A Rare Case Report

Gummadapu Sarat, Nuthalapati Priyanka, Meka Purna Venkata Prabhat, Chintamaneni Raja Lakshmi, Sujana Mulk Bhavana, and Dharmavaram Ayesha Thabusum

Department of Oral Medicine & Radiology, Drs. Sudha and Nageswara Siddhartha Institute of Dental Sciences, Chinoutpalli, Gannavaram Mandal, Andhra Pradesh 521286, India

Correspondence should be addressed to Nuthalapati Priyanka; dr.priyanka1724@gmail.com

Academic Editor: Yousef S. Khader

Hypophosphatemic rickets (HR) is a type of hereditary rickets characterized by persistent hypophosphatemia and hyperphosphaturia. The most predominant type is inherited in an X-linked fashion and caused by mutation in the gene encoding the phosphate-regulating endopeptidase homolog, X-linked (PHEX), identified in 1995. The X-linked hypophosphatemic (XLH) rickets is a rare hereditary metabolic disorder with a prevalence of 1 in 20,000 and causes deficient calcification of mineralized structures such as bones and teeth resulting in dental problems in terms of delayed eruption, spontaneous periapical infections, and exfoliation. We report one such unique case of hypophosphatemic vitamin D-resistant rickets in siblings exhibiting classical features of rickets with emphasis on its treatment and dental considerations.

1. Introduction

Rickets, a disease that occurs in children, is the failure of mineralization of osteoid commonly associated with either vitamin D deficiency or decrease of serum phosphate levels leading to hypophosphatemia. The condition, hypophosphatemic rickets, first described by Albright et al. [1] in 1937, with a prevalence of 1 in 20,000 [2], may be hereditary or acquired. Among these familial hypophosphatemia conditions is a rare inherited disorder [3]. It is most often inherited as X-linked trait with dominant transmission; however autosomal dominant and recessive forms also occur [4].

The case report describes the clinical, radiological, and biochemical features of hypophosphatemic rickets in siblings who came to the clinic with a chief complaint of missing teeth.

2. Case Report

A 10-year-old girl (Case 1) presented to the department of oral medicine with a chief complaint of missing teeth in the upper front region of the jaw for 7 years. There was history of trauma to the upper front region of jaw at about 3 years of age resulting in loss of deciduous teeth and delay in the eruption of permanent teeth.

2.1. Case 1. The patient is the second offspring after a full term normal uneventful pregnancy.

General examination (Case 1) revealed the height and weight as 45 inches and 14 kgs, which are less when compared with average height and weight of an age-matched Indian girl (average height: 54.4 inches, average weight: 32.5 kgs). There were frontal bossing, depressed nasal bridge (Figure 1), and knock knees (Figure 3). No signs of rachitic rosary (Figure 2), enlargement of wrist (Figure 3) and ankle joints, and bowed legs (Figure 4) were observed.

On intraoral examination, caries-free mixed dentition was present with missing permanent maxillary centrals and laterals with fair oral hygiene (Figure 5).

Radiographic Findings. Chest radiograph, radiograph of hip with femur and tibia, wrist radiograph, and orthopantomograph (OPG) were advised.

Radiographic findings of chest radiograph, radiograph of hip with femur and tibia, and wrist radiograph were interpreted by a general radiologist with 30-year experience.

(1) Chest radiograph (Figure 6) revealed mild scoliosis.

(2) Radiograph of hip with femur and tibia (Figure 7) revealed coxavara deformity.

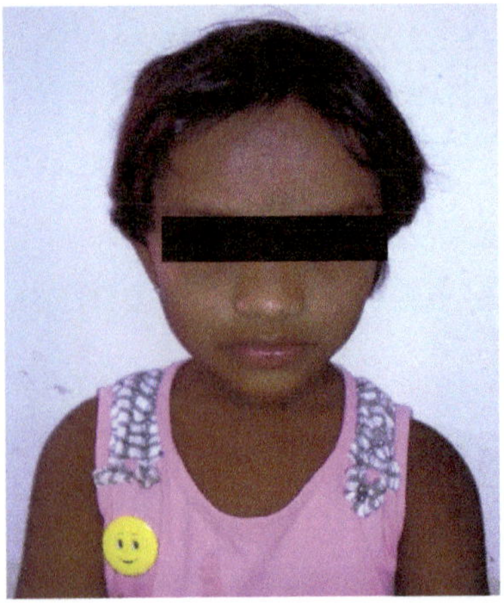

FIGURE 1: Showing frontal bossing and depressed nasal bridge.

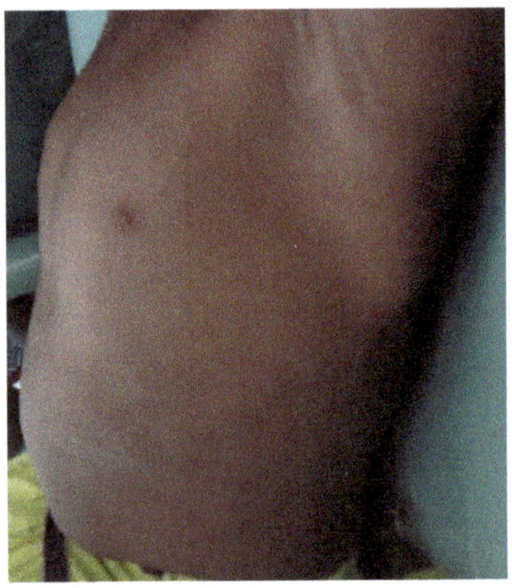

FIGURE 2: Showing no signs of rachitic rosary and Harrison's groove.

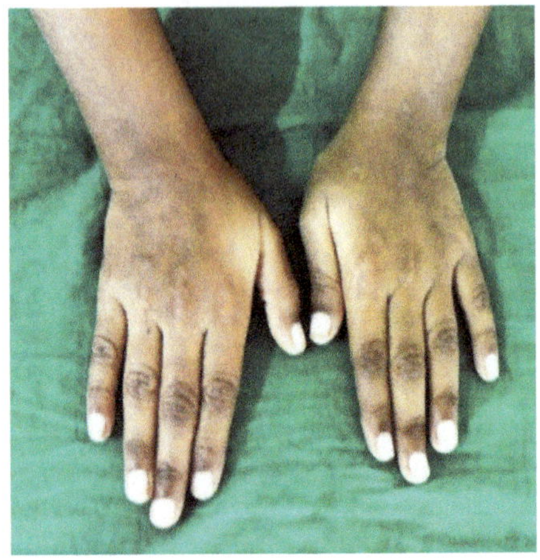

FIGURE 3: Showing no signs of widening of metaphysis.

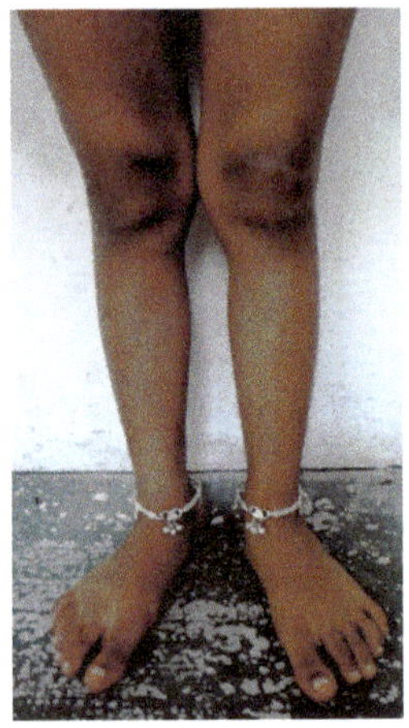

FIGURE 4: Showing knock knees.

(3) Wrist radiograph (Figure 8) revealed (a) epiphysis for radius noted but epiphysis for ulna not yet visualised, (b) few growth arrest lines noted in the lower end of radius, and (c) skeletal age found to be 5 yrs.

(4) OPG (Figure 9) revealed (a) the presence of deciduous teeth 53, 54, 62, 63, and 65, (b) presence of all the permanent teeth, and (c) enlarged pulp chambers with highly placed pulp horns extending to the dentinoenamel junction.

2.2. Case 2. On further investigation, the patient's mother revealed history of consanguineous marriage and that her younger daughter (Case 2), who is 7 years old, also showed similar features.

General examination revealed the height and weight as 23 inches and 10 kgs, which are less when compared with average height and weight of an age-matched Indian girl (average height: 47.4 inches, average weight: 21.8 kgs). Further examination revealed the clinical characteristics of base diagnosis given: There was bowing of legs (Figure 13) and enlargement at the wrist (Figure 12) and ankle joints (Figure 13). The presence of rachitic rosary (Figure 10) and Harrison's groove (Figure 11) was also noted.

On intraoral examination, incompetent lips, macroglossia (Figure 10), and caries-free mixed dentition were present with missing maxillary centrals, canines, and mandibular lateral incisors with fair oral hygiene (Figure 14).

Radiographic Findings. Chest radiograph, radiograph of hip with femur and tibia, wrist radiograph, and intraoral periapical (IOPA'S) radiographs were advised.

(1) Chest radiograph (Figure 15) revealed (a) mild scoliosis, (b) both humeral metaphyses showing fraying of bones with resorption in their proximal ends, and (c) ribs being broadened and anterior ends of ribs appearing to be widened which is the classical feature of rickets.

(2) Radiograph of hip with femur and tibia (Figure 16) revealed (a) cupping/fraying in both lower end of femur and upper end of tibia in both hips, (b) cortical thinning, (c) bowing of legs, (d) growth arrest lines, (e) epiphyseal widening, and (f) femoral ossific nuclei

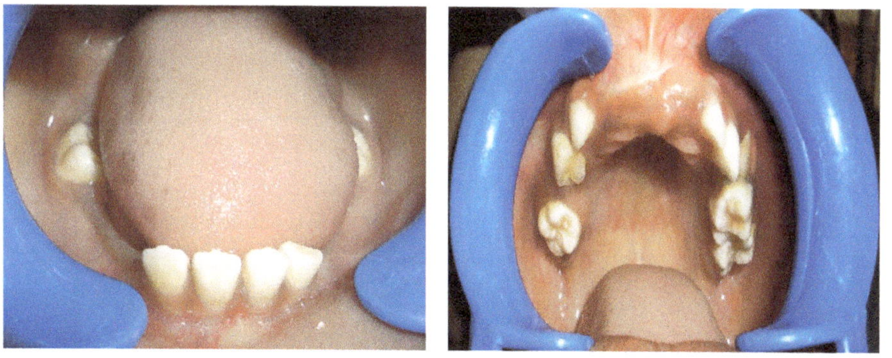

FIGURE 5: Showing missing teeth in relation to upper and lower anterior ends and mixed dentition.

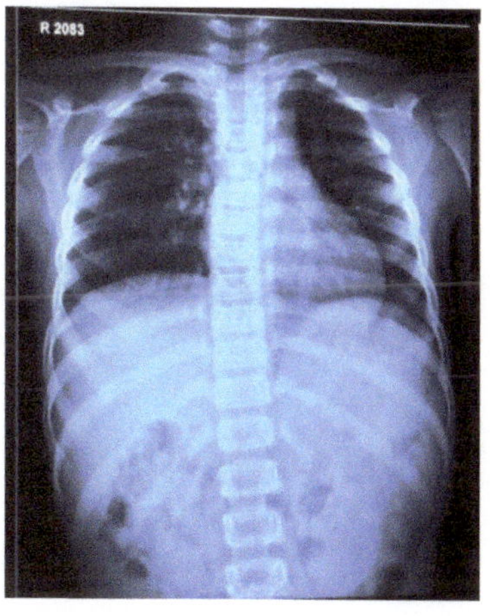

FIGURE 6: Chest radiograph.

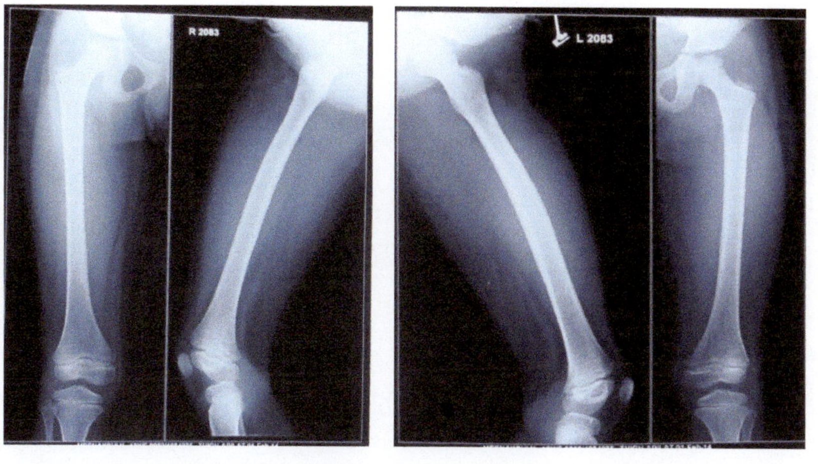

FIGURE 7: Radiograph of hip with femur and tibia.

not fully developed and appearing to be superiorly migrated.

(3) Wrist radiograph (Figure 17) revealed (a) widening and cupping/fraying of metaphysis in the lower ends of radius and ulna, (b) significant osteoporosis, (c) epiphysis for radius visible but epiphysis for ulna not yet visualised, (d) evidence of periostitis in metacarpals, (e) resorption of bones seen, and (f) skeletal age found to be 2 yrs.

(4) IOPA'S (Figure 18) shows the presence of deciduous teeth 52, 54, 55, 62, 65, 74, and 84 and all the permanent teeth.

TABLE 1: Depicting the laboratory investigations of both the siblings.

Serial number	Investigation	Normal levels	Levels in Case 1	Levels in Case 2
1	Serum inorganic phosphorus	4.5–5.5 mg/dL	3 mg/dL	2.8 mg/dL
2	Serum alkaline phosphatase	100–644 IU/L	1143 IU/L	1378 IU/L
3	Vitamin D	20–50 ng/mL	15 ng/mL	12 ng/mL
4	Serum chloride	98–106 mMol/L	113 mMol/L	89 mMol/L
5	Serum potassium	3.4–5.2 mMol/L	3.2 mMol/L	2.5 mMol/L
6	Serum bicarbonate	19–25 mMol/L	15 mMol/L	11 mMol/L
7	Serum calcium	8.8–10.8 mg/dL	9.1 mg/dL	7.3 mg/dL

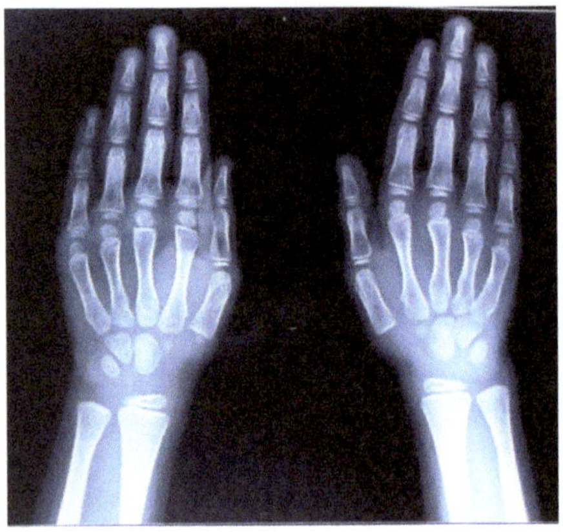

FIGURE 8: Wrist radiograph.

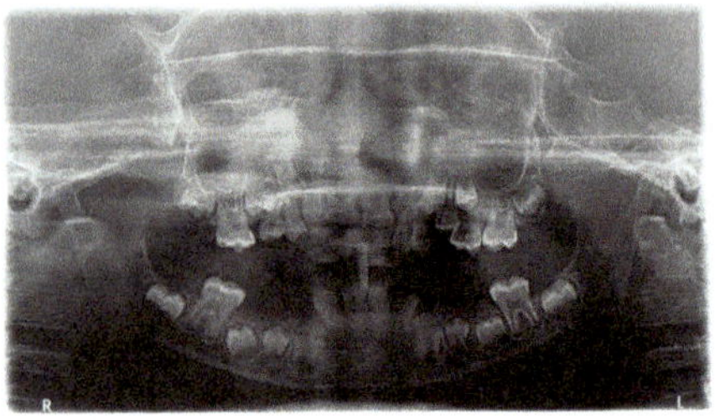

FIGURE 9: OPG.

Laboratory investigations of both Cases 1 and 2 are presented in Table 1. The ultrasound report of kidneys revealed early renal disease and complete blood picture revealed leucocytosis and thrombocytosis in both siblings.

3. Treatment

The general management is taking care by using neutral phosphate and calcitriol supplements for both siblings. As the patient's chief complaint was delayed eruption of teeth, Case 1 was given denture (Figure 19) so that it causes a stimulating effect on the underlying permanent teeth and causes its eruption along with fulfillment of esthetics. Case 2 was kept under observation for eruption of permanent teeth and if not, the same treatment as in Case 1 was planned.

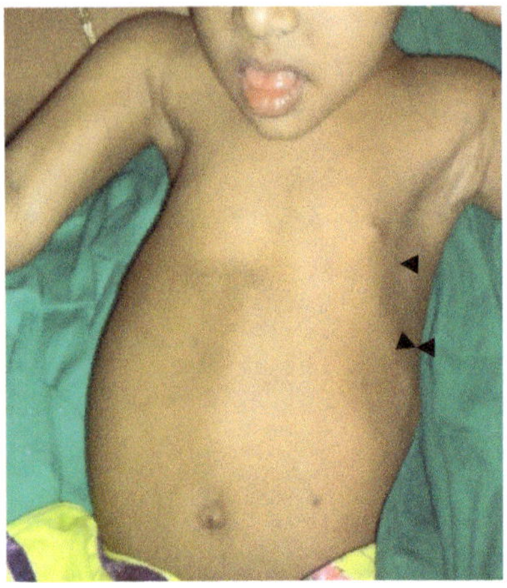

FIGURE 10: Showing rachitic rosary, incompetent lips, and macroglossia.

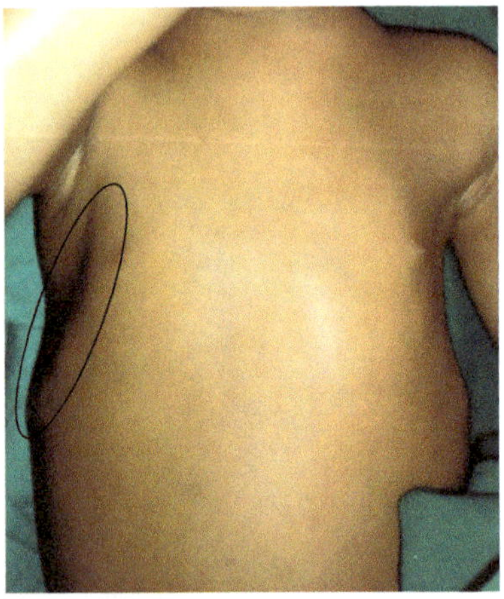

FIGURE 11: Showing Harrison's groove on the chest region.

4. Outcome and Follow-Up

The siblings were advised for periodical follow-ups for prevention of formation of abscesses along with fluoride and pit and fissure sealants application. Regular blood investigations were done to rule out the complications of medications used such as secondary hyperparathyroidism and nephrocalcinosis. On long term follow-up, of about 1 year, they

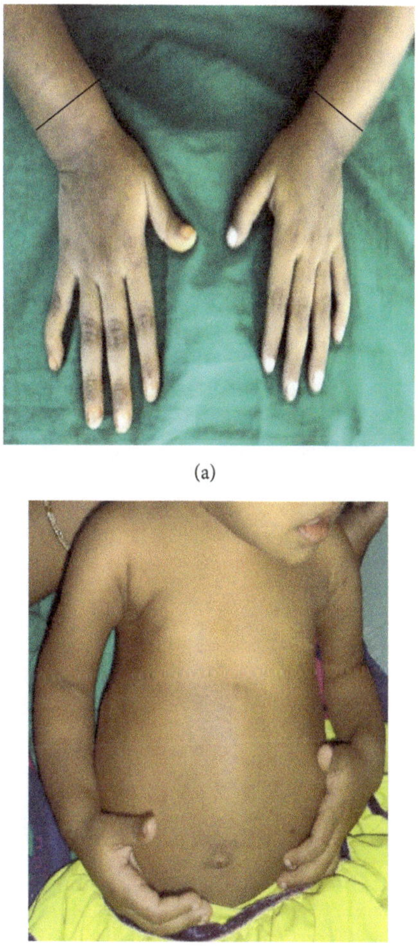

(a)

(b)

FIGURE 12: Showing widening of metaphysis.

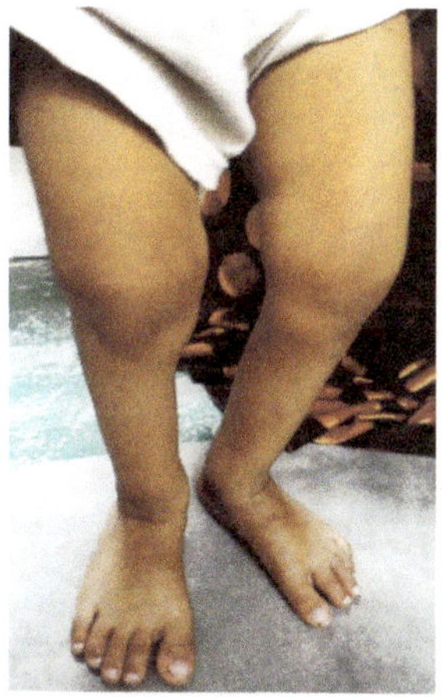

FIGURE 13: Showing bowed legs and enlargement of ankles.

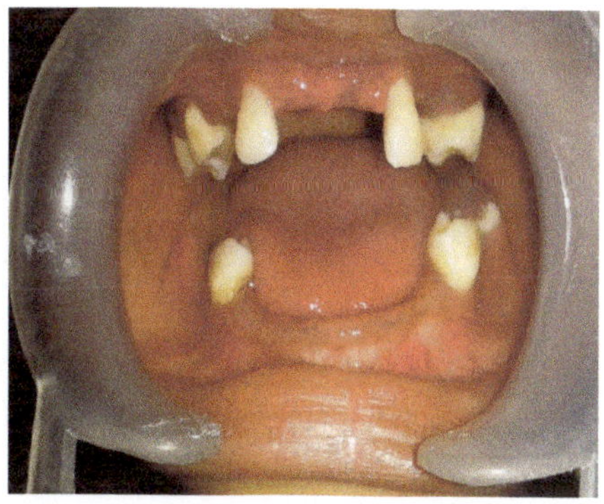

FIGURE 14: Showing mixed dentition and missing teeth in relation to upper and lower anterior ends.

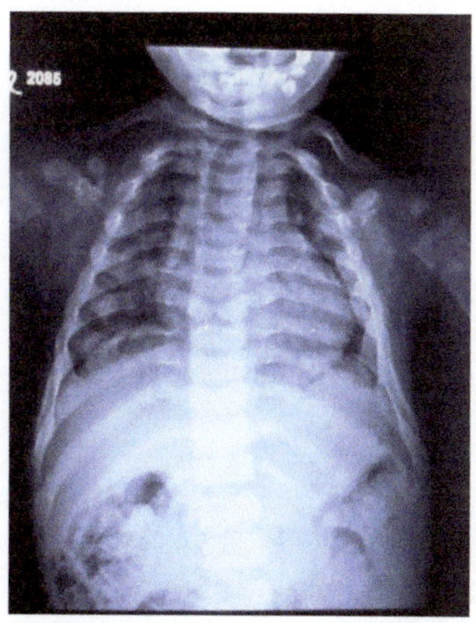

FIGURE 15: Chest radiograph.

showed improvement in gait physical activity and eruption of permanent teeth.

5. Discussion

The term rickets is derived from an old English word "wrickken," which means "to twist," and a Greek word "rachitis," which means inflammation of the spine. When the demineralized osteoid accumulates at the sites of bone formation, bones gradually soften leading to deformities in association with weight-bearing sites.

Initially, environmentally caused rickets was very common; however, when it was treated and prevented by public health measures, the vitamin D-resistant rickets came into picture. Econs and Francis [5] highlighted that some of the patients with rickets did not respond to physiological doses of vitamin D and named the condition as vitamin D-resistant rickets.

Inorganic phosphate plays a major role in many biological systems, including cell membrane functions, energy metabolism, cell signalling, and oxygen transport. In hypophosphatemic rickets, renal proximal tubular resorption is compromised due to mutations in PHEX gene which is a phosphate-regulating gene. It encodes a zinc metalloendopeptidase which is predominantly expressed in osteoblast and odontoblast [3, 5]. So the patient presents with hypophosphatemia along with a relative 1,25-(OH)2 vitamin D deficiency leading to the manifestations of rickets.

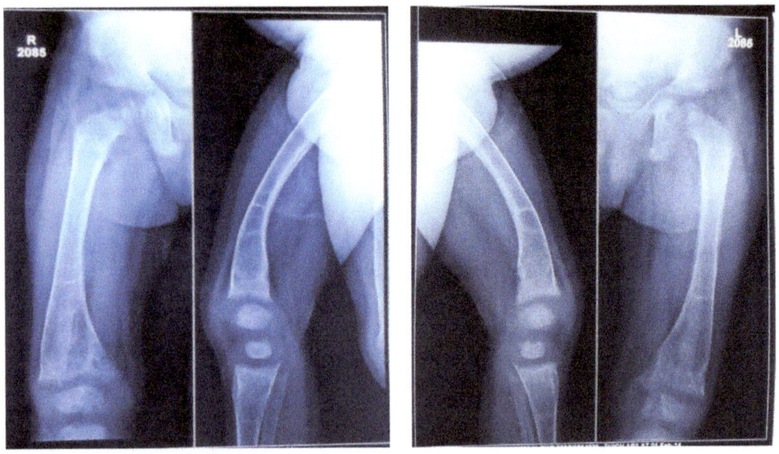

FIGURE 16: Radiograph of hip with femur and tibia.

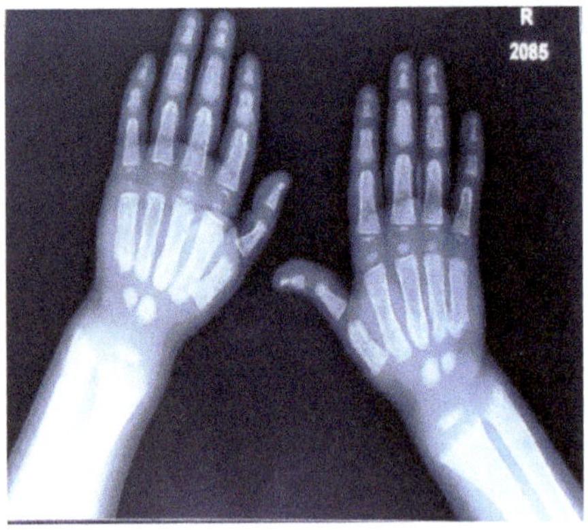

FIGURE 17: Wrist radiograph.

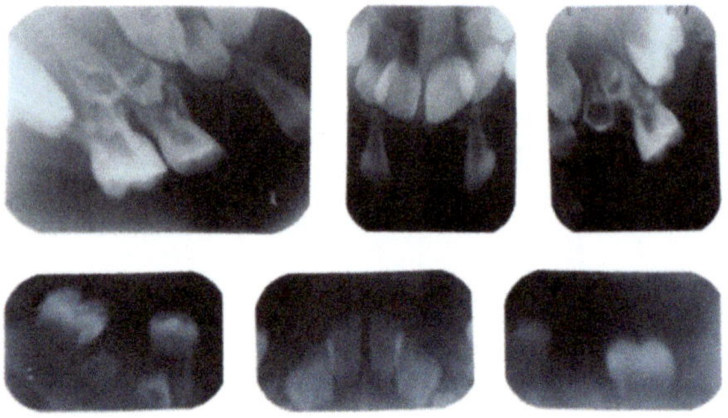

FIGURE 18: Intraoral periapical radiographs.

Familial hypophosphatemic rickets, in most patients, appears in a familial line of X-linked, dominant inheritance with the same prevalence in both sexes; however, it may also occur sporadically [6, 7]. Hypophosphatemic rickets is identified by clinical and radiological features such as decreased vertical height, craniotabes, rachitic rosary, bowing leg deformity (genu varum) or knock knee (genu valgum), double malleoli sign of ankles, metaphyseal hyperplasia of wrist, and Harrison's groove on the chest [8, 9]. Bowing deformity is common in the femur and tibia. The femur shows the coxa vara type of deformity, in which the neck makes an angle of less than 120° with the shaft of the femur [10].

Hypophosphatemic rickets has been related to several primary and permanent teeth alterations. The most commonly reported ones include normal but thin enamel and globular dentin and enlarged pulp chambers with pulp horns extending up to the dentinoenamel junction [11]. In this report, we did not observe specific enamel defects or hypoplasia in the case, but enamel and dentin layer were quite thin, with highly positioned pulp horns according to the radiographic and clinical evaluation. The aggregation of all these factors contributes to the formation of dental abscesses in cases when enamel is lost due to attrition or incipient caries and pulp infection takes place through poorly calcified dentin leading to multiple periodontal abscesses [12, 13] which is interestingly not found in the present case. The early exfoliation of deciduous teeth in rickets can be attributed to poorly defined lamina dura, dysplastic roots, and hypoplastic alveolar ridge [12]. In the present cases loss of deciduous teeth might have been due to trauma as well in both siblings. Hypophosphatemic rickets may be associated directly with increased prevalence of dental taurodontism [8, 14], an increase in the length of the body at the expense of the root.

Laboratory findings including low serum phosphate concentration and reduced tubular resorption of phosphate corrected for glomerular filtration rate (TmP/GFR) are characteristic. Serum calcium and 25-hydroxy vitamin D are within the normal range or decreased; parathyroid hormone is normal to slightly elevated. Alkaline phosphatase is characteristically elevated. In Case 2, all findings were positive along with low calcium and vitamin D levels whereas in Case 1 there were elevated alkaline phosphatase activity and decreased serum inorganic phosphorus levels. Additionally, the normal physiologic response of hypophosphatemia with supplementation of vitamin D is absent in these siblings suggestive of vitamin D-resistant hypophosphatemic rickets.

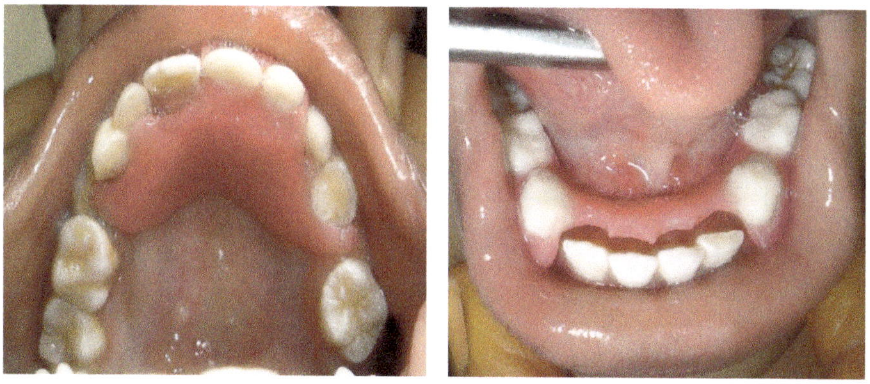

FIGURE 19

A family history of short stature, orthopedic abnormalities, poor dentition, and parental consanguinity may signify inherited rickets and the diagnostic criteria of X-linked hypophosphatemic rickets globally are based on history, clinical examination, and biochemical and radiological evaluation which are significant in these siblings.

The treatment of hypophosphatemic rickets is done by the oral administration of phosphorus and vitamin D. Currently, growth hormone [15] and KRN23 [16] a recombinant human monoclonal antibody targeting FGF23 are under investigation for hypophosphatemic rickets.

In our cases, general management is taking care by using neutral phosphate and calcitriol supplements. Regarding dental complaint Case 1 was given denture (Figure 19) and Case 2 was kept under observation for eruption of permanent teeth.

6. Learning Points

(i) Hypophosphatemic rickets is a rare disorder with dental manifestations seen in spectrum of severity, ranging from very severe, with involvement of nearly the entire dentition, to very mild with normal appearance of the teeth.

(ii) Being dentists, we hardly come across this rare variety of rickets in our clinics. Dental abscess in clinically normal teeth, early spontaneous exfoliation of clinically intact primary teeth, and the numerous teeth missing were the characteristics of patients with hypophosphatemic rickets.

(iii) So early detection, treatment, and proper adherence to treatment provide a good dental future to the patients limiting delayed eruption, spontaneous dental necrosis, and dental diseases classically associated with hypophosphatemic rickets.

Competing Interests

The authors declare that there are no competing interests regarding the publication of this paper.

References

[1] A. Sattur, V. G. Naikmasur, R. Shrivastava, and M. Babshet, "Familial hypophosphatemic rickets," *Journal of Indian Society of Pedodontics and Preventive Dentistry*, vol. 28, no. 4, pp. 302–306, 2010.

[2] G. G. Hernández and F. B. Laguna, "Dental characteristics of hypophosphatemic rickets. Case report," *Revista Odontológica Mexicana*, vol. 17, no. 2, pp. 101–108, 2013.

[3] J. Walton, "Familial hypophosphatemic rickets: a delineation of its subdivisions and pathogenesis," *Clinical Pediatrics*, vol. 15, no. 11, pp. 1007–1012, 1976.

[4] P. S. N. Rowe, C. L. Oudet, F. Francis et al., "Distribution of mutations in the PEX gene in families with X-linked hypophosphataemic rickets (HYP)," *Human Molecular Genetics*, vol. 6, no. 4, pp. 539–549, 1997.

[5] M. J. Econs and F. Francis, "Positional cloning of the PEX gene: new insights into the pathophysiology of X-linked hypophosphatemic rickets," *American Journal of Physiology—Renal Physiology*, vol. 273, no. 4, pp. F489–F498, 1997.

[6] D. Fraser and C. R. Scriver, "Familial forms of vitamin D-resistant rickets revisited. X-linked hypophosphatemia and autosomal recessive vitamin D dependency," *American Journal of Clinical Nutrition*, vol. 29, no. 11, pp. 1315–1329, 1976.

[7] J. R. Goodman, M. J. Gelbier, J. H. Bennett, and G. B. Winter, "Dental problems associated with hypophosphataemic vitamin D resistant rickets," *International Journal of Paediatric Dentistry*, vol. 8, no. 1, pp. 19–28, 1998.

[8] M. Larmas, E. L. Hietala, S. Similä, and U. Pajari, "Oral manifestations of familial hypophosphatemic rickets after phosphate supplement therapy: a review of the literature and report of case," *ASDC Journal of Dentistry for Children*, vol. 58, no. 4, pp. 328–334, 1991.

[9] G. J. Vasilakis, V. K. Nygaard, and D. M. DiPalma, "Vitamin D resistant rickets. A review and case report of an adolescent boy with a history of dental problems," *Journal of Oral Medicine*, vol. 35, no. 1, pp. 19–26, 1980.

[10] W. K. Seow and S. C. Latham, "The spectrum of dental manifestations in vitamin D-resistant rickets: implications for management," *Pediatric Dental Journal*, vol. 8, no. 2, pp. 245–250, 1986.

[11] C. M. Pereira, C. R. de Andrade, P. A. Vargas, R. D. Coletta, O. P. de Almeida, and M. A. Lopes, "Dental alterations associated

with X-linked hypophosphatemic rickets," *Journal of Endodontics*, vol. 30, no. 4, pp. 241–245, 2004.

[12] E. N. Tulloch and F. F. Andrews, "The association of dental abcesses with vitamin D resistant rickets," *British Dental Journal*, vol. 154, pp. 136–138, 1983.

[13] S. T. Tournis, P. V. Giannikou, I. N. Paspati, E. A. Katsalira, I. C. Voskaki, and G. P. Lyritis, "Co-existence of X-linked hypophosphatemic rickets (XLH) and primary hyperparathyroidism. Case report and review of the literature," *Journal of Musculoskeletal Neuronal Interactions*, vol. 5, no. 2, pp. 150–154, 2005.

[14] E. C. Tumen, I. Yavuz, D. S. Tumen, and F. Atakul, "Dental and histologic findings of X-linked hypophosphataemic vitamin D-resistant rickets: a case report," *International Dental and Medical Disorders*, vol. 1, pp. 37–42, 2008.

[15] D. Haffner, R. Nissel, E. Wühl, and O. Mehls, "Effects of growth hormone treatment on body proportions and final height among small children with X-linked hypophosphatemic rickets," *Pediatrics*, vol. 113, no. 6, pp. e593–e596, 2004.

[16] T. O. Carpenter, E. A. Imel, M. D. Ruppe et al., "Randomized trial of the anti-FGF23 antibody KRN23 in X-linked hypophosphatemia," *The Journal of Clinical Investigation*, vol. 124, no. 4, pp. 1587–1597, 2014.

40

Blade of Grass as an Unusual Cause of Recurrent Facial Cutaneous Sinus Tract: A Clinical Case

Resmije Ademi-Abdyli,[1] Feriall Perjuci,[1] Teuta Bicaj,[2] and Yll Abdyli[3]

[1] *Department of Oral Surgery, Medical Faculty, University of Prishtina, Dental Branch, 10000 Prishtina, Kosovo*
[2] *Department of Prosthetic Dentistry, Medical Faculty, University of Prishtina, Dental Branch, 10000 Prishtina, Kosovo*
[3] *Medical Faculty, University of Prishtina, Dental Branch, 10000 Prishtina, Kosovo*

Correspondence should be addressed to Teuta Bicaj; teutab68@yahoo.com

Academic Editor: Tommaso Lombardi

The presence of an embedded foreign body in the oral and maxillofacial region is not unusual, but the impaction of a foreign body with vegetative nature is rare. Prompt diagnosis and surgical removal of these foreign bodies will minimize their associated complications. This case report presents a patient with recurrent submandibular abscess and persistent facial cutaneous sinus tract caused by a retained blade of grass inside the facial soft tissue. The fact that the plain radiograph misdiagnosed the presence of a foreign body meant that the pathology persisted for about three months, and the patient underwent hospitalization, surgical procedures, and antibiotic regimens; however all of these failed until the foreign body was detected and removed. *Conclusion.* To avoid misdiagnosis of foreign body presence in the orofacial region, notably suspected foreign bodies with low radiopacity, the clinician must perform careful clinical examination and use the ultrasonography. Also, in the uncertain cases where the pathology persists, despite having undertaken surgical procedures and antibiotic regimens, the clinician should pay more attention to the patient's history which may suggest the presence of the foreign body.

1. Introduction

The cutaneous sinus tract in the orofacial region as a sequel of dental origin is a common condition, and its diagnosis is usually easy, if the clinician considers the possibility of its dental origin. However, cutaneous sinus tract can also be a sequel of a retained occult foreign body (FB) in soft tissues [1].

The entry of foreign bodies (FBs) into the orofacial region and their inculpation is not unusual. Their entrance could be accidental due to trauma or iatrogenic factors [2–4].

FBs may remain dormant in the soft tissue for years without causing damage to adjacent structures [1]; however, some FBs can be a source of chronic inflammatory reactions and infection [5, 6].

Although most of the impacted FBs in oral and perioral tissue are of inorganic nature such as parts of surgical instruments or burs and filling materials (amalgams, composites, cements, or gutta-percha points) [4, 7, 8], the researched literature reveals few cases with FB impaction of a vegetative nature [1, 6, 9–12].

Detection of FBs inside the soft tissue is often very difficult because the ingrained FBs induce a reparative granuloma formation which surrounds them, making their detection by eye difficult, even during surgical treatment [1]. The early detection and diagnosis of FBs is usually based on the patients' history, clinical examination, and the various radiographic imaging methods such as plain radiographs, CT (computed tomography), and ultrasound.

The visibility of FBs on plain radiographs depends on their ability to absorb X-rays, their density and the difference in density between them and the tissue in which they are embedded, therefore conventional plain radiography is helpful only in cases of radiopaque FBs.

When common radiographs, patient history and clinical examinations fail to reveal the presence of retained FBs with low radiopacity, they can be detected using CT scans and ultrasonography [1, 4, 12–18].

Based on the study of Javadrashid et al. [17], wood could only be detected using an ultrasound as it is highly sensitive and more effective than CT for identifying the superficial FBs with low radiopacity.

When the history is dubious and radiographic analyses are inconclusive, surgical exploration remains the diagnostic choice in conjunction with therapeutic modality.

2. The Objective of the Study

To alert clinicians that in the process of FB diagnosis, in addition to clinical, radiographic, and other available examination methods, the patient's history should be considered essential, especially in the uncertain cases where the pathology persists, despite performed surgical procedures and antibiotic regimens.

3. Clinical Case

A 28-year-old male reported to the Department of Oral Surgery with a history of complaints such as pain, recurrent swelling of the cheek, and cutaneous sinus tract, over a period of three months.

Based on patient's history, more than two months earlier, he attended to the Maxillofacial Surgery Department with complaints as pain and recurrent swelling of the cheek. The maxillofacial surgeon performed an extraoral incision and drainage of the pus from the submandibular region and suggested surgical extraction of the impacted wisdom tooth, documented by lateral radiography, as the cause of complaints. According to patient's data, although the oral surgeon performed the surgical removal of the wisdom tooth, he still had the same complaints. Consequently, he returned to the Department of Oral Surgery. Since a postsurgical wound infection was suspected, the oral surgeon performed the curettage of the surgical wound and prescribed antibiotics.

After a month, despite the previously performed treatments (tooth extraction, repeated tooth sockets curettages, and antibiotic regimens), the same symptoms returned, so he attended again to the Oral Surgery Department, the last dental visit. The complaints presented as dull pain, recurrent swelling, and purulent discharge from the cutaneous sinus tract at the incisional site of the involved region.

4. Clinical Findings and Diagnosis

Upon extraoral inspection of the right submandibular region, cutaneous sinus tract covered with scrub was noted at the incisional site, resulting in purulent discharge under pressure. Intraoral examination revealed a postoperative wound (postextraction tooth socket) of the right wisdom tooth, which did not heal completely after two months of tooth extraction. The patient's past medical history, dental history, and clinical examination were not helpful for any diagnosis. Since as evidence for patient's preoperative dental situation we had at our disposal only patient's lateral radiography (Figure 1), which showed a right mandibular impacted wisdom tooth, a retroalveolar radiograph was requested (Figure 2) with the aim of searching for the cause of delayed wound healing and persistent cutaneous sinus tract.

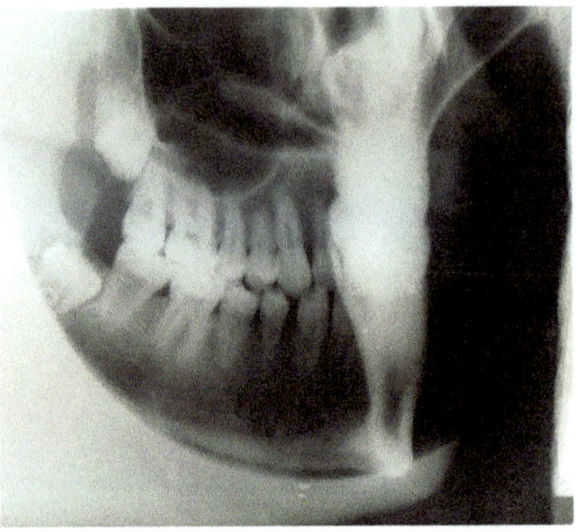

FIGURE 1: Preoperative lateral radiography of right side mandibular wisdom tooth.

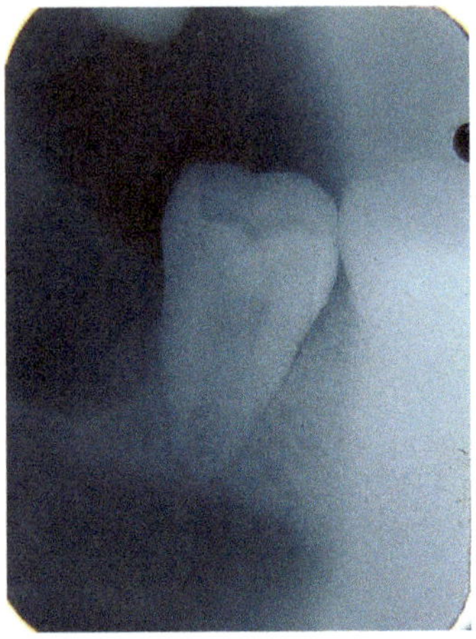

FIGURE 2: Postoperative retroalveolar radiography of postextraction tooth socket (wisdom tooth).

As the conventional retroalveolar radiography did not reveal anything suspicious (Figure 2), it was decided to perform the revision of the postoperative tooth socket and curettage of the extraoral cutaneous sinus tract, under local anesthesia. During intraoral curettage of the tooth socket, only granulations were dislodged, while, during extraoral curettage of cutaneous sinus tract canal, a short and thin FB, similar to that of a tooth brush fiber, appeared unexpectedly (Figure 3).

It was difficult to determine the nature of this FB, but the patient eagerly exclaimed "*It's grass. It's a blade of grass which I used to clean my tooth three months ago.*"

Upon our request for an explanation as to the way in which inoculation of this occult FB occurred, the patient recited the history of this blade of grass. The patient disclosed that, three months earlier, he had a soft tissue inflammation around the right mandibular wisdom tooth. In order to clean the pocket between the inflamed soft tissue and the tooth, he used the long blade of grass, a part of which unstrapped and disappeared somewhere in his mouth.

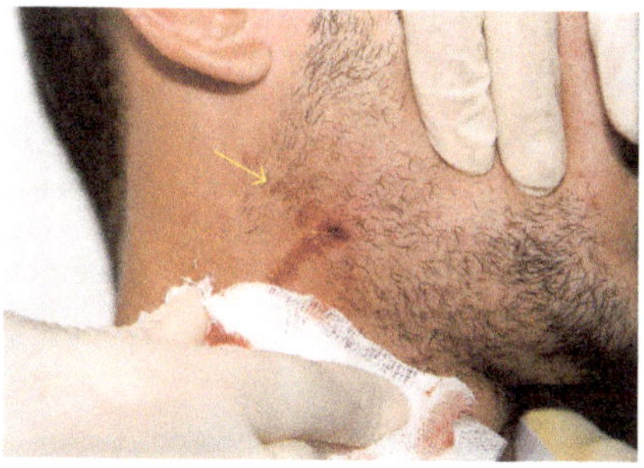

(a)

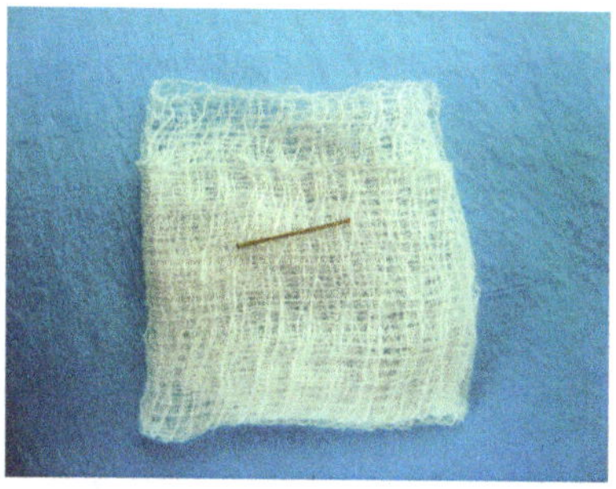

(b)

FIGURE 3: (a) Blade of grass revealed during curettage of cutaneous sinus tract. (b) Blade of grass.

That same night, the first complaints of severe pain at the right side of the lower jaw began, followed by complaints of swelling of the cheek on the same side on the very next day. He visited the regional general dentist twice within two weeks. Although he used the prescribed antibiotics by general dentist, his condition was worsening, so the patient asked for help from a general practitioner who suggested hospitalization in the Department of Infectious Diseases, where he was treated for infectious parotitis for approximately ten days.

According to patient's history, he was well for almost two weeks following hospitalization, but later on the pain and swelling recurred, so he was referred to the Maxillofacial Surgery Department where he was initially diagnosed, extraoral incision was performed, and he was referred to the Oral Surgery Department for impacted tooth extraction. Despite surgical removal of the impacted wisdom tooth, he still had the same complaints; therefore, he returned to the Department of Oral Surgery several times including this last visit.

In response to why he did not mention the blade of grass when he first attended the Maxillofacial and Oral Surgery Department, the patient revealed that during his initial complaints (pain and swelling) at his first visit to the general dentist, and during hospitalization at the Clinic for Infectious Diseases, he emphasized the incident with the blade of grass but the clinicians neglected this history, making him cast away his bad experience with the blade of grass as he deemed it to be insignificant information. Following the patient's explanation about the history of the blade of grass and careful examination of the retained FB, the case was finally diagnosed as

Recurrent facial cutaneous sinus tract of submandibular region secondary to the retained blade of grass inside the orofacial soft tissues.

5. Discussion

Based on the literature, the impaction of foreign bodies (FBs) with vegetative nature is rare [1, 5, 9–11]. They can induce an intense inflammatory reaction in the surrounding tissues and may get a secondary infection, so the patient may present with recurrent, nonhealing sinus on the orofacial region [1, 4]. FBs sometimes migrate within the tissues and become symptomatic after a certain period of time. In these cases, it is very difficult to discern the direct relationship between the suspected FBs with the clinical symptoms presented [10].

Their detection is often very difficult, especially the radiolucent vegetative FBs lodged deep in the tissue, because plain radiographs are unable to detect them. These vegetative FBs can go undetected, causing significant morbidity, repeated visits, high cost, and extensive surgery if another imaging is not considered [12, 13, 19].

To avoid misdiagnosis, especially in uncertain cases where the pathology persists even after conventional management, the clinician must consider an impacted FB as a possible cause of recurrent abscess or sinus tract [9]. Therefore, the clinician should perform careful examination and pay close attention to the patient's history which may suggest the presence of the FB. Furthermore, prompt diagnosis and surgical removal of FBs will minimize their associated complications [4].

The course of our presented case show the similarity with the cases presented in the literature [4, 10]. But actual presented case related with a short, thin blade of grass, initially inoculated intraorally, which migrated extraorally within the soft tissue of the face; relatively far from its primary inoculation, complicated with pain, recurrent swelling and cutaneous sinus discharge were bigger diagnostic challenge, because of the fact that patient's history at Maxillofacial and Oral Surgery Department did not offer any data regarding FB presence. Also the inoculated vegetative FB with low density structure was impossible to visualize with disposal conventional radiographs, such as lateral and retroalveolar radiography (Figures 1 and 2)

The presented case, respectively, patient's bad experience with the misdiagnosed, retained FB inside the soft tissue of the face, its consequences, and many follow-up treatments including surgical tooth extraction, incision, drainage, antibiotic therapy, and repeated curettages, can be explained, blamed, or even somehow justified with the following facts:

(1) The general dentist, general practitioner, and specialist of infectious diseases misdiagnosed the case because of erroneous taking of the patient's history and clinical examination and negligence with regard to the patient's history in relation to the problems with his wisdom tooth and his experience with the blade of

grass. Thus, unfortunately, the patient was mistakenly treated for infective parotitis.

(2) The maxillofacial surgeon's misdiagnosis arouses from the fact that, throughout the dental history, the patient did not offer any indication of foreign body presence, and hence the maxillofacial surgeon appointed all of the patient's complaints to the impacted wisdom tooth as the possible cause of symptoms (recurrent infection with swelling and pain). So he accordingly performed the extraoral incision and preferred surgical tooth extraction.

(3) The case was also misdiagnosed at his first two visits to the Oral Surgery Department, because again the patient did not offer any indication for FB presence, and the conventional lateral radiography did not show a vegetative FB being radiolucent, so the oral surgeon performed the extraction of the impacted tooth, suspected as the cause of the patient's problems.

So on the patient's last (third) visit to the Oral Surgery Department, we were both fortunate and surprised to retrieve the blade of grass as an occult FB during the curettage of the facial sinus tract, as we did not suspect to find anything suchlike, because of wanting patients history about the inoculated blade of grass and lacking of the retroalveolar radiography to visualize the FB with low density structure. Thus finally, the case was diagnosed as "*recurrent facial cutaneous sinus tract of submandibular region secondary to the retained blade of grass inside the orofacial soft tissues*" after the removal to which the patient responded well and the cutaneous sinus tract healed uneventfully.

6. Conclusion

To avoid misdiagnosis of all pathologies and notably the misdiagnosis of FB presence, as well as performing clinical examinations, the clinician must pay attention to the patient's history which may be suggestive of FB presence; especially in uncertain cases where the pathology persists even after surgical procedures and antibiotic regimens. In cases where strong suspicion for a retained FB exists based on the patient's history, although not seen on a plain radiograph, the alternative route of investigation should be the use of an ultrasound or surgical exploration.

Abbreviations

CT: Computed tomography
FB: Foreign body.

Disclosure

Resmije Ademi-Abdyli is the first author.

Competing Interests

The authors declare that they have no competing interests.

References

[1] A. Auluck, A. G. Behanan, K. M. Pai, and C. Shetty, "Recurrent sinus of the cheek due to a retained foreign body: report of an unusual case," *British Dental Journal*, vol. 198, no. 6, pp. 337–339, 2005.

[2] R. V. McKinney Jr., G. L. Brady, and B. B. Singh, "Metallic foreign body embedded in the cheek for 20 years," *The Journal of the American Dental Association*, vol. 102, no. 3, pp. 331–333, 1981.

[3] D. Quiamud, "Foreign bodies in maxillofacial region," *Journal of the Pakistan Dental Association*, vol. 10, no. 3, pp. 153–157, 2001.

[4] S. B. Aregbesola and V. I. Ugboko, "Unusual foreign bodies in the orofacial soft tissue spaces: a report of three cases," *Nigerian Journal of Clinical Practice*, vol. 16, no. 3, pp. 381–385, 2013.

[5] W. D. Martins, D. M. Fávaro, and F. H. Westphalen, "Emergency maxillofacial radiology. Foreign body localization: report of cases," *Dentomaxillofacial Radiology*, vol. 34, no. 3, pp. 189–192, 2005.

[6] M. N. Spengos, "Roentgeno-oddities: a pea in the cheek," *Oral Surgery, Oral Medicine, Oral Pathology*, vol. 43, no. 2, pp. 320–321, 1977.

[7] E. Cataldo and H. Santis, "Response of the oral tissue to exogenous foreign materials," *Journal of Periodontology*, vol. 45, no. 2, pp. 93–106, 1974.

[8] D. R. Weathers and R. M. Fine, "Amalgam tattoo of oral mucosa," *Archives of Dermatology*, vol. 110, no. 5, pp. 727–728, 1974.

[9] A. Sethi, A. Sabherwal, S. K. Basu, and D. Sareen, "An unusual cause of recurrent cheek abscess: a clinical case," *Brazilian Journal of Oral Sciences*, vol. 5, no. 16, pp. 982–984, 2006.

[10] S. Mohanavalli, J. David, and A. Gnanam, "Rare foreign bodies in oro-facial regions," *Indian Journal of Dental Research*, vol. 22, no. 5, pp. 713–715, 2011.

[11] S. E. Sobol, I. N. Jacobs, L. Levin, and R. F. Wetmore, "Pistachio nutshell foreign body of the oral cavity in two children," *International Journal of Pediatric Otorhinolaryngology*, vol. 68, no. 8, pp. 1101–1104, 2004.

[12] D. D. Graham Jr., "Ultrasound in the emergency department: detection of wooden foreign bodies in the soft tissues," *Journal of Emergency Medicine*, vol. 22, no. 1, pp. 75–79, 2002.

[13] K. S. Oikarinen, T. M. Nieminen, H. Mäkäräinen, and J. Pyhtinen, "Visibility of foreign bodies in soft tissue in plain radiographs, computed tomography, magnetic resonance imaging, and ultrasound: an in vitro study," *International Journal of Oral & Maxillofacial Surgery*, vol. 22, no. 2, pp. 119–124, 1993.

[14] M. Tahmasebi, H. Zareizadeh, and A. Motamedfar, "Accuracy of ultrasonography in detecting radiolucent soft-tissue foreign bodies," *Indian Journal of Radiology and Imaging*, vol. 24, no. 2, pp. 196–200, 2014.

[15] D. E. Manthey, A. B. Storrow, J. M. Milbourn, and B. J. Wagner, "Ultrasound versus radiography in the detection of soft-tissue foreign bodies," *Annals of Emergency Medicine*, vol. 28, no. 1, pp. 7–9, 1996.

[16] M. Orlinsky, P. Knittel, T. Feit, L. Chan, and D. Mandavia, "The comparative accuracy of radiolucent foreign body detection using ultrasonography," *The American Journal of Emergency Medicine*, vol. 18, no. 4, pp. 401–403, 2000.

[17] R. Javadrashid, D. F. Fouladi, M. Golamian et al., "Visibility of different foreign bodies in the maxillofacial region using plain radiography, CT, MRI and ultrasonography: an in vitro study," *Dentomaxillofacial Radiology*, vol. 44, no. 4, 2015.

[18] M. H. Aras, O. Miloglu, C. Barutcugil, M. Kantarci, E. Ozcan, and A. Harorli, "Comparison of the sensitivity for detecting foreign bodies among conventional plain radiography, computed tomography and ultrasonography," *Dentomaxillofacial Radiology*, vol. 39, no. 2, pp. 72–78, 2010.

[19] M. A. Anderson, W. L. Newmeyer III, and E. S. Kilgore Jr., "Diagnosis and treatment of retained foreign bodies in the hand," *The American Journal of Surgery*, vol. 144, no. 1, pp. 63–67, 1982.

41

A Rare Case of Concomitant Maxilla and Mandible Brown Tumours, Papillary Thyroid Carcinoma, Parathyroid Adenoma, and *Osteitis Fibrosa Cystica*

Thaís Borguezan Nunes,[1] Sheyla Batista Bologna,[1] Andréa Lusvarghi Witzel,[1] Marcello Menta Simonsen Nico,[2] and Silvia Vanessa Lourenço[1]

[1]*Department of Stomatology, School of Dentistry, University of São Paulo, Avenida Professor Lineu Prestes 2227, Cidade Universitária, 05508-000 São Paulo, SP, Brazil*
[2]*Department of Dermatology, Medical School, University of São Paulo, Avenida Dr. Enéas de Carvalho 255, 3o Andar, Sala 3068, 05403-000 São Paulo, SP, Brazil*

Correspondence should be addressed to Thaís Borguezan Nunes; thaborg@gmail.com

Academic Editor: Tommaso Lombardi

Objective. The brown tumour of hyperparathyroidism is a result of a metabolic disorder caused by primary hyperparathyroidism. *Report.* We described a case of a 37-year-old female patient presenting bimaxillary intraoral lesions and swelling in the neck. Incisional biopsy of the oral lesion was performed and histopathological examination revealed a central giant cell lesion composed by intense haemorrhagic exudate, abundant presence of giant cells, and areas with hemosiderin pigment. The patient also presented high levels of serum calcium and parathyroid hormone, hyperfunctioning parathyroid tissue, bilateral parenchymal nephropathy, and densitometry lower than expected, showing an advanced stage of *osteitis fibrosa cystica*. Synchronous parathyroid adenoma and papillary thyroid carcinoma were confirmed by imaging exams and histopathologically. *Conclusion.* The composition of all the clinical, pathological, and imaging findings led to the final diagnosis of brown tumour of hyperparathyroidism. The occurrence of parathyroid adenoma, papillary thyroid carcinoma, and brown tumours of hyperparathyroidism in their late stage (*osteitis fibrosa cystica*) associated with oral brown tumours involving the mandible and maxilla is extremely rare.

1. Introduction

Severe parathyroid bone disease is rare. *Osteitis fibrosa cystica* is the end-stage manifestation of primary hyperparathyroidism. The bone lesions are the result of a metabolic disorder caused by the altered parathyroid, mainly due to adenomas in 85% of the patients [1]; the overproduction of parathyroid hormones (PTH) causes imbalance in osteoclast activity resulting in bone destruction [2]. Histologically, the lesions are characterised by the presence of osteoclasts associated with areas of irregular bone resorption, which is replaced by fibrous vascularised tissue (fibrous cysts) and osteoclast-like giant cells. Accumulation of red blood cells and their pigments give a reddish/brown hue to the lesions, hence the name "brown tumour" [3].

Brown tumours of hyperparathyroidism are infrequent today due to improved medical technology that enables early diagnoses and correction of PTH levels [4]. The classical bone lesions are most frequently found in long bones, pelvis, and ribs. Facial involvement is only exceptional and, when present, usually involves the mandible. The occurrence of parathyroid adenoma, papillary thyroid carcinoma, and brown tumours of hyperparathyroidism involving the mandible and maxilla is extremely rare [5, 6].

We report herein a very rare case of concomitant maxilla and mandible brown tumours, thyroid carcinoma, parathyroid adenoma, and *osteitis fibrosa cystica*.

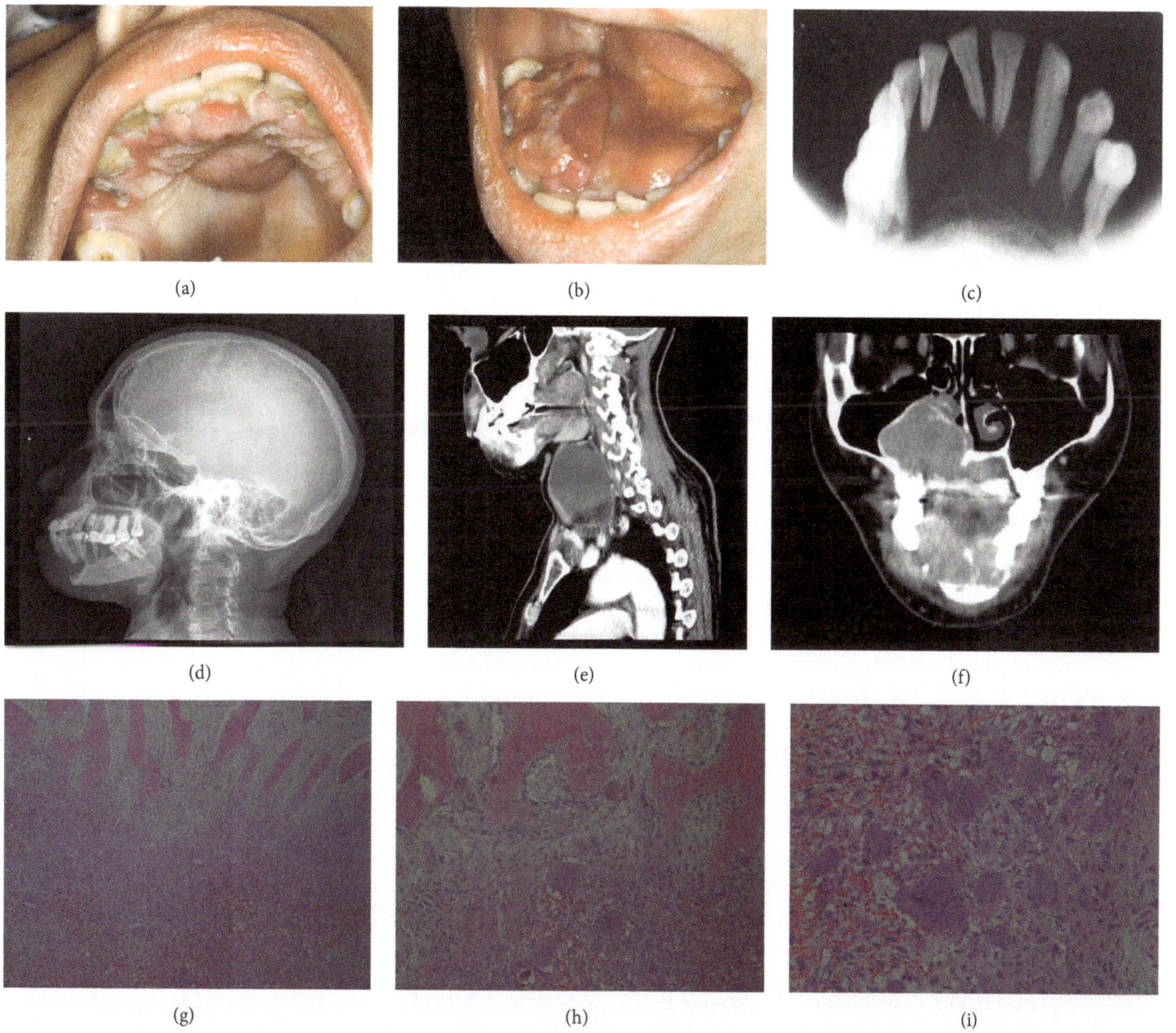

FIGURE 1: (a)-(b) Clinical aspects of the maxilla and mandible lesions: haemorrhagic tumour masses involving the vestibular and lingual/palatal gingiva. (c) Radiographic aspects of the occlusal X-ray: large radiolucent area involving the teeth roots, with resorption (floating teeth). (d) Radiographic aspects of the lateral skull X-ray: evidence of an extensive bone loss in the mandible, resulting in a floating teeth appearance. (e) Sagittal CT scan image: expansive lesion with anterior displacement of the thyroid lobe and posterior contact with prevertebral muscles. (f) Coronal CT scan image: expansive lesions with central soft parts components and involvement of medial right maxillary sinus wall, alveolar and palatine processes up to the floor of the nasal fossa; the lesion is also seen in the right mandibular ramus and on the mentonian region, with involvement of the anterior teeth. (g)–(i) Histopathological aspects of the mandible lesion: the mass of multinucleated giant cells permeated by haemorrhagic infiltration next to the mandibular compact bone trabeculae (g); detail of multinucleated giant cells, fibroblasts, blood cells, and inflammatory infiltrate close to compact bone trabeculae (h); multinucleated giant cells and blood cells that compose the mandibular lesion (i). Haematoxylin and eosin, original magnification ×40, ×200, and ×400, respectively.

2. Case Report

A 37-year-old woman presented to the Clinics of the Dental School, University of São Paulo, complaining of oral pain and facial deformity. The patient reported bleeding and painful oral lesions over the last 6 months.

The physical examination revealed a consistent cervical mass on the left side of the neck. Intraoral inspection showed an exophytic mass extending from the right mandibular lateral incisor to the molars. The associated teeth were mobile and enclosed by the tissue growth. In the maxilla, a swelling was seen across the palatal midline, extending from anterior region to posterior right side. Both maxilla and mandible lesions were soft in consistency and tender on palpation (Figures 1(a)-1(b)).

The patient's past medical and family history were non-contributory. Due to the severity of the case, the patient was referred to the Clinics Hospital, Medical School, University of São Paulo (HCFMUSP), for systemic investigation and medical management.

The X-rays images revealed an ill-defined osteolytic lesion causing expansion of the affected mandible, loss of lamina dura, and roots resorption of the anterior teeth (Figures 1(c)-1(d)). Computed Tomography (CT) was used to scan sites suspected to be affected by the brown tumours. Bone rarefaction focuses were also observed in the proximal phalanx of the third toe and the ribs. In the cervical region a massive septated cystic-solid lesion was located posteriorly to the left thyroid lobe besides the presence of thyroid nodules (Figures 1(e)-1(f)).

The bone densitometry values were below the expected limits for the patient's age and parathyroid scintigraphy showed hyperfunctioning parathyroid tissue on the left side.

An incisional biopsy was performed in the mandible lesion and histopathological examination was consistent with central giant cell lesions, composed of intense hemorrhagic exudate, abundant presence of multinucleated giant cells, and areas with haemosiderin pigment (Figures 1(g)–1(i)).

The biochemical investigations were carried out and showed marked hypercalcaemia (15.70 mg/dL, range 8.60–10.20 mg/dL) and an elevated parathyroid hormone (PTH) concentration (1472.00 pg/mL, range 16–87 pg/mL) in the blood.

The patient had partial thyroidectomy and parathyroidectomy on the left side. The PTH concentration taken 1 hour after the adenoma had been removed confirmed a level within the normal range. The diagnosis of papillary thyroid carcinoma and parathyroid adenoma was confirmed histologically (serial paraffin sections).

The serum calcium and inorganic phosphorus levels were estimated daily after surgery. The postoperative hypocalcemia was administered by calcium carbonate orally in addition to vitamin D until stable levels. Thyroid hormone replacement therapy was instituted.

At 6-month follow-up, there was only a modest improvement of oral pain, but the oral lesions had remained. The patient interrupted her clinical follow-up despite the efforts of the medical team.

3. Discussion

The occurrence of brown tumours in both jaws concomitant with the presence of hyperparathyroidism, parathyroid adenoma, and synchronous papillary thyroid carcinoma is very rare according to the literature [7, 8]. The brown tumour of hyperparathyroidism results from a metabolic disorder that affects long bones, ribs, and pelvis. The disease is most common in adults aged 50 years and over and affects 3 females to 1 male [4]. The facial involvement, though rare, manifests itself mainly in the mandible [3].

There is a great variation in the clinical expression of hyperparathyroidism. Hyperparathyroidism may be caused primarily by excessive secretion of PTH or secondarily due to kidney disease. The resultant hypercalcemia causes various metabolic problems, such as kidney stones, gastrointestinal disturbances, and muscular weakness [1, 2]. Our patient was below the average age and due to a very low grade of educational instruction, she did not seek treatment until she presented severe deformities and metabolic disorders that impacted her life quality. Additionally, the patient reported that she was diagnosed with a "thyroid cyst" two years before, but no treatment was performed due to difficulties in assessing public health system hospitals.

Radiographically, the present case was similar to those previously reported by other authors [9]. The progressive loss of bone mineral content due to the increased PTH secretion may produce radiolucent bone lesions of ill-defined margins, as those that were seen in our patient.

The destructive bone lesions of brown tumour show similar histological features to those viewed in central giant cell lesions, aneurysmal bone cyst, and cherubism and these are considered as differential diagnosis [4, 7]. The histopathological examination was consistent with a central giant cell lesion, but the composition of all the clinical, pathological, and imaging findings enabled us to reach the final diagnosis of brown tumour of hyperparathyroidism.

The pathogenesis of this disease is caused by the marked increase in osteoclastic bone resorption followed by replacement of marrow spaces with fibrovascular tissue and increased formation of osteoid. The cystic spaces are populated with clusters of giant cells as well as with hemosiderin-filled macrophages and plump fibroblasts. Clinically, these areas appear as red-brown friable mass, hence the term brown tumour [3, 10].

Brown tumours are the late manifestation of severe hyperparathyroidism; this clinical situation is also known as *osteitis fibrosa cystica*. Occasionally, *osteitis fibrosa cystica* can be mistaken for a malignant lesion, even though it is reactive and clearly nonneoplastic [8].

Primary hyperparathyroidism is characterized by hypersecretion of PTH, which is caused by adenomas in 85% of all cases. The presence of brown tumours is recognized in less than 5% of these cases [1].

According to the literature, concomitant thyroid disease is present in 3.1% of patients with primary hyperparathyroidism [11], but the reason of this association remains unclear. Although this situation is unusual, the diagnosis of coexisting diseases should be considered. The investigation of the thyroid is recommended to identify the presence of nodules. They also must be removed during parathyroid surgical approach in patients with primary hyperparathyroidism [5, 12]. In fact, our patient was diagnosed with parathyroid adenoma and papillary thyroid carcinoma. The early identification of cancer and appropriate resection of the affected glands quickly permitted the metabolic control, as noted in the assessment of serum levels of inorganic phosphorus and PTH after the surgery.

It was not possible to evaluate whether surgical excision of parathyroid adenoma and papillary thyroid carcinoma allowed the regression of oral lesions in our patient. After 6-month follow-up, she showed discrete improvement in pain, but she did not perform imaging tests that were previously requested for bone evaluation, and after this appointment she interrupted the treatment.

Some authors report that the excision of parathyroid lesions results in controlled serum levels leading to a gradual decrease in the maxillary tumours; therefore, treatment is directed to the correction of hyperparathyroidism instead of any local intervention in bone affected by brown tumours. Once hormonal dysfunction is corrected, the bones tend to mineralize completely, resulting in the regression of the osteolytic lesions [13, 14]. Brown tumours should only be removed if they persist even after removal of parathyroid adenoma [7], when functional problems are detected [1], or if tumours are too large [15]. Although the regression of brown tumours can take several months, conservative management can avoid more invasive procedure in facial bones, preventing further deformities [14].

4. Conclusion

The composition of all the clinical, pathological, and imaging findings led to the final diagnosis of brown tumour of hyperparathyroidism. The occurrence of parathyroid adenoma, papillary thyroid carcinoma, and brown tumours of hyperparathyroidism in the last stage (*osteitis fibrosa cystica*) with oral manifestation involving the mandible and maxilla is extremely rare. The appropriate resection of the affected glands leads to the metabolic control of serum levels of calcium and PTH. Exuberant cases, as the one reported, still occur in developing countries due to poor and inefficient governmental health and education policies.

Conflict of Interests

The authors declare that there is no conflict of interests regarding the publication of this paper.

References

[1] K. Triantafillidou, L. Zouloumis, G. Karakinaris, E. Kalimeras, and F. Iordanidis, "Brown tumors of the jaws associated with primary or secondary hyperparathyroidism. A clinical study and review of the literature," *American Journal of Otolaryngology—Head and Neck Medicine and Surgery*, vol. 27, no. 4, pp. 281–286, 2006.

[2] M. R. Rubin, V. A. Livolsi, F. Bandeira, G. Caldas, and J. P. Bilezikian, "Tc99m-sestamibi uptake in osteitis fibrosa cystica simulating metastatic bone disease," *Journal of Clinical Endocrinology and Metabolism*, vol. 86, no. 11, pp. 5138–5141, 2001.

[3] F. Jebasingh, J. J. Jacob, A. Shah, T. V. Paul, and M. S. Seshadri, "Bilateral maxillary brown tumours as the first presentation of primary hyperparathyroidism," *Oral and Maxillofacial Surgery*, vol. 12, no. 2, pp. 97–100, 2008.

[4] S. Chowdhury, A. Aggarwal, N. Mittal, and A. Shah, "Brown tumor of hyperparathyroidism involving craniomaxillofacial region: a rare case report and literature review," *Minerva Stomatologica*, vol. 62, no. 9, pp. 343–348, 2013.

[5] S. Vysetti, P. Sridhar, B. Theckedath, J. L. Gilden, and P. Morawiecki, "Synchronous papillary thyroid carcinoma and primary hyperparathyroidism: diagnosis and management issues," *Hospital Practice*, vol. 40, no. 4, pp. 16–19, 2012.

[6] W. Pawlak, A. Bohdanowicz-Pawlak, M. Bolanowski, J. Szymczak, G. Bednarek-Tupikowska, and K. Łuczak, "Primary hyperparathyroidism presenting as a giant cell tumor of the jaws," *Neuro Endocrinology Letters*, vol. 34, no. 2, pp. 107–110, 2013.

[7] H. Yamazaki, Y. Ota, T. Aoki, and K. Karakida, "Brown tumor of the maxilla and mandible: progressive mandibular brown tumor after removal of parathyroid adenoma," *Journal of Oral and Maxillofacial Surgery*, vol. 61, no. 6, pp. 719–722, 2003.

[8] F. Selvi, S. Cakarer, R. Tanakol, S. D. Guler, and C. Keskin, "Brown tumour of the maxilla and mandible: a rare complication of tertiary hyperparathyroidism," *Dentomaxillofacial Radiology*, vol. 38, no. 1, pp. 53–58, 2009.

[9] P. Polat, M. Kantarc, F. Alper, M. Koruyucu, S. Suma, and O. Onbaş, "The spectrum of radiographic findings in primary hyperparathyroidism," *Clinical Imaging*, vol. 26, no. 3, pp. 197–205, 2002.

[10] N. Soundarya, P. Sharada, N. Prakash, and G. L. Pradeep, "Bilateral maxillary brown tumors in a patient with primary hyperparathyroidism: report of a rare entity and review of literature," *Journal of Oral and Maxillofacial Pathology*, vol. 15, no. 1, pp. 56–59, 2011.

[11] S. Y. Morita, H. Somervell, C. B. Umbricht, A. P. B. Dackiw, and M. A. Zeiger, "Evaluation for concomitant thyroid nodules and primary hyperparathyroidism in patients undergoing parathyroidectomy or thyroidectomy," *Surgery*, vol. 144, no. 6, pp. 862–867, 2008.

[12] H. Javadi, S. Jallalat, S. Farrokhi et al., "Concurrent papillary thyroid cancer and parathyroid adenoma as a rare condition: a case report," *Nuclear Medicine Review*, vol. 15, no. 2, pp. 153–155, 2012.

[13] S. Gangidi, R. Dyer, and D. Cunliffe, "Not all radiolucencies of the jaw require enucleation: a case of brown tumour," *British Journal of Oral and Maxillofacial Surgery*, vol. 50, no. 3, pp. e33–e35, 2012.

[14] J. A. Reséndiz-Colosia, S. A. Rodríguez-Cuevas, R. Flores-Díaz et al., "Evolution of maxillofacial brown tumors after parathyroidectomy in primary hyperparathyroidism," *Head & Neck*, vol. 30, no. 11, pp. 1497–1504, 2008.

[15] A. Praveen and R. Thriveni, "Maxillary and mandibular hyperparathyroidism," *National Journal of Maxillofacial Surgery*, vol. 3, no. 1, pp. 51–54, 2012.

42

Iatrogenic Inflammatory Fibrosis of Hard Palate in a 13-Year-Old Female Patient

Shanthan Mettu,[1] Radhika Muppa,[1] G. Siva Prasad Reddy,[2] Srinivas Nallanchakrava,[1] and Sri Veda Gurugubelli[1]

[1] *Department of Pediatric Dentistry, Panineeya Institute of Dental Sciences, Kamalanagar, Dilsukhnagar, Hyderabad, Andhra Pradesh 500060, India*
[2] *Department of Oral and Maxillofacial Surgery, Panineeya Institute of Dental Sciences, Kamalanagar, Dilsukhnagar, Hyderabad, Andhra Pradesh 500060, India*

Correspondence should be addressed to Shanthan Mettu; mettushanthanreddy@gmail.com

Academic Editors: V. Brailo and U. Zilberman

Palatal swellings are rare in children and the incidence differs from that of the adult counterparts. When the palatal swellings do arise in children, they usually are palatal abscess from periapical region, and few cases like pleomorphic adenoma in young adults have also been reported. But inflammatory fibrosis of palate in children is a rare occurrence. Inflammatory fibrosis is formation of excess fibrous connective tissue in an organ or tissue, as a reparative or reactive process. This report describes an unusual case of iatrogenic inflammatory fibrosis on the palate due to extraction of tooth number 22 in a 13-year-old female patient. The patient presented with a single large well-circumscribed oval palatal swelling that was soft, fluctuant, not fixed, and nontender. Surgical excision of the lesion was done and it was sent for histopathological assessment. The biopsy showed fibrous tissue with collagen fibers, spindle shaped fibroblasts, neovascularization, RBCs, chronic inflammatory cells, and traces of salivary gland and nerve tissue.

1. Introduction

Rapidly growing, aggressive palatal swellings are relatively rare in children when compared to adults. Among all the palatal swellings, pleomorphic adenoma is the most frequently encountered lesion in young adults [1]. Cases of iatrogenically caused inflammatory fibrosis have not been reported or explored to a large extent in the literature, especially in children. Tooth extraction is one of the most frequent dental procedures performed in a dental office and is sometimes accompanied by intra- and postsurgical complications. Fibrosis is a rare complication after extraction and is characterized by formation of excess fibrous connective tissue in an organ or tissue, which can be reparative, reactive, benign, or pathological [2]. We hereby report a case of a 13-year-old girl with inflammatory fibrosis on the hard palate caused as a complication after extraction of tooth number 22.

2. Case Report

A 13-year-old female patient reported to the Department of Pediatric Dentistry, Panineeya Dental College, Hyderabad with a complaint of swelling in the palate region for the last 15 days. When detailed history was obtained, patient gave no history of systemic disease or allergies. Patient presented with congenitally missing tooth number 21. She observed a swelling for which she reported to an undisclosed private dental office where tooth number 22 was extracted. The nodular swelling on the buccal aspect of tooth number 22 disappeared and a swelling on the palatal aspect appeared within two days of extraction and rapidly increased to the present size, for which the patient reported to our institution.

Patient presented with a $4.5 \times 2.7 \times 0.8$ cm linear swelling, oval in shape, towards the left side extending from the palatal aspect of tooth number 21 to tooth number 26 (Figure 1). The

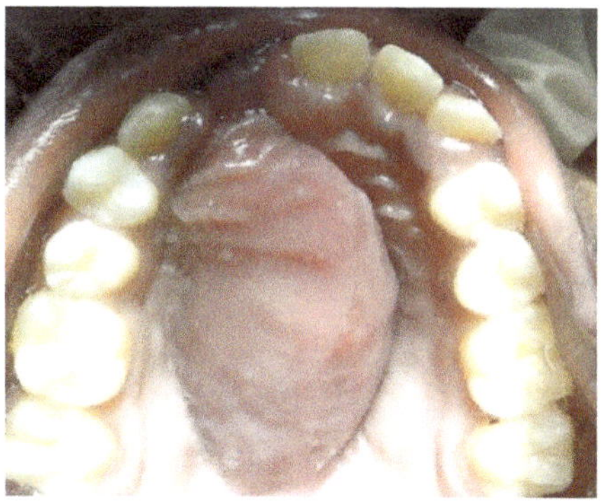

FIGURE 1: Intraoral preoperative photograph showing palatal swelling.

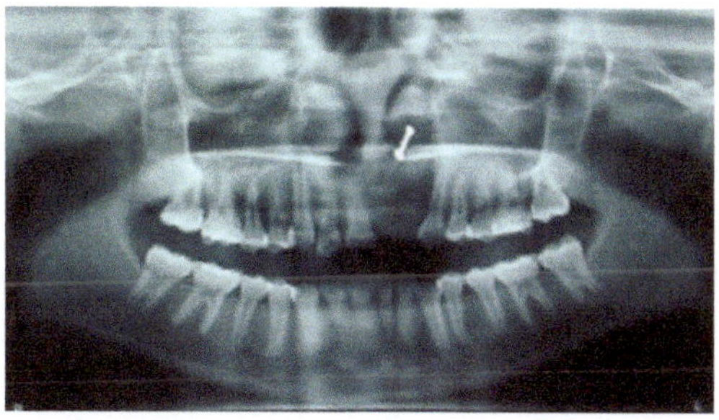

FIGURE 2: Orthopantomograph showing missing tooth number 21 and tooth number 22.

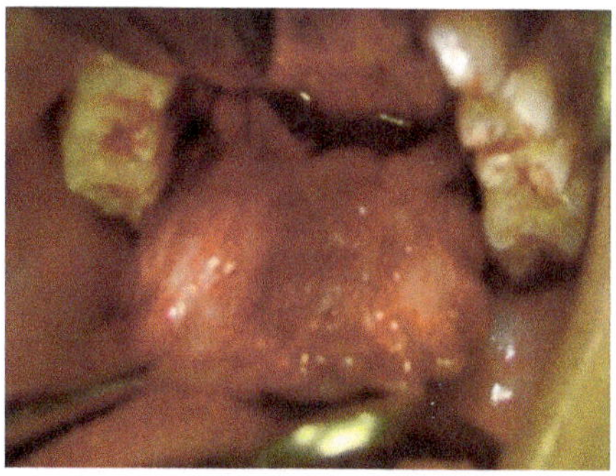

FIGURE 3: Intraoperative photograph showing excision of the lesion.

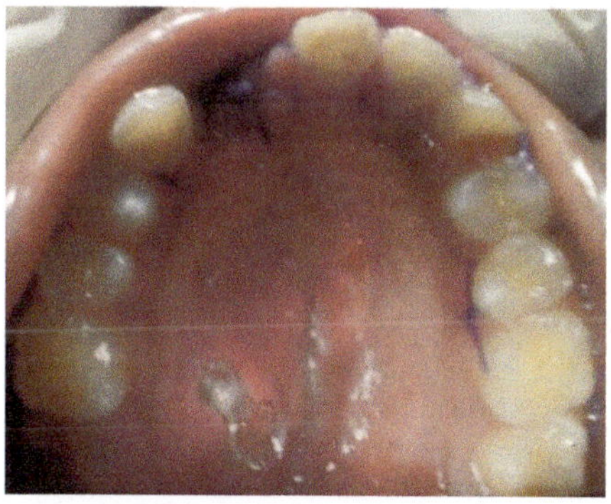

FIGURE 4: 1 week postoperative photograph showing palatal healing.

swelling presented as soft, fluctuant, sessile, and nontender. The orthopantomograph and the maxillary occlusal view radiograph revealed a diffuse radiolucency with relation to the extracted tooth number 22 (Figure 2). During the first visit fine needle aspiration cytology (FNAC) was done and the microscopic features showed mixed inflammatory cell infiltrate chiefly lymphocytes and neutrophils within a fibrous background, suggestive of infected cystic fluid. The patient was prescribed broad-spectrum antibiotics for five days and was recalled at regular intervals.

It was observed that there was no difference in the size of the swelling, even after one week, so enucleation of the lesion was planned under general anaesthesia (GA). Complete haematological tests along with a radiograph of chest PA view were ordered as a preoperative protocol and the case was posted for treatment under GA. Nasotracheal intubation was done and nerve block with 2% lignocaine was given around the lesion. Crevicular incision was performed around the gingival margin on the palatal aspect extending from the regions of 16 to 26, anteroposteriorly. A full thickness mucoperiosteal flap was raised and complete dissection of the lesion was done separating it from the palatal mucosa (Figure 3). Wound closure was done using 3-0 Vicryl and the acrylic feeding plate was placed, which was fabricated prior to the surgery. Extubation of the nasotracheal tube and recovery of patient were uneventful. Patient was recalled after one week for review and subsequently advised to discontinue the acrylic plate after 10 days (Figure 4).

The excised specimen was sent for biopsy and microscopy revealed fibrous connective tissue consisting of plump, spindle shaped fibroblasts neovascularization with extravasated red blood cells. It also showed infiltrate of chronic inflammatory cells with no evidence of salivary gland tissue or nerve tissue, thus suggestive of inflammatory fibrosis (Figure 5). The patient has been under followup for the last 6 months and no evidence of reoccurrence appeared (Figure 6).

3. Discussion

Damage to the surrounding soft tissues is easily inflicted during negligently performed local anesthetic technique and extraction procedures. In this present case, it could have been any of the two. More serious complications are caused when deeper structures are traumatized when the procedure is done without good knowledge of technique and the anatomy of the tissues. These complications can appear during or after the procedure. The complications may range from infection inflammation trauma to nerves resulting in variable nerve dysfunctions [3].

Inflammatory fibrosis manifests as a postextraction complication caused by possible localized iatrogenic trauma to the soft tissues, deregulating the wound healing process at either the proliferative or remodeling stages. It may also be caused if the irritant persists in the tissues continually during the process of healing. Fibrosis can occur with or without inflammation [4].

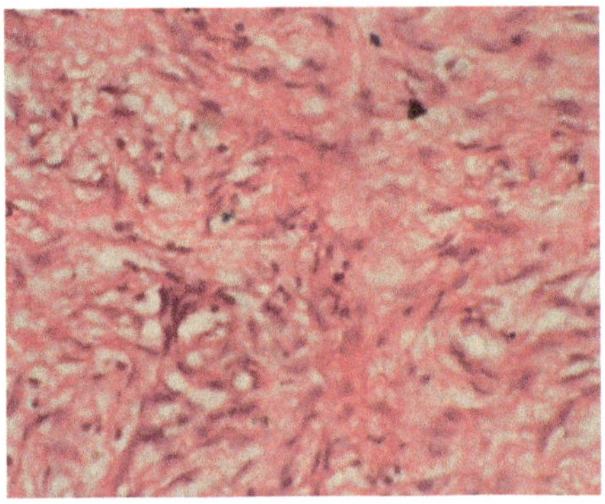

FIGURE 5: Photomicrograph showing fibrous connective tissue consisting of plump, spindle shaped fibroblasts.

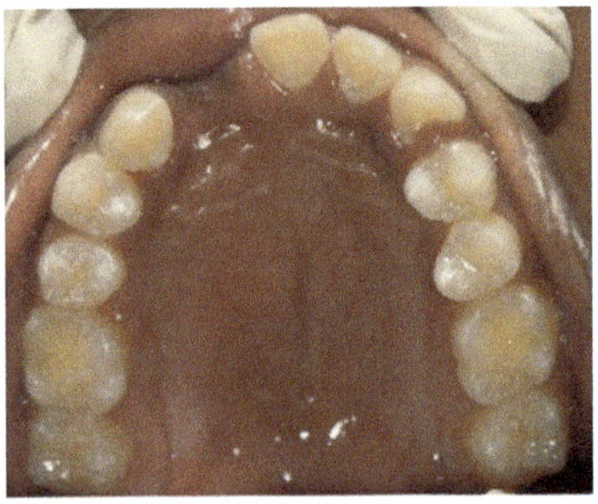

FIGURE 6: 6-month postoperative photograph showing good healing of the palate with no recurrence of the lesion.

Fibrosis is similar to the process of scarring, which involves immigration, proliferation of fibroblasts, and also extracellular matrix deposition by these fibroblasts, which is followed by collagen synthesis. Researchers have suggested that NLRP3 inflammasome is a key cellular sensor that results in generation of an inflammatory response. This inflammasome mediates the activation and recruitment of inflammatory cells to the site of injury as an initial response. Many observations suggest that tissue remodeling and fibrosis are similar, but a delicate alteration in the biosynthetic pathway of reconstruction of extracellular matrix may affect the balance [5].

Complications resulting from rapid palatal injection of local anesthetic solutions, particularly those containing a vasoconstrictor, have been reported, which include ischemia, allergic reactions, epithelial desquamations, traumatic injuries, ulcerations, fibrosis, and also necrosis [6].

Here in the present case, the clinical, radiographic, and histological features were correlated to arrive at a final diagnosis of iatrogenic inflammatory fibrosis.

4. Conclusion

Though a rare occurrence, inflammatory fibrosis of hard palate may result as a complication of tooth extraction due to iatrogenic factors. So a thorough knowledge of the clinical, radiographic, and histological features of fibrosis is essential for a proper diagnosis. In spite of the fact that the complications are sometimes inevitable, comprehensive knowledge about the technique and anatomy is necessary for preventing iatrogenic challenges during tooth extraction.

Conflict of Interests

The authors declare that they have no conflict of interests.

References

[1] K. Dhanuthai, K. Sappayatosok, and K. Kongin, "Pleomorphic adenoma of the palate in a child: a case report," *Medicina Oral, Patologia Oral y Cirugia Bucal*, vol. 14, no. 2, pp. E73–E75, 2009.

[2] B. Shreedhar, M. Kamboj, N. Kumar, and S. Shamim Khan, "Fibrous dysplasia of the palate: report of a case and review of palatal swellings," *Case Reports in Pediatrics*, vol. 2012, Article ID 179853, 4 pages, 2012.

[3] H. S. Batal and G. Jacob, "Surgical extractions," in *Manual of Minor Oral Surgery For the General Dentist*, K. R. Koerner, Ed., pp. 19–48, Blackwell, Munksgaard, Danmark, 2006.

[4] T. A. Wynn, "Integrating mechanisms of pulmonary fibrosis," *Journal of Experimental Medicine*, vol. 208, no. 7, pp. 1339–1350, 2011.

[5] T. A. Wynn, "Cellular and molecular mechanisms of fibrosis," *Journal of Pathology*, vol. 214, no. 2, pp. 199–210, 2008.

[6] R. S. Roda and P. L. Blanton, "The anatomy of local anesthesia," *Quintessence international*, vol. 25, no. 1, pp. 27–38, 1994.

43

Early Loading of Single-Piece Implant for Partially Edentulous Posterior Arch: A Prospective One-Year Case Report

Amol Beldar,[1] Manohar L. Bhongade,[2] Girish Byakod,[3] and Chandrashekar Buregoni[1]

[1] *Department of Periodontics and Implant Dentistry, Mahatma Gandhi Vidyamandir's KBH Dental College, Panchavati, Nashik 422003, Maharshtra, India*
[2] *Department of Periodontics and Implant Dentistry, Sharad Pawar Dental College and Hospital Of Deemed University, Sawangi (Meghe), Wardha, Maharashtra, India*
[3] *Department of Periodontics and Implant Dentistry, Rangoonwala Dental College, Pune, Maharashtra, India*

Correspondence should be addressed to Amol Beldar; amol_b007@yahoo.com

Academic Editors: C. N. Elias, A. V. Ritter, and E. F. Wright

Implant therapy is now well established, and there is an increasing need for shorter rehabilitation time. Original prerequisites of osseointegration have been reassessed to satisfy continuously increasing patient's expectation of reduced treatment time, improved esthetics, and increased comfort. Shorter healing time may be appropriate in some circumstances, and examples of early loading have been reported in animal and human studies. However, to date there are insufficient data to determine a universally acceptable opinion on early loading of implants for single-tooth replacement. This case report involves early loading, combined with construction of a restoration, inserted directly after 6 weeks of implant surgery and followup of one year.

1. Introduction

Implants used for single-tooth replacement represent a more recent evolution of implant dentistry. As far greater number of patients are edentulous in a single-tooth gap or partial-arch space than completely edentulous. The opportunity to provide implant-supported tooth replacement for these patients significantly exceeds the opportunity for those who are completely edentulous [1]. The biomechanics of implants in these situations are significantly more different than in completely edentulous conditions, particularly in the context of early restoration of these implants. Abundant evidence clearly exists to support early loading of implants under full-arch clinical conditions. One of the unraveled parameters predicting osseointegration is micromotion at the implant-tissue interface not surpassing the threshold of 50–150 microns during the postimplantation healing phase. The most prerequisite for immediate loading and early loading is the achievement of high implant stability. Limiting implants micromotion below the threshold that could interfere with osseointegration, despite occlusal function, has been well documented and elucidated by means of authors [2].

Several long-term studies on single-tooth replacement have shown excellent results over a 5-year period [3]. To achieve successful bone-to-implant contact (osseointegration), oral implants placed according to a 2-stage surgical protocols have been advocated to remain unloaded for a healing period of 3–6 months [3]. A reanalysis of this original experimental design has questioned the necessity for a long implant healing period [3]. The current scientific literature supports the concept that implants can be loaded early or immediately. Recently, healing time of 6 weeks for implants placed in good quality bone has been recommended [4]. These recommendations resulted from a better understanding of the bone implant healing interface [5] and improved implant surface technology [6]. Studies regarding different types of prosthesis have shown that early loading of implants can provide treatment outcomes comparable to those achieved using standard healing periods before loading [7]. The early loading of implant supporting a full arch

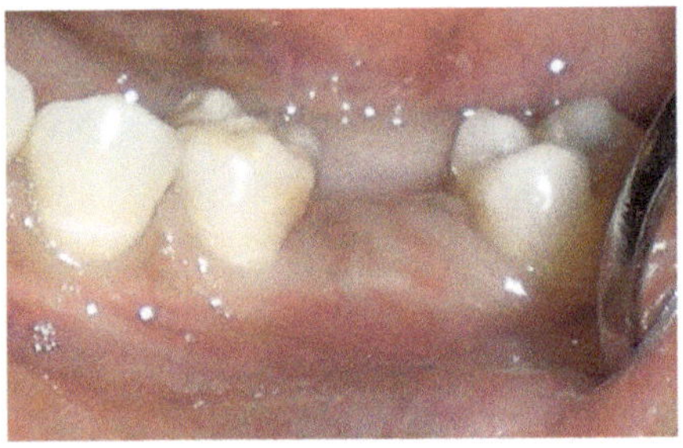

FIGURE 1: Preoperative view of the posterior left first molar, number 36.

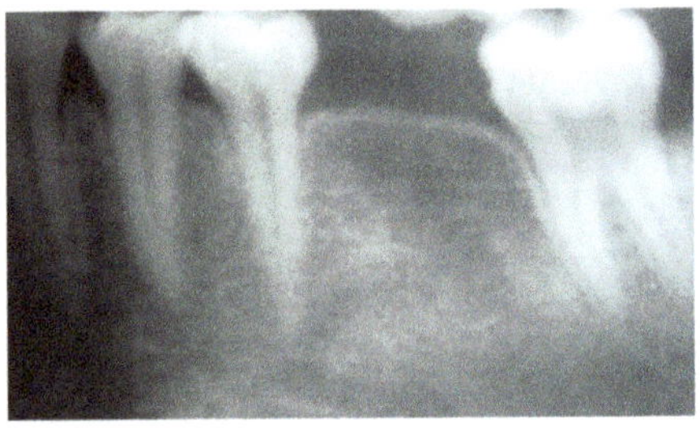

FIGURE 2: Preoperative radiograph of tooth, number 36, note the good height of the alveolar bone.

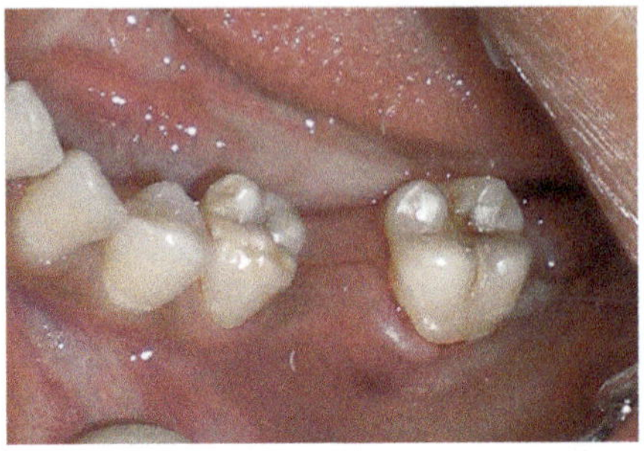

FIGURE 3: Crestal incision made along the crest of the ridge.

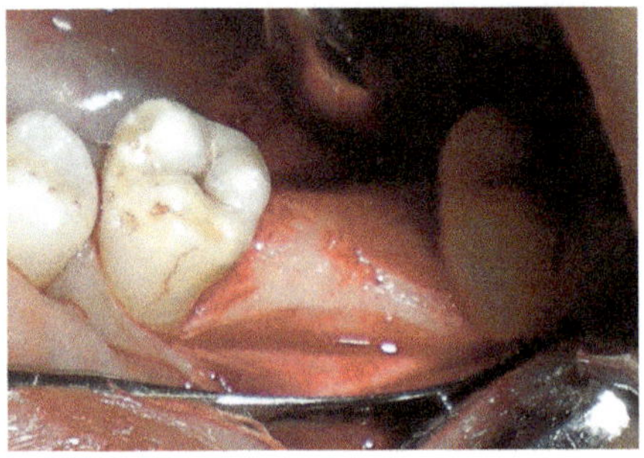

FIGURE 4: Broad buccolingual width of the residual ridge.

prosthesis in the edentulous mouth has also been studied. The studies regarding early loading of implant supported single tooth crowns in anterior arch are available in the literature but case reports and studies on early loading replacing single-tooth implant in posterior arch have not been reported. The purpose of the investigation was to know whether the early loading of single-tooth implant deleteriously affects the implant survival in the posterior arch.

2. Case Report

A 20-year-old female patient presented with a request to discuss the options for prosthetic replacement of mandibular left first molar which was extracted 6 months back. Clinical examination revealed a mesioangular impacted tooth third molar which was advised to be extracted. After two months, the patient reported back again for the prosthetic replacement of the molar (Figures 1 and 2). There was no significant past or present medical history and oral hygiene was acceptable. Prior to the surgical procedure, the patient was instructed to rinse with 0.2% chlorhexidine gluconate (Hexidine, ICPA Health Products Ltd., India) for one minute. The surgical protocols emphasized complete asepsis and infection control. The type of implant used was an acid-etched, tapered self threaded implant (HI-Tec) of diameter 4.5 × 13 mm. Briefly, after induction of local anesthesia, a crystal incision was made along the crest of the ridge using Bard-Parker number 12 surgical blade, bisecting the existing keratinized mucosa (Figure 3). A full thickness mucoperiosteal flap was raised buccally and lingually to the level of mucogingival junction, exposing the underlined ridge of the implant site, and a ridge alveoplasty was performed with the help of 0.2 mm round bur to achieve a flat bone surface of sufficient width (Figure 4). A surgical drill guide was used for the precise placement of the pilot drill. After pilot drill application, the implant site was prepared with the corresponding size of parallel drill (Figure 5). The implants were placed in the recipient site by means of an insertion device, and a torque driver set at 35 N cm which was used to evaluate primary stability of implant (Figure 6). It was the level of torque that the manufacturer recommended to be applied to the implant. To detect and prevent unfavorable rotation of implant, the implant was secured through a mounting sleeve that allowed manual detection of rotation. The appropriate position of the implant neck in both the vertical and horizontal dimensions was decisive. The implant neck was positioned at the crystal bone level or slightly submerged (Figure 7). Immediately after implant placement, the flap was replaced in its original position and sutured with nonresorbable suture (4-0) using a combination of inverted mattress and interrupted sutures. The inverted mattress sutures kept the bleeding edges of the flap close together, while the interrupted sutures sealed the edges. Intraoral periapical radiograph was taken immediately after surgery (Figure 8).

3. Prosthetic Reconstruction

After surgical intervention, the prefabricated temporary crown with acrylic resin was trimmed, polished, and cemented 24 hours after surgery. Compared to natural teeth, the temporary restoration was of a narrow occlusal surface without any contacts in functional occlusion. In maximum

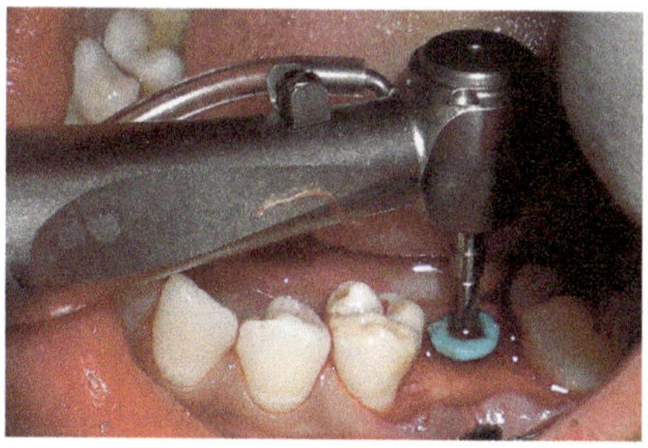

FIGURE 5: Pilot drill is used to increase the osteotomy site to confirm position and angulation.

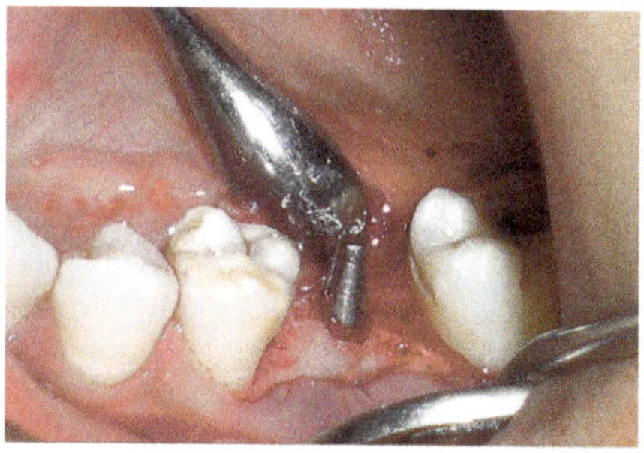

FIGURE 7: Implant placed into the osteotomy site.

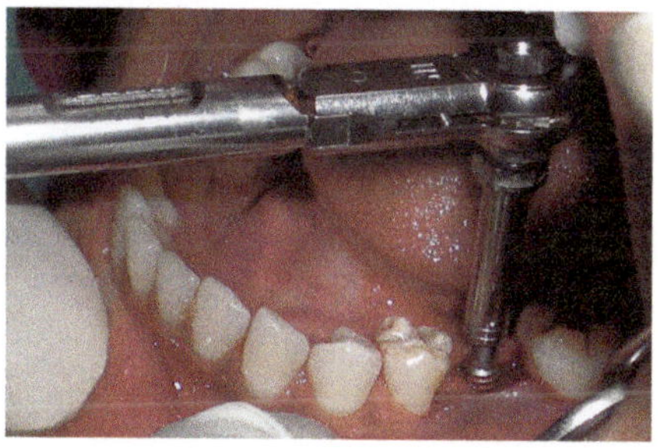

FIGURE 6: Wrench used for tightening implant.

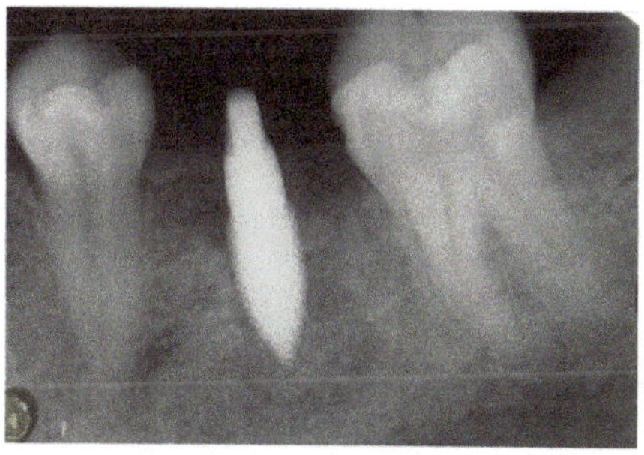

FIGURE 8: Radiographic view of the implant after surgery.

intercuspation, only point occlusal contacts were provided. The interproximal contacts were designed as broader contact areas to distribute the forces of mastication and to provide support. Depending on the gingival thickness, the crown margin was located from 0.5 to 1 mm below the gingiva. The temporary restoration was replaced with permanent restoration after six weeks (Figure 9). The definitive restoration was fabricated with a metal ceramic crown. The morphology of the occlusal surfaces of restoration was similar to that of the natural teeth with occlusal contact in maximum intercuspation and physiologic cusp inclination. The premature contacts during lateral and protrusive movement were avoided. The crown restoration was cemented and followup of one year of implant survival was assessed (Figure 10).

4. Discussion

Most standard protocols in implant dentistry suggest a healing period of 3 months for mandible and 6 months for maxilla [8], but the time required for treatment, need for additional surgical procedures, and indefinite periods of temporization are obstacles that sometimes prevent the patients from implant treatments. To remove these obstacles, it would be beneficial to load implants within the few weeks after implant placement. Studies regarding different types of prostheses have shown that early loading of mandibular implants can provide treatment outcomes comparable to those achieved using standard healing periods before loading [9]. The long-term success of early loaded implant has been investigated in animal and human studies. Brånemark et al. [9] assessed peri-implant conditions of early loaded implants in a prospective split mouth controlled study and suggested that implant may very well be suitable for early loading at 6 weeks. Recently, Cochran et al. [10] in a prospective multicenter cohort study involving 133 patients with 383 implants found that implants could be successfully restored after 6 weeks of loading and yielded a success rate greater than 99%, two years after prosthetic restoration. The early loading of implants supporting a full arch prosthesis in edentulous mandible has also been studied. However, to the author's knowledge, studies regarding early loading of implants-supported single-tooth crowns in the mandible are not reported in the literature.

The basic concept behind the present case report was that early loading is not an absolute contraindication, but rather a relative one. Most available studies on the subject have offered solutions for full-arch reconstruction [11]. In such cases, the occlusal load is maximal and therefore requires maximal initial stability and support. For full-arch restorations, intra-arch stabilization is possible, and cross-arch stabilization is a recommended guideline to minimize micromovement, which can be a principal cause of early implant failure. For single-tooth restorations, the adjacent teeth can withstand a major part of the occlusal forces. In the present case report, acrylic resin temporary crowns were used to prevent transmission of some of the load directly to the implant and thicker acrylic resin occlusal width, but no more than 2 to 3 mm was used to further diminish the occlusal forces. Several factors influence stability: the potential bone-implant surface area (as dictated by length, width, and screw type versus cylinder, and microtexture); bone quality; initial bone-implant contact.

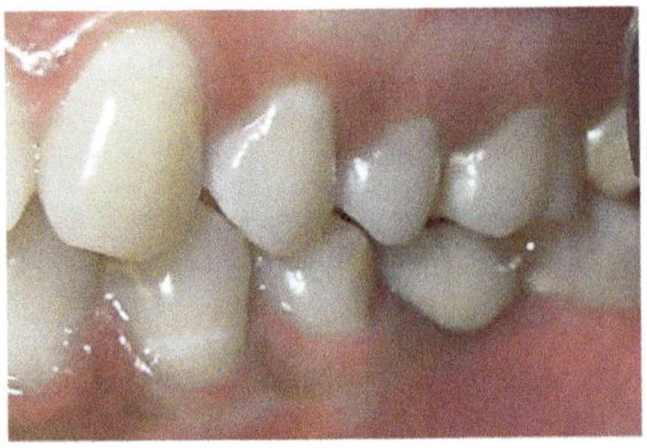

Figure 9: Clinical view of the final restoration at six weeks after surgery.

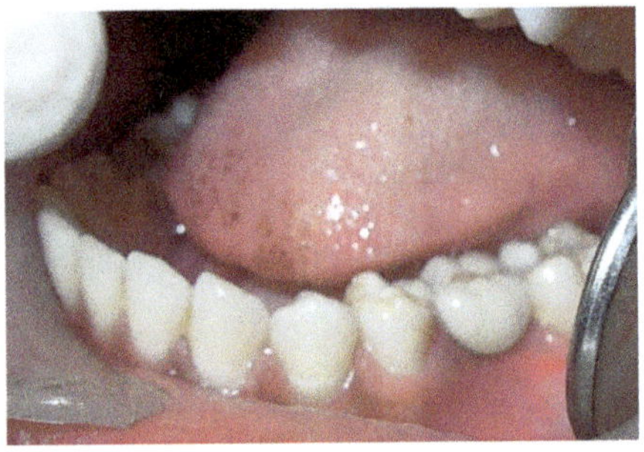

Figure 10: Clinical view of the final restoration at 12 months after surgery.

Early publications on immediate restoration of single, unsplinted implants in the esthetic zone were presented as case reports and series. Kupeyan and May [12] reported on series of 10 and 14 immediately restored implants, respectively, in the maxillary anterior region. Kupeyan and May [12] performed their study in healed ridges with machined titanium Brånemark System implants (Nobel Biocare), and all implants clinically integrated and remained stable for the observation periods of 6 months to 3 years. Additional case reports of small series of patients by Andersen and coworkers [13] and Cannizzaro and Leone (2003) [14] confirmed the observations of 100% survival of single-tooth replacement in the maxillary anterior region. All authors advocated maximization of implant stability by using long implants and eliminating occlusal contact in centric and excursive movements.

In the present case report, sandblasted acid etched (SLA) implant was used for early loading procedure. The advantages of SLA include faster osseointegration, proportionally greater bone-implant contact, and greater reverse-torque resistance compared to noncoated implants. It was also demonstrated that when single-tooth implant is placed in partially edentulous arch and loaded early (6 weeks), did not appear to jeopardize the osseointegration healing process in the posterior mandible. The primary and the secondary stability were also achieved. The primary implant stability at placement is the mechanical phenomenon related to the quality and quantity of the bone at the recipient site, the type and design of the implant used and the surgical technique used. The secondary implant stability increased in stability attributable to the bone formation and remodeling at the implant tissue interface in the surrounding bone. Piattelli et al. [15] compared the histology of nonsubmerged unloaded and early loaded titanium screw implants in monkeys. They found a tight contact of new bone to implant surfaces in all the samples examined. However, around the necks of early loaded implants, they observed lamellar cortical bone that was thicker than that in the unloaded implant. Engquist et al. [16] found less marginal bone loss in early loaded implants as compared to conventional implants. If implants are placed in soft bone, initial stabilization can be compromised leading to micromotion and failure. Immediate/early stabilization and splinting of implants help to reduce excessive micromotion of implants.

Excellent short-term data have been presented for early loaded implants in partially edentulous jaws. However, it must be remembered that most of the papers reviewed are produced by practitioners who are highly trained in dental implant placement. Few long-term multicenter studies are available. Most studies on patient benefits are also needed. Besides shorter treatment time for the doctor/patients with early loaded implants, there are psychological factors for the patients that warrant more attention. Based on this case report, it is suggested that the immediate loading/early method should be limited to healed sites. Further clinical and histologic studies are necessary to promote routine clinical application of this technique.

5. Conclusions

Implants with high initial primary stability seem to function well under the influence of immediate and early loading. Available bone quality needs to be evaluated to ensure the proper implant diameter. By using surgical methods capable of enhancing primary implant stability, the placement of early loaded implants in less dense bone can result in a successful outcome. A successful integration of early loaded implants may require a final torque exceeding 35 N cm and an implant stability quotient value above 60. No difference in bone remodeling seems to exist between early loaded and two-stage implants. Within the limits of the present investigation, early loading of single-tooth implants placed in healed sites was a possible treatment alternative. Obviously, long-term data are needed to fully evaluate the benefits and risks of early loaded implants.

Conflict of Interests

The authors declare no conflict of interests.

References

[1] U.S. Department of Health and Human Services, "Oral health in America: a report of surgeon general," NIH Publication 00-4713, U.S. Department of Health and Human services, and Craniofacial Research, Rock-Ville, Md, USA, 2000.

[2] S. Szmukler-Moncler, A. Piattelli, G. A. Favero, and J. H. Dubruille, "Considerations preliminary to the application of

early and immediate loading protocols in dental implantology," *Clinical Oral Implants Research*, vol. 11, no. 1, pp. 12–25, 2000.

[3] W. Becker and B. E. Becker, "Replacement of maxillary and mandibular molars with single endosseous implant restorations: a retrospective study," *The Journal of Prosthetic Dentistry*, vol. 74, no. 1, pp. 51–55, 1995.

[4] D. L. Cochran, "The scientific basis for and clinical experiences with Straumann implants including the ITI Dental Implant System: a consensus report," *Clinical Oral Implants Research*, vol. 11, pp. 33–58, 2000.

[5] J. E. Davies, "Understanding peri-implant endosseous healing," *Journal of Dental Education*, vol. 67, no. 8, pp. 932–949, 2003.

[6] D. L. Cochran, R. K. Schenk, A. Lussi et al., "Bone response to unloaded and loaded titanium implants with a sand blasted and acid etched surface: a histometric study in the canine mandible," *Journal of Biomedical Materials Research*, vol. 40, no. 1, pp. 1–11, 1998.

[7] A. G. T. Payne, A. Tawse-Smith, W. D. Duncan, and R. Kumara, "Conventional and early loading of unsplinted ITI implants supporting mandibular overdentures two-year results of a prospective randomized clinical trial," *Clinical Oral Implants Research*, vol. 13, no. 6, pp. 603–609, 2002.

[8] R. Adell, U. Lekholm, B. Rockler, and P. I. Branemark, "A 15-year study of osseointegrated implants in the treatment of the edentulous jaw," *International Journal of Oral Surgery*, vol. 10, no. 6, pp. 387–416, 1981.

[9] P. I. Brånemark, B. O. Hansson, R. Adell et al., "Osseointegrated implants in the treatment of the edentulous jaw. Experience from a 10-year period," *Scandinavian Journal of Plastic and Reconstructive Surgery*, vol. 16, pp. 1–132, 1977.

[10] D. L. Cochran, D. Buser, C. M. Ten Bruggenkate et al., "The use of reduced healing times on ITI® implants with a sandblasted and acid-etched (SLA) surface: early results from clinical trials on ITI® SLA implants," *Clinical Oral Implants Research*, vol. 13, no. 2, pp. 144–153, 2002.

[11] I. Ericsson, K. Randow, K. Nilner, and A. Peterson, "Early functional loading of Brånemark dental implants: 5-year clinical follow-up study," *Clinical Implant Dentistry and Related Research*, vol. 2, no. 2, pp. 70–77, 2000.

[12] H. K. Kupeyan and K. B. May, "Implant and provisional crown placement: a one stage protocol," *Implant Dentistry*, vol. 7, no. 3, pp. 213–219, 1998.

[13] E. Andersen, H. R. Haanæs, and B. M. Knutsen, "Immediate loading of single-tooth ITI implants in the anterior maxilla: a prospective 5-year pilot study," *Clinical Oral Implants Research*, vol. 13, no. 3, pp. 281–287, 2002.

[14] G. Cannizzaro and M. Leone, "Restoration of partially edentulous patients using dental implants with a microtextured surface: a prospective comparison of delayed and immediate full occlusal loading," *International Journal of Oral and Maxillofacial Implants*, vol. 18, no. 4, pp. 512–522, 2003.

[15] A. Piattelli, M. Corigliano, A. Scarano, and M. Quarante, "Bone reactions to early occlusal loading of two-stage titanium plasma-sprayed implants: a pilot study in monkeys," *International Journal of Periodontics and Restorative Dentistry*, vol. 17, no. 2, pp. 163–169, 1997.

[16] B. Engquist, P. Åstrand, B. Anzén et al., "Simplified methods of implant treatment in the edentulous lower jaw: a 3-year follow-up report of a controlled prospective study of one-stage versus two-stage surgery and early loading," *Clinical Implant Dentistry and Related Research*, vol. 7, no. 2, pp. 95–104, 2005.

44

Multiple Cementoblastoma: A Rare Case Report

G. Iannaci,[1] R. Luise,[1] G. Iezzi,[2] A. Piattelli,[2] and A. Salierno[3]

[1] *Department of Pathology, Incurabili Hospital ASLNAPOLI1 Centro, Via Maria Longo, 50-80138 Napoli, Italy*
[2] *Department of Medical, Oral and Biotechnological Sciences, University of Chieti-Pescara, Chieti, Italy*
[3] *Department of Oral Medicine, School of Dentistry of the Second University of the Study of Naples, Naples, Italy*

Correspondence should be addressed to G. Iannaci; giuseppe.iannaci@tin.it

Academic Editors: M. B. D. Gaviao, J. A. Shibli, and R. Sorrentino

Benign cementoblastoma is a rare ectomesenchymal odontogenic tumor that originates from the root of the tooth and that is characterized by the formation of cementum-like tissue. A 60-year old man was referred to us complaining of pain in his right jaw. The patient underwent TC dental scan of the mandible, which highlighted the presence of three well-circumscribed, round, unilocular neoformations of radiopaque appearance with a radiotransparent edge, one of which was in close contact with the roots of the lower right second molar. Microscopic examination of the greater sample consisted, in its central portion, of dense mineralized acellular trabeculae of basophilic tissue cement-like, devoid of vessels, adhering to the root of the tooth, while peripherally was observed a zone of vascularized osteoid surrounded, occasionally, by a thin rim of cementoblasts mixed with fibrous tissue and inflammatory elements. This lesion was diagnosed as cementoblastoma. The second lesion appeared radiologically and histologically entirely identical to cementoblastoma, but it did not show the intimate association with the root of involved tooth. After a careful review of the literature, the diagnosis of residual cementoblastoma was made. The clinicopathologic features, treatment, and prognosis of this rare tumor are here discussed for the young dental practitioner.

1. Introduction

Benign cementoblastoma is a rare lesion of the oral cavity, currently classified by the World Health Organization (WHO 2005) as an ectomesenchymal odontogenic tumor that originates from the root of the tooth and that is characterized with the formation of cementum-like tissue [1, 2]. It usually arises in the first permanent molars in their mandibular region but can also be associated with multiple teeth, deciduous teeth, or unerupted molars [3, 4]. The caucasians race and male sex are more commonly affected than black race and female (ratio 2.1 : 1), with a very wide age range and a peak incidence between the second and third decade of life. Clinically, the lesion presents as a nodular formation, hard-elastic in consistency producing swelling in the alveolar ridge area. Paresthesias of the lower lip or a pathologic fracture of the jaw have been rarely reported. The radiological findings show a well-defined radiopaque mass surrounded with a thin, radiolucent rim of nonmineralized tissue, in intimate association of the root of the involved tooth. The resorption of the tooth root, the loss of the regular outline with the obliteration of the periodontal ligament are clinical and radiological features that can be frequently found [5, 6]. We describe a rare case of multiple cementoblastoma: a classic cementoblastoma in direct *continuity* with the *root* of the *tooth* (true cementoma) and a residual cementoblastoma localized in the *edentulous area* post-extraction.

2. Case Report

A 60-years-old man was referred to us complaining of pain in his right jaw. The *examination of the patient's medical history revealed* good general health, absence of systemic diseases, and smoking habit (10 cigarettes\day). The clinical examination showed discrete oral hygiene, thick and flat periodontal biotype, class II malocclusion with marked loss of vertical size, multiple missing teeth in the site 1.4-1.5-3.5-3.6-3.7-4.5-4.6., presence of swelling, hard elastic consistency, and crepitus on palpation in the region corresponding to the elements 4.4-4.7 and in the edentulous area 4.6, 4.5. The orthopantomography revealed on the upper jaw radicular

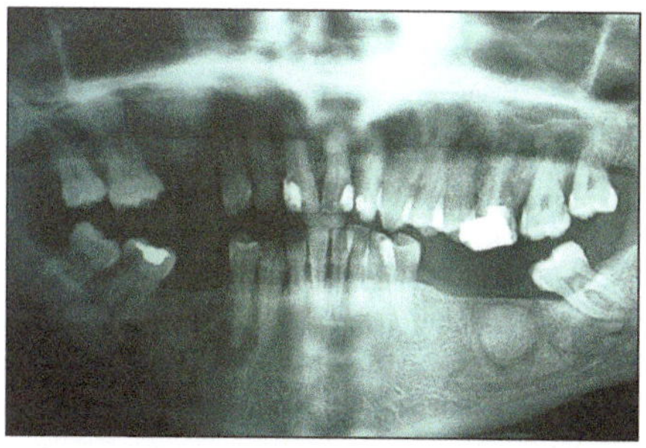

FIGURE 1: The first orthopantomography revealed the presence of three well-circumscribed, round, unilocular neoformations of radiopaque appearance with a radiotransparent edge, one of which was in close contact with the roots of the lower right second molar.

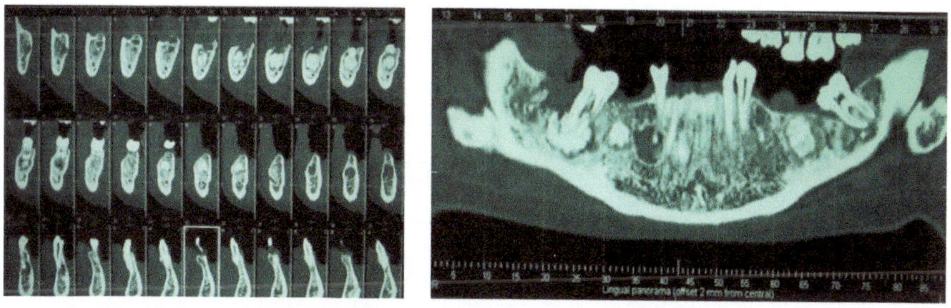

FIGURE 2: TC dental scan of the mandible.

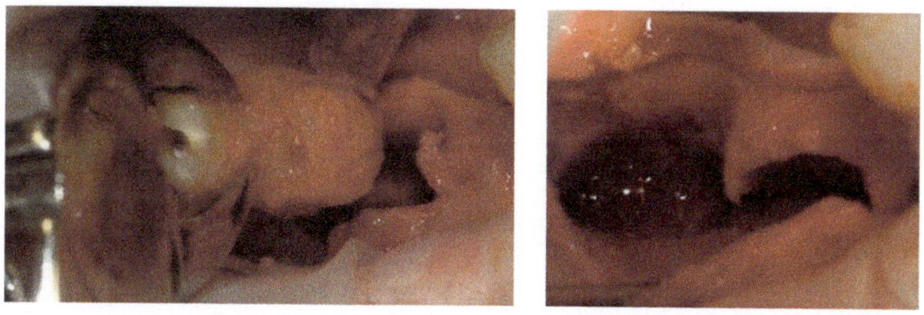

FIGURE 3: The surgical treatment included the full enucleation of the lesion on site 4.7 with the annexed dental element on the right jaw and the lesion corresponding to the edentulous area 4.6.

element in 1.4 region, conservative restoration in 1.1-2.1-2.2-2.6, the presence of radiopaque unilocular lesion adjacent to the root apex of the element 1.6 while the lower arch showed a carious radiolucency at the crown of element 4.7 and other lesions spread to the mandibular body. Particularly, these lesions were thus located: three unilocular round shaped radiopaque lesions with a perilesional radio transparent rib next to the edentulous sites 3.6-4.6 and in contact with the roots of the element 4.7, whose appearance is suggestive for a neoformation (Figure 1); a rounded radiolucent lesion with radiopaque perilesional flange at the root apex of the element 4.4 whose appearance argued for a radicular cyst of endodontic origin. The test thermal pulp vitality with ethyl chloride, performed on elements 4.4 and 4.7, was negative.

The initial treatment plan included the implementation of an etiological instrumental therapy (motivation to oral hygiene, periodontal probing, scaling, and radicular smoothing), extraction of root element in endodontic treatment on site 1.4, a conservative endodontic treatment of the element 4.4 in order to resolve endodontically periapical radiolucent lesion and endodontic treatment of 4.7 to cure the acute pulpitis. After two months, following the resolution of acute symptomatology, in order to better analyze the lesions that were evident in the orthopantomography, the patient underwent TC dental scan of the mandible (Figure 2), which highlighted the presence of three well-circumscribed, round, unilocular neoformations of radiopaque appearance with a radiotransparent edge, one of which was in close contact with the roots of the lower right second molar.

The surgical treatment that included the enucleation of the only two lesions on the right jaw, the ones involved in the acute pain, was performed in local and regional *anaesthesia* with a full-thickness flap, osteotomy using rotating tools, *enucleation* of the lesion corresponding to the edentulous area 4.6 and the full enucleation on site 4.7 with the annexed dental element (Figure 3) because the indissociability of the lesion from the root of the dental element has not allowed a more conservative approach "apicoectomy." Finally after a cleaning of the residual cavity, the flap suture with continuous suture ethicon "3–0" was performed.

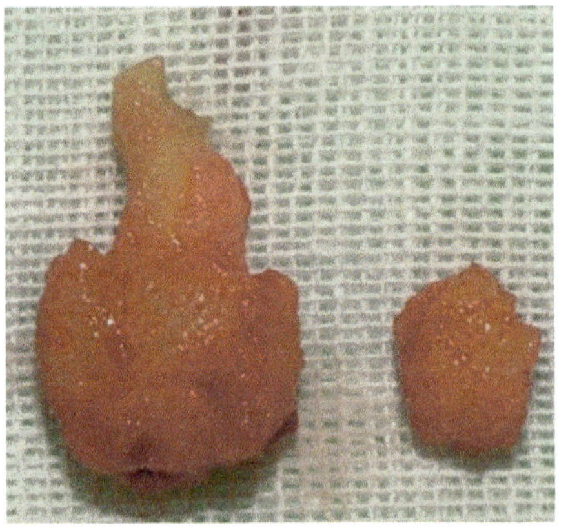

FIGURE 4: Macroscopically the two samples presented as a nodular, hard-elastic in consistency, the largest of which was adherent to the dental element.

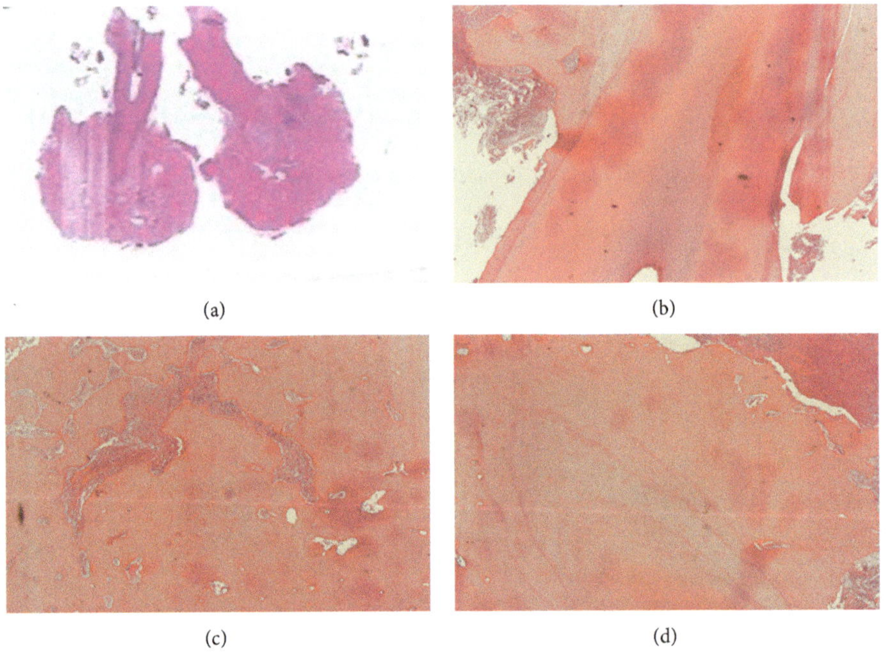

(a) (b) (c) (d)

FIGURE 5: ((a) and (b)) H&E (4x\10x) cementoblastoma closely connected with the tooth root; ((c) and (d)) H&E 20x. Cementoblastoma and residual cementoblastoma revealed the same histological appearance: dense mineralized acellular trabeculae of basophilic tissue cement-like, devoid of vessels, adhering to the root of the tooth.

The specimens were sent to surgical pathology for definitive diagnosis. Both lesions were examined in toto (Figure 4) and the two samples, macroscopically, presented as a nodular, hard-elastic in consistency, color greyish white of 2 × 1 cm and 1 × 1 cm, the largest of which was adherent to the dental element. The tissue samples were fixed in 10% formalin, decalcified with formic acid, and then routinely processed and embedded in paraffin, with cut sections of 3-4 micron. The sections were stained with haematoxylin-eosin. Microscopic examination of the greater sample consisted, in its central portion, of dense mineralized acellular trabeculae of basophilic tissue cement-like, devoid of vessels, adhering to the root of the tooth, while peripherally was observed a zone of vascularized osteoid surrounded, occasionally, by a thin rim of cementoblasts mixed with fibrous tissue and inflammatory elements. The largest lesion, closely connected with the tooth root, was diagnosed as cementoblastoma (Figure 5). The second lesion appeared radiologically and histologically entirely identical to cementoblastoma, but it did not show the intimate association with the root of involved tooth, and, so, it posed the differential diagnosis between osteoblastoma and residual cementoblastoma because both lesions may arise in the edentulous area after extraction. Therefore, after a careful review of the literature and considering the epidemiological and clinical data, the diagnosis of residual cementoblastoma rather than osteoblastoma was made. The clinicopathologic

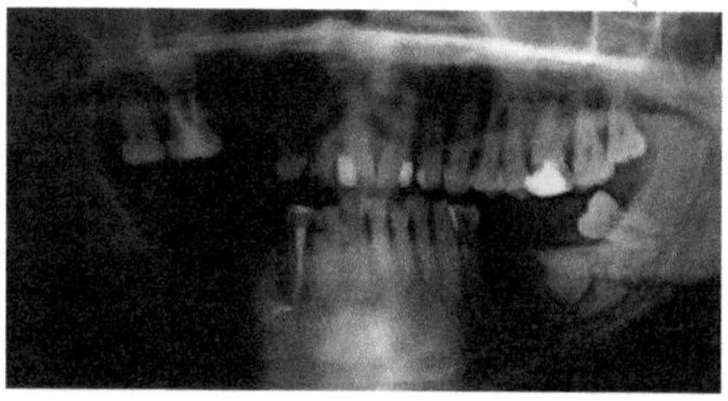

FIGURE 6: The follow-up after one year of both tumors was negative for disease recurrence.

features, treatment, and prognosis are discussed. It is in general agreement with observations emerging from the international scientific literature, which claims that, if the cementoblastoma is properly treated, it does not recur. The follow-up after one year of both tumors was negative for disease recurrence. The features of the lesion remained in site were unchanged (Figure 6). Although this neoplasm is rare, the dental practitioner should be aware of the clinical and radiographic features that will lead to its early diagnosis and treatment.

3. Discussion

The location and the histological presentation of benign cementoblastoma is totally identical to osteoblastoma [7, 8]. The osteoblastoma is a rare benign tumor that produces bone, in which the rim of osteoblasts surrounds the trabeculae forming a well-circumscribed lesion, usually greater than 2 cm in diameter. This neoplasm affects young patients; in 90% of cases, they are males under 30 years and the most typical localization includes the mandible: preferentially in the body rather than in the middle portion or in the coronoid process. Radiologically as a well-circumscribed lesion with a mixed pattern, lytic, and sclerotic appears, which reflects the different degree of mineralization of the matrix. It is believed that the two lesions are manifestations of the same process and that the use of a term rather than another is a purely academic exercise [9–11]. Indeed, according to the recent literature, the only difference consists in the fact that osteoblastoma does not melt at the root of the involved tooth as in the case of cementoblastoma that, sometimes, can also involve the periodontal ligament. Other authors, such as Slootweg, classify as osteoblastoma the lesion correlated with root canal but not fused with it. In our case, the second lesion posed further problems of differential diagnosis: in fact it is not possible to value the relationship with the tooth root because the tumour arises in the edentulous area after extraction. Benign cementoblastoma must be, also, differentiated from nonneoplastic processes such as osteoid osteoma that, however, is easily distinguished from a microscopic point of view because it presents a reversed architecture compared to it, presenting dense trabeculae of osteoid in the center rather than peripheral area [12]. After evaluating the site, the patient's age, and rarity in the literature of synchronous association cementoblastoma with osteoblastoma, we opted for the diagnosis of multiple cementoblastoma.

References

[1] L. Barnes, J. W. Eveson, P. Reichart, and D. Sidransky, *Pathology & Genetics Head and Neck Tumours WHO Classification of Tumours*, 2005.

[2] R. A. Cawason, W. H. Binnie, P. M. Speight, A. W. Barrett, and J. M. Wright, *Lucas's Pathology of Tumors of the Oral Tissues*, 5th edition, 1998.

[3] A. Piattelli, L. Di Alberti, A. Scarano, and M. Piattelli, "Benign cementoblastoma associated with an unerupted third molar," *Oral Oncology*, vol. 34, no. 3, pp. 229–231, 1998.

[4] J. A. Baart, C. Lekkas, and I. Van der Waal, "Residual cementoblastoma of the mandible," *Journal of Oral Pathology and Medicine*, vol. 20, no. 6, pp. 300–302, 1991.

[5] L. Pacifici, M. Tallarico, A. Bartoli, A. Ripari, and A. Cicconetti, "Benign cementoblastoma: a clinical case of conservative surgical treatment of the involved tooth," *Minerva Stomatologica*, vol. 53, no. 11-12, pp. 685–691, 2004.

[6] F. T. Monks, J. C. Bradley, and E. P. Turner, "Central osteoblastoma or cementoblastoma? A case report and 12 year review," *British Journal of Oral Surgery*, vol. 19, no. 1, pp. 29–37, 1981.

[7] P. J. Slootweg, "Cementoblastoma and osteoblastoma: a comparison of histologic features," *Journal of Oral Pathology and Medicine*, vol. 21, no. 9, pp. 385–389, 1992.

[8] E. J. Cundiff II, "Developing cementoblastoma: case report and update of differential diagnosis," *Quintessence International*, vol. 31, no. 3, pp. 191–195, 2000.

[9] B. R. Pynn, T. D. Sands, and G. Bradley, "Benign cementoblastoma: a case report," *Journal of Canadian Dental Association*, vol. 67, no. 5, pp. 260–262, 2001.

[10] S. Leena Sankari and K. Ramakrishnan, "Benign cementoblastoma," *Journal of Oral and Maxillofacial Pathology*, vol. 15, no. 3, pp. 358–360, 2011.

[11] M. Sumer, K. Gunduz, A. P. Sumer, and O. Gunhan, "Benign cementoblastoma: a case report," *Medicina Oral, Patología Oral y Cirugía Bucal*, vol. 11, no. 6, pp. E483–E485, 2006.

[12] A. R. Huber and G. S. Folk, "Cementoblastoma," *Head and Neck Pathology*, vol. 3, no. 2, pp. 133–135, 2009.

45

Dental Treatment of a Child with Pallister-Killian Syndrome

Serhan Didinen,[1] Didem Atabek,[2] Gülay Kip,[2,3]
Aslı Patır Münevveroğlu,[1] and Özlem Tulunoğlu[4]

[1] *Department of Pediatric Dentistry, Faculty of Dentistry, Istanbul Medipol University, Turkey*
[2] *Department of Pediatric Dentistry, Faculty of Dentistry, Gazi University, Turkey*
[3] *Department of Anesthesia and Reanimation, Faculty of Medicine, Gazi University, Turkey*
[4] *Department of Pediatric Dentistry, School of Dental Medicine, Case Western Reserve University, Cleveland, OH, USA*

Correspondence should be addressed to Aslı Patır Münevveroğlu; apatir@medipol.edu.tr

Academic Editor: Michael J. Wahl

The Pallister-Killian syndrome (PKS) is an extremely rare genetic disorder with an incidence estimated around 1/25000. PKS is a multiple congenital anomaly deficit syndrome caused by mosaic tissue limited tetrasomy for chromosome 12p. The presented report is the first confirmed case with PKS in Turkey. This report focuses on the orofacial clinical manifestations of an 6-year-old boy with PKS who was referred to the Department of Paediatric Dentistry clinic, Gazi University. It has been learned that the PKS was diagnosed 1 year after birth. Due to intellectual disability, it was decided to make the dental treatments under moderate sedation. Although significant tongue thrust and anterior open bite were determined, any oral appliances could not be applied because of the 2 epilepsy seizures in the last 2 years. The aim was to treat decayed teeth and set good oral hygiene in the patient's mouth. Still, there is a probability for epilepsy seizures. If epileptic seizures stop permanently, we can apply an oral appliance to block tongue thrust. The patient is now under control. In cases of systemic and oral findings such as PKS, conducting medical and dental approaches together will increase the life quality of patients.

1. Background

The Pallister-Killian syndrome (PKS) is an extremely rare genetic disorder with an incidence estimated around 1/25000. PKS is a multiple congenital anomaly complex mosaic genetic duplication syndrome caused by mosaic tissue limited tetrasomy for chromosome 12p. It is defined as a mosaic condition as a result of not all cells having an extra chromosome [1, 2]. When genetic changes occur somatically, the individual exhibits cells with at least two different genotypes, and this state is known as mosaicism [3]. Somatic mosaicism is defined as the presence of two or more populations of cells with different genotypes in an individual who has developed from a single fertilized egg [2].

PKS has variable clinical manifestations and the syndrome may affect different organs and body systems. Although none of the features is pathognomonic for this chromosomal disorder, the more consistent anomalies include craniofacial dysmorphism (prominent forehead, sparse anterior scalp hair, flat occiput, hypertelorism, short nose with anteverted nostrils, flat nasal bridge, and malformed ears), short neck, limb deformities, pigmentary skin anomalies, and nail hypoplasia [4–6]. Progressive psychomotor developmental delay, severe hypotonia, deafness, and seizures become more prominent with age. In contrast, in perinatally diagnosed cases, a much higher incidence of internal organ anomalies, like congenital diaphragmatic hernia, cardiovascular anomalies, and anorectal anomalies, is noted [7]. This age-dependent phenotype expression is another characteristic of PKS [4].

Frequency of seizures, age of onset, typical seizure types, response to treatment, and prognosis of epilepsy are hardly known in PKS [8]. Epileptic seizure prevalence in PKS is in the vicinity of 42–59% as shown by case series and meta-analysis studies [9, 10].

This report provides the dental treatment of a 6-year-old boy with two sessions of deep sedation. To our knowledge,

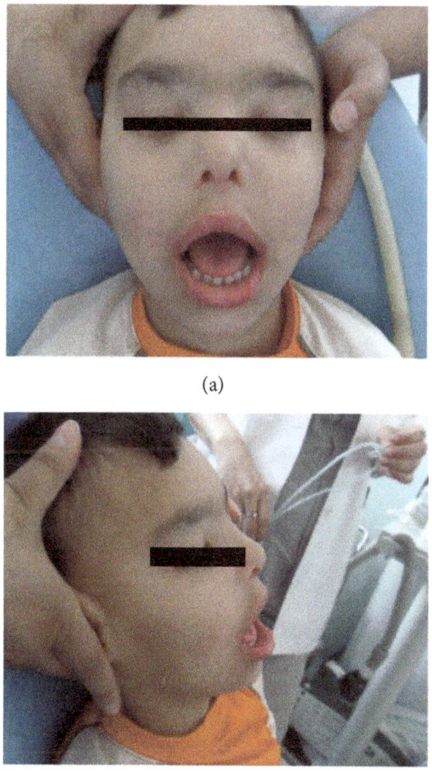

(a)

(b)

FIGURE 1: Orofacial clinical manifestations of a 6-year-old boy with PKS.

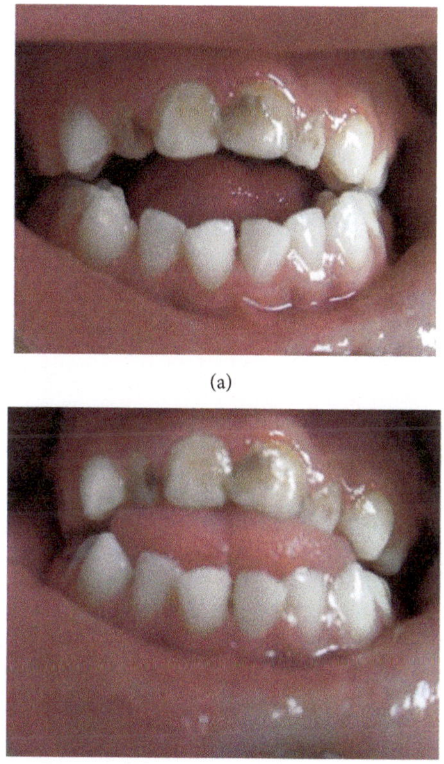

(a)

(b)

FIGURE 2: Oral findings related to PKS: oral breathing, anterior open bite, tongue thrust, mandibular prognathism, and macroglossia.

the presented case is the first confirmed dental patient with PKS in Turkey.

2. Procedure

This report focuses on the orofacial clinical manifestations of a 6-year-old boy with PKS who was referred to the Department of Pediatric Dentistry clinic, Faculty of Dentistry, Gazi University (Figures 1(a) and 1(b)). It has been learned that the PKS was diagnosed 1 year after birth.

Orbital hypertelorism and esophoria, bitemporal alopecia, bilateral hearing loss, open posture of mouth, prominent and large forehead, flat nose bridge, and short nose are observed extraorally.

During the clinical examination, some oral findings related to PKS were diagnosed as follows (Figures 2(a) and 2(b)): oral breathing, anterior open bite, tongue thrust, mandibular prognathism, and macroglossia. It was observed that there are shallow caries in teeth #55 and #65 and profound caries in teeth #51, #52, #61, #62, #36, #46, #74, #75, #84, and #85. Considering the patient's mental retardation and lack of cooperation on dental chair, it was decided to make the dental treatments under moderate sedation. During the first session of sedation, teeth #51, #52, #61, #62, #74, #75, and #84 were extracted and #85, #36, and #46 were restored with amalgam restoration (Cavex, Haarlem, Netherlands) (Figures 3(a), 3(b), and 3(c)).

After the dental treatments under sedation, the patient's family were advised to clean their child's teeth regularly and visit our clinic every 6 months, for follow-ups. However, the patient returned to the clinic 3 years after treatment again with pain in his teeth. Due to lack of routine controls, newly decayed teeth were observed and a new treatment plan was established for second session of moderate sedation. Under sedation, teeth #55 and #46 were restored with composite, resin (Tetric-N-Ceram, Ivoclar Vivadent, Schaan, Liechtenstein) (Figures 4(a) and 4(b)).

After this session, the patient's parents changed their phone number without declaration. Also, they have not visited our clinic again, for follow-up controls or any other complaints.

3. Discussion

Severe to profound developmental delay is observed in most individuals with PKS, although there have been an increasing number of mildly affected individuals with PKS reported [11]. Average ages for achieving motor milestones in PKS include 10.8 months (rolling), 21.2 months (sitting independently), and 38.8 months (walking). Although there are many individuals with PKS who do not attain speech, initiation of speech often starts at 36 months [12]. Repetitive hand and body movements were frequently noticed (75%), and this condition makes the dental treatment impossible under

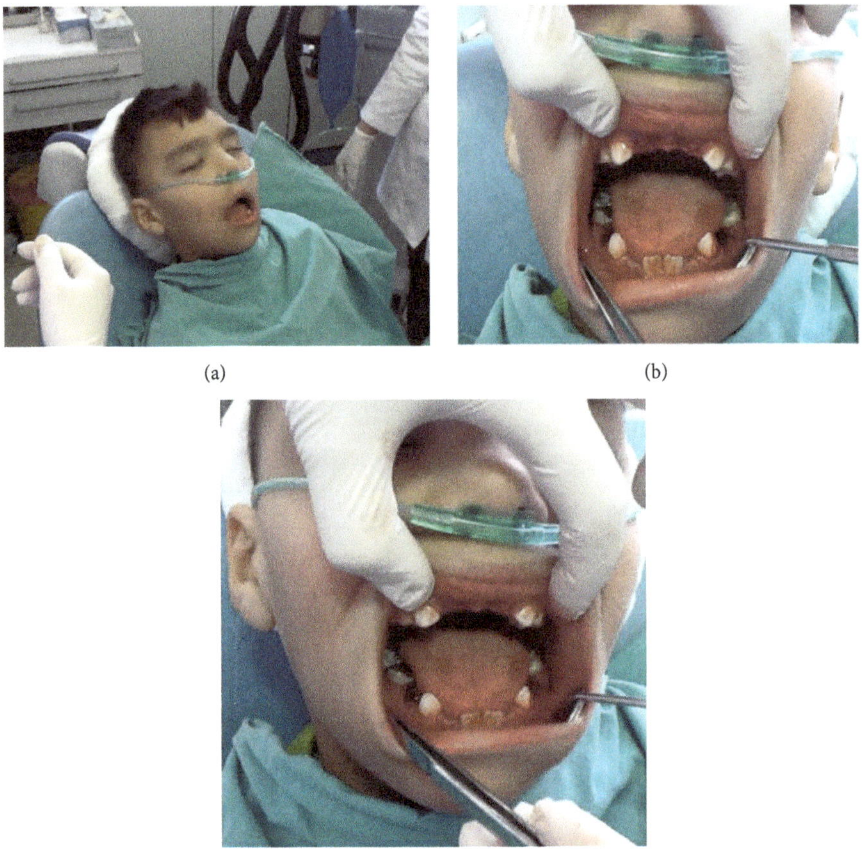

(a) (b) (c)

FIGURE 3: Considering the patient's mental retardation and lack of cooperation on dental chair, it was decided to make the dental treatments under moderate sedation.

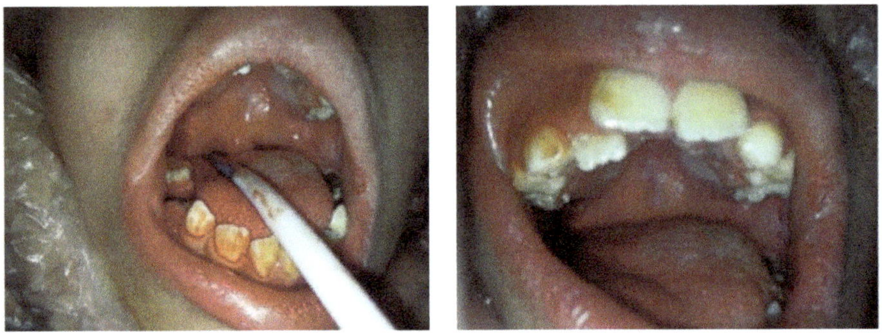

(a) (b)

FIGURE 4: Newly decayed teeth were observed and a new treatment plan was established for second session of moderate sedation.

full-consciousness situation [2]. General anesthesia and deep sedation was observed as an effective dental treatment option for these types of patients who have involuntary movements. Also, hear loss and cataract are other rough factors to communicate with the patient.

Routine dental procedures can be successfully performed under sufficient precautions [13]. Treatment of oral habits in children with special care poses a challenge for dentists. Reminder therapy and use of a reward system should be attempted prior to the placement of any dental appliance [14]. Dentists should use corrective intraoral appliances to treat thumb-sucking if the habit is chronic, if the child above 4 years old, and if the child requests help in stopping the habit [15]. Although the use of fixed appliances is indicated in a child with epilepsy, due to the risk of dislodgement and potential airway obstruction [16], the neurologist advised us not to apply a fixed or removable oral appliance, till seizures totally stop.

Mouth breathing and tongue thrusting can be counted as factors for future caries and malocclusion [17]. Chronic mouth breathing occurs with the obstruction of the nasal airway which is caused by chronic allergy and the excessive lymphoid tissue proliferation [18]. Mouth breathing was shown as an etiological factor for tongue thrusting and anterior dental open bite in current studies [19]. When the malocclusion remains for a long period of time, the tongue fills the oral cavity and makes lips lose their tonus [20–22]. The presented case exhibits mouth opening since he was born and open bite due to this habit.

4. Conclusion

Pallister-Killian syndrome is an extremely rare syndrome and dentists are unfamiliar with how to manage it. Dentists should warn the parents about preventive issues and regular dental visit to save children from caries. However, if the patient is seen in a bad oral situation, deep sedation is a beneficial way to treat all teeth in one session.

Conflict of Interests

The authors declare that there is no conflict of interests regarding the publication of this paper.

References

[1] M. Murakami, T. Iwasa, Y. Takahashi, and M. Morine, "Amniocentesis can be useful during the third trimester of pregnancy for antenatal diagnosis of Pallister-Killian syndrome: a case report," *Clinical and Experimental Obstetrics and Gynecology*, vol. 38, no. 3, pp. 269–271, 2011.

[2] K. Izumi and I. D. Krantz, "Pallister-Killian syndrome," *American Journal of Medical Genetics. Part C: Seminars in Medical Genetics*, vol. 166, no. 4, pp. 406–413, 2014.

[3] N. B. Spinner and L. K. Conlin, "Mosaicism and clinical genetics," *American Journal of Medical Genetics C*, vol. 166, no. 4, pp. 397–405, 2014.

[4] M. Baglaj, J. King, and R. Carachi, "Pallister-Killian syndrome: a report of 2 cases and review of its surgical aspects," *Journal of Pediatric Surgery*, vol. 43, no. 6, pp. 1218–1221, 2008.

[5] J. F. Reynolds, A. Daniel, T. E. Kelly et al., "Isochromosome 12p mosaicism (Pallister mosaic aneuploidy or Pallister-Killian syndrome): report of 11 cases," *American Journal of Medical Genetics*, vol. 27, no. 2, pp. 257–274, 1987.

[6] G. Horneff, F. Majewski, B. Hildebrand, T. Voit, and H.-G. Lenard, "Pallister-Killian syndrome in older children and adolescents," *Pediatric Neurology*, vol. 9, no. 4, pp. 312–315, 1993.

[7] P. A. Mowery-Rushton, M. P. Stadler, S. J. Kochmar, E. McPherson, U. Surti, and W. A. Hogge, "The use of interphase FISH for prenatal diagnosis of Pallister-Killian syndrome," *Prenatal Diagnosis*, vol. 17, no. 3, pp. 255–265, 1997.

[8] M. S. Candee, J. C. Carey, I. D. Krantz, and F. M. Filloux, "Seizure characteristics in Pallister-Killian syndrome," *American Journal of Medical Genetics Part A*, vol. 158, no. 12, pp. 3026–3032, 2012.

[9] H. J. Stalker, B. A. Gray, A. Bent-Williams, and R. T. Zori, "High cognitive functioning and behavioral phenotype in Pallister-Killian syndrome," *American Journal of Medical Genetics—Part A*, vol. 140, no. 18, pp. 1950–1954, 2006.

[10] M. M. Bielanska, M. M. Khalifa, and A. M. V. Duncan, "Pallister-Killian syndrome: a mild case diagnosed by fluorescence in situ hybridization. Review of the literature and expansion of the phenotype," *American Journal of Medical Genetics*, vol. 65, no. 2, pp. 104–108, 1996.

[11] A. Kostanecka, L. B. Close, K. Izumi, I. D. Krantz, and M. Pipan, "Developmental and behavioral characteristics of individuals with Pallister-Killian syndrome," *American Journal of Medical Genetics Part A*, vol. 158, no. 12, pp. 3018–3025, 2012.

[12] A. Wilkens, H. Liu, K. Park et al., "Novel clinical manifestations in Pallister-Killian syndrome: comprehensive evaluation of 59 affected individuals and review of previously reported cases," *American Journal of Medical Genetics—Part A*, vol. 158, no. 12, pp. 3002–3017, 2012.

[13] P. L. Jacobsen and O. Eden, "Epilepsy and the dental management of the epileptic patient," *Journal of Contemporary Dental Practice*, vol. 9, no. 1, pp. 54–62, 2008.

[14] S. Greenleaf and J. Mink, "A retrospective study of the use of the Bluegrass appliance in the cessation of thumb habits," *Pediatric Dentistry*, vol. 25, no. 6, pp. 587–590, 2003.

[15] N. Chhabra, A. Chhabra, and S. Bansal, "An innovative approach to cessation of thumb-sucking in a child with epilepsy: a case report," *Special Care in Dentistry*, vol. 32, no. 6, pp. 270–273, 2012.

[16] C. K. Vorkas, M. K. Gopinathan, A. Singh, O. Devinsky, L. M. Lin, and P. A. Rosenberg, "Epilepsy and dental procedures. A review," *The New York State Dental Journal*, vol. 74, no. 2, pp. 39–43, 2008.

[17] M. D. Indira, K. S. Dhull, B. Nandlal, P. S. Praveen Kumar, and R. S. Dhull, "Biological restoration in pediatric dentistry: a brief insight," *International Journal of Clinical Pediatric Dentistry*, vol. 7, no. 3, pp. 197–201, 2014.

[18] W. G. Watson, "Open-bite-a multifactorial event," *American Journal of Orthodontics*, vol. 80, no. 4, pp. 443–446, 1981.

[19] G. M. Greenlee, G. J. Huang, S. S.-H. Chen, J. Chen, T. Koepsell, and P. Hujoel, "Stability of treatment for anterior open-bite malocclusion: a meta-analysis," *American Journal of Orthodontics and Dentofacial Orthopedics*, vol. 139, no. 2, pp. 154–169, 2011.

[20] S. B. Haralur and A. S. Al-Qahtani, "Replacement of missing anterior teeth in a patient with chronic mouth breathing and tongue thrusting," *Case Reports in Dentistry*, vol. 2013, Article ID 759162, 5 pages, 2013.

[21] N. E. Ahmad, A. E. Sanders, R. Sheats, J. L. Brame, and G. K. Essick, "Obstructive sleep apnea in association with periodontitis: a case-control study," *Journal of Dental Hygiene*, vol. 87, no. 4, pp. 188–199, 2013.

[22] B. M. Pennel and J. G. Keagle, "Predisposing factors in the etiology of chronic inflammatory periodontal disease," *Journal of Periodontology*, vol. 48, no. 9, pp. 517–532, 1977.

46

Resection and Reconstruction of Maxillary Class IIIc Defect in a Case of Adenoid Cystic Carcinoma: Cost-Sensitive Technique without Microvascular Grafts

Dwarkadas Adwani,[1] Anirudh Bhattacharya,[1,2] Rajender Singh Arora,[3] Ramawatar Soni,[4] and Nitin Adwani[1]

[1] *Department of Oral & Maxillofacial Surgery, VYWS Dental College & Hospital, Amravati 444601, India*
[2] *Adwani Multispeciality Dental Hospital, Ambapeth, Amravati 444601, India*
[3] *Department of Head & Neck Oncology, Amravati Cancer Hospital, Amravati 444601, India*
[4] *Department of Pathology, Dr. PDMMC Hospital, Amravati 444601, India*

Correspondence should be addressed to Anirudh Bhattacharya; dranirudhb@gmail.com

Academic Editors: Y.-K. Chen and R. Crespi

ACC is a rare malignant tumor that affects most commonly the major and minor salivary glands and rarely the paranasal sinuses, lacrimal gland, larynx, ear, vulva, and so forth. The maxillary sinus when affected is considered having a poor prognosis due to delayed diagnosis and delayed treatment credited to its slow spread, late symptoms, and complex anatomy which hampers surgical resection. The expressions of tumor markers too have a significant role in determining the prognosis. The treatment of choice consists of wide radical resection of the tumor followed by radiotherapy. Rehabilitation options in cases with huge maxillary defects still need further exploration.

1. Introduction

Adenoid cystic carcinoma (ACC) is a rare malignancy, accounting for less than 5% of all head and neck cancers [1]. ACC arises within secretory glands, most commonly the major and minor salivary glands of the head and neck. ACC can also originate from sites other than the salivary glands, such as the lacrimal gland, external ear, paranasal sinuses, larynx, tracheobronchial tree, breast, and vulva, and such ACC is called nonsalivary ACC [2]. ACC of the maxillary antrum is frequently overlooked, and therefore, patients with this tumour usually come at an advanced stage making radical resection unlikely. Difficult access and anticipated surgical morbidity are other major barriers in treatment. Biological markers Ki-67, cyclineD1, E-cadherin, and p16 also have an important impact on prognosis [3, 4]. Older age, advanced stage, positive resection margin, high histological grade, and higher expression of Ki-67 were also associated with poor outcomes.

2. Case Report

A 40-year-old male patient reported to the Department of Oral and Maxillofacial Surgery with a chief complaint of painless swelling on the left side of the face and obstruction in nasal breathing since 3 years. The swelling was slow growing, painless, and persistent in growth. There was no reduction in size of the swelling since the patient had noticed it. Personal history was negative for any detrimental habits. On extra oral examination, a large swelling was seen on left side of face, extending superoinferiorly from medial canthus of left eye till left commissure of lips and anteroposteriorly from the left lateral surface of nasal septal cartilage till 4 cm short of tragus of left ear. On nasal examination, there was severe deviation of nasal septum seen towards the right side, along with thick polyp-like mucosal obstruction in the left nostril. On eye examination, the left eye was virtually closed and raised due to the pressure from the swelling over orbit inferiorly and

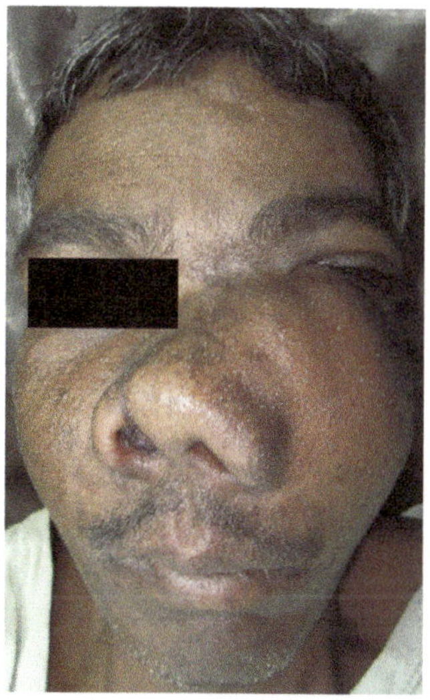

Figure 1

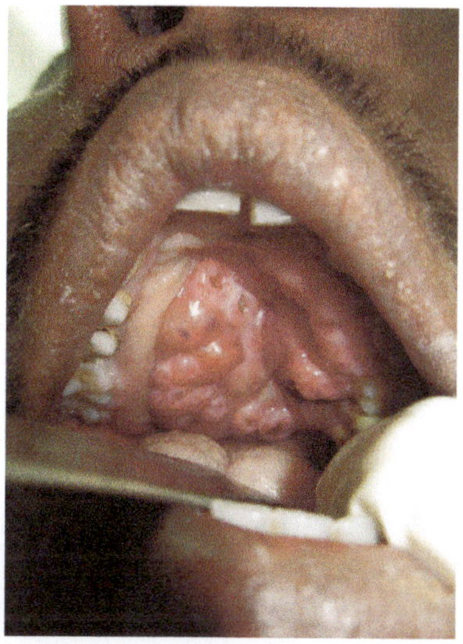

Figure 2

medially (Figure 1). Eyeball movements in all directions were normal with intact vision. Direct and consensual pupillary reflexes were present. No cervical lymphadenopathy was discernible. Intraoral examination revealed a well-defined nodular swelling covering the whole hard palate. The overlying mucosa was ulcerated on some areas and reddish in colour. It was nonfluctuant, noncompressible, and nontender. On hard tissue examination, all the permanent teeth were present, without any related dental problems (Figure 2). Laboratory blood and other serological investigations as well as ultrasonography of neck were noncontributory. Chest X-ray revealed no pleural or parenchymal abnormalities. Radiographic investigations including pantomogram, PNS Water's view, and high resolution computed tomography (HR-CT) scan were carried out. CT scan of paranasal sinuses revealed

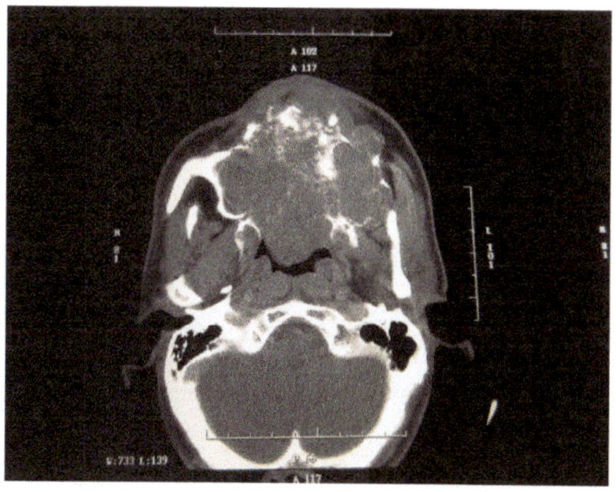

Figure 3

a large heterogenous mass in the left maxillary sinus, destroying all its walls crossing the midline and extending into the adjacent right nasal cavity, anterosuperiorly extending into left orbit and left ethmoidal sinus, anteroinferiorly into the hard palate and alveolar ridge, and posteroinferiorly extending into nasopharynx (Figure 3). Later, fine needle aspiration cytology was performed, and serosanguineous fluid was aspirated. Smear showed many clusters of glandular epithelial cells and eosinophilic globules along with blood cells. Findings were suggestive of a secretory gland tumor. Based on a provisional diagnosis of malignant tumor, an incisional biopsy was performed from palate near the left maxillary canine tooth. The microscopic examination of the tumour revealed features of Grade II adenoid cystic carcinoma (grading as per Szanto et al.). On immunohistochemistry examination, the tumour cells were positive for E-cadherin (Grade I, 10% of the tumour cells), positive for cyclinD1 (Grade 1+, 15% of tumour cells), showing low positivity (1%) for Ki-67, and negative for p16. Finally, based on the confirmatory diagnosis of adenoid cystic carcinoma arising from maxillary sinus, total maxillectomy along with left infraorbital rim was carried out, creating a class IIIc defect (Figures 4(a) and 4(b)). Immediate reconstruction options were very limited due to poor socioeconomic condition of the patient; therefore, we went with an unconventional method. For the loss of left infraorbital rim and floor, pedicled temporalis myofascial flap was harvested and was transpositioned into the mucosa of nasopharynx to provide an inferior base for the left globe and reduce enophthalmos. Next, to compensate for hard tissue loss, a titanium 2.5 mm continuous reconstruction plate was fixed over the body of zygoma (4 screws on either side) bilaterally to support the midfacial soft tissue structures from collapsing and threatening airway (Figure 5). The postsurgical histopathology reports confirmed the tumor-free surgical margins and the preoperative biopsy findings. Patient was sent for radiotherapy (RT), 60 gray (Gy) for a period of 45 days. After 4 weeks, a customized acrylic obturator was provided to conceal the remaining defect and to ease phonation and deglutition (Figure 6). Patient was quite comfortable with that, and his speech was pretty clear. He is in followup for the past 12 months, without any signs of recurrence or other functional difficulties except loss of masticatory ability (Figure 7).

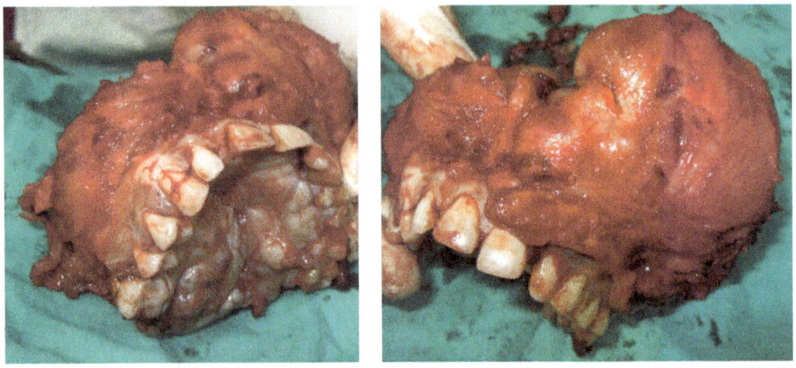

(a) (b)

Figure 4

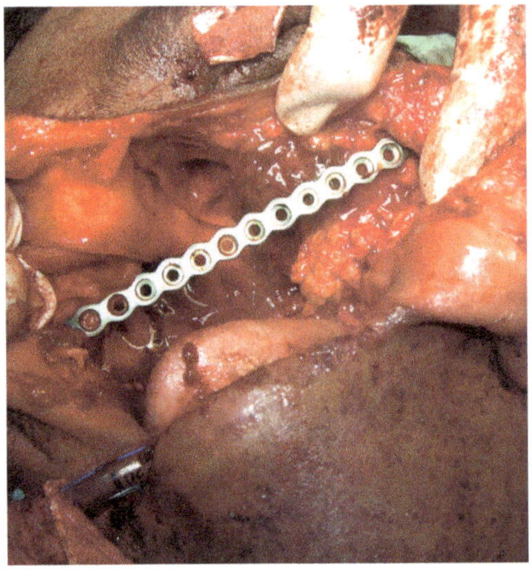

Figure 5

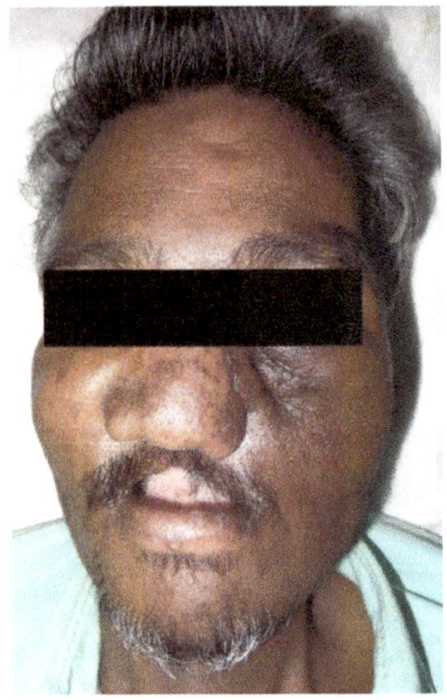

Figure 7

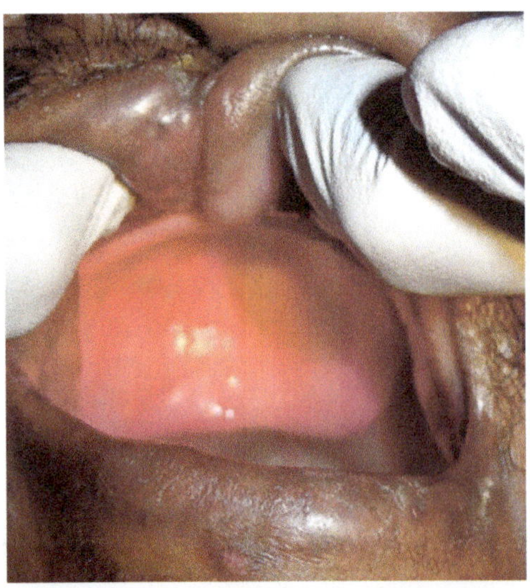

Figure 6

3. Discussion

Malignancies of the nasal cavity and paranasal sinuses represent only 3% to 5% of all head and neck carcinomas [5–7]. After bone invasion, the complex anatomy of the region, associated with invasion of adjacent structures and its proximity to vital structures, such as eyes, brain, and cranial nerves, has a significant direct negative impact on prognosis and survival [6, 8]. Destruction of maxillary sinus bone walls with local spreading of the tumor is common, making it difficult to reach adequate complete resection and tumor-free margins, which leads to high local recurrence rates [9]. Surgery is the treatment of choice for maxillary sinus carcinomas, and prognosis is better for patients managed by surgery followed by RT rather than for patients submitted to RT and/or chemotherapy (CT) alone [6]. Among the glandular tumors, ACC is considered to have the worst prognosis, but some authors have claimed that overall 5-year survival for maxillary sinus ACC is 57% [5, 10]. Prognosis and survival rates also depend on the histological grading of the tumour and expression of biological markers like Ki-67, cyclinD1, p16, and E-cadherin. Further, the reconstruction options in huge class IIIc defects of maxilla are limited. The conventional most favoured reconstruction modalities like free tissue transfer or the Zygoma implants are too technique sensitive and high cost bearing which cannot be executed for a part of Indian population with low socioeconomic status. In the best interest of the patient, a new cost-effective and least invasive method of supporting midfacial soft tissue structures, globe, and an obturator was tried. By this technique we were able to provide good phonation and deglutition capability to the patient, but in spite of trying our best, mastication could not be restored with such limited resources. This was the best which could be done for our patient with maxillary class IIIc defect, as in the published literature; also this type of maxillary defect is stated to be the most controversial [11]. The demand for an acceptable, very cost-effective, and least morbid technique diverted our efforts in creating something for every needy patient of such kind who cannot afford high cost and technique-sensitive microvascular tissue transfers.

References

[1] D. R. Gomez, B. S. Hoppe, S. L. Wolden et al., "Outcomes and prognostic variables in adenoid cystic carcinoma of the head and neck: a recent experience," *International Journal of Radiation Oncology Biology Physics*, vol. 70, no. 5, pp. 1365–1372, 2008.

[2] A. G. Lee, P. H. Phillips, N. J. Newman et al., "Neuro-ophthalmologic manifestations of adenoid cystic carcinoma," *Journal of Neuro-Ophthalmology*, vol. 17, no. 3, pp. 183–188, 1997.

[3] K. Triantafillidou, J. Dimitrakopoulos, F. Iordanidis, and D. Koufogiannis, "Management of adenoid cystic carcinoma of minor salivary glands," *Journal of Oral and Maxillofacial Surgery*, vol. 64, no. 7, pp. 1114–1120, 2006.

[4] L. Norberg-Spaak, I. Dardick, and T. Ledin, "Adenoid cystic carcinoma: use of cell proliferation. BCL-2 expression, histologic grade, and clinical stage as predictors of clinical outcome," *Head and Neck*, vol. 22, no. 5, pp. 489–497, 2000.

[5] L. L. Myers, B. Nussenbaum, C. R. Bradford, T. N. Teknos, R. M. Esclamado, and G. T. Wolf, "Paranasal sinus malignancies: an 18-year single institution experience," *Laryngoscope*, vol. 112, no. 11, pp. 1964–1969, 2002.

[6] P. Dulguerov, M. S. Jacobsen, A. S. Allal, W. Lehmann, and T. Calcaterra, "Nasal and paranasal sinus carcinoma: are we making progress? A series of 220 patients and a systematic review," *Cancer*, vol. 92, no. 12, pp. 3012–3029, 2001.

[7] T. Norlander, J. Frödin, C. Silfverswärd, and A. Änggard, "Decreasing incidence of malignant tumors of the paranasal sinuses in Sweden: an analysis of 141 consecutive cases at Karolinska Hospital from 1960 to 1980," *Annals of Otology, Rhinology and Laryngology*, vol. 112, no. 3, pp. 236–241, 2003.

[8] J. N. Waldron, O. 'Sullivan B, P. Gullane et al., "Carcinoma of the maxillary antrum: a retrospective analysis of 110 cases," *Radiotherapy and Oncology*, vol. 57, no. 2, pp. 167–173, 2000.

[9] L. Tran, J. Sidrys, D. Horton, A. Sadeghi, and R. G. Parker, "Malignant salivary gland tumors of the paranasal sinuses and nasal cavity. The UCLA experiences," *The American Journal of Clinical Oncology*, vol. 12, no. 5, pp. 387–392, 1989.

[10] N. Bhattacharyya, "Survival and staging characteristics for non-squamous cell malignancies of the maxillary sinus," *Archives of Otolaryngology—Head and Neck Surgery*, vol. 129, no. 3, pp. 334–337, 2003.

[11] J. Brown, "Maxillary reconstruction," *Indian Journal of Plastic Surgery*, vol. 40, no. 12, pp. S35–S43, 2007.

Permissions

All chapters in this book were first published in CRID, by Hindawi Publishing Corporation; hereby published with permission under the Creative Commons Attribution License or equivalent. Every chapter published in this book has been scrutinized by our experts. Their significance has been extensively debated. The topics covered herein carry significant findings which will fuel the growth of the discipline. They may even be implemented as practical applications or may be referred to as a beginning point for another development.

The contributors of this book come from diverse backgrounds, making this book a truly international effort. This book will bring forth new frontiers with its revolutionizing research information and detailed analysis of the nascent developments around the world.

We would like to thank all the contributing authors for lending their expertise to make the book truly unique. They have played a crucial role in the development of this book. Without their invaluable contributions this book wouldn't have been possible. They have made vital efforts to compile up to date information on the varied aspects of this subject to make this book a valuable addition to the collection of many professionals and students.

This book was conceptualized with the vision of imparting up-to-date information and advanced data in this field. To ensure the same, a matchless editorial board was set up. Every individual on the board went through rigorous rounds of assessment to prove their worth. After which they invested a large part of their time researching and compiling the most relevant data for our readers.

The editorial board has been involved in producing this book since its inception. They have spent rigorous hours researching and exploring the diverse topics which have resulted in the successful publishing of this book. They have passed on their knowledge of decades through this book. To expedite this challenging task, the publisher supported the team at every step. A small team of assistant editors was also appointed to further simplify the editing procedure and attain best results for the readers.

Apart from the editorial board, the designing team has also invested a significant amount of their time in understanding the subject and creating the most relevant covers. They scrutinized every image to scout for the most suitable representation of the subject and create an appropriate cover for the book.

The publishing team has been an ardent support to the editorial, designing and production team. Their endless efforts to recruit the best for this project, has resulted in the accomplishment of this book. They are a veteran in the field of academics and their pool of knowledge is as vast as their experience in printing. Their expertise and guidance has proved useful at every step. Their uncompromising quality standards have made this book an exceptional effort. Their encouragement from time to time has been an inspiration for everyone.

The publisher and the editorial board hope that this book will prove to be a valuable piece of knowledge for researchers, students, practitioners and scholars across the globe.

List of Contributors

Shivani Utneja, Gaurav Garg and Sangeeta Talwar
Department of Conservative Dentistry and Endodontics, Maulana Azad Institute of Dental Sciences, Bahadurshah Zafar Marg, New Delhi 110002, India

Shipra Arora
Department of Periodontics, Maulana Azad Institute of Dental Sciences, Bahadurshah Zafar Marg, New Delhi 110002, India

Simel Ayyildiz
Department of Prosthodontics, Center of Dental Sciences, Gulhane Military Medical Academy, Etlik, 06018 Ankara, Turkey

Cem Sahin
School of Dental Technology, Hacettepe University, 06100 Ankara, Turkey

Özlem Marti Akgün and Feridun Basak
Department of Pediatric Dentistry, Center of Dental Sciences, Gulhane Military Medical Academy, 06018 Ankara, Turkey

Ali S. Aljhani
Division of Orthodontics, College of Dentistry, King Saud University for Health Sciences and National Guard Health Affairs, P.O. Box 22490, Riyadh, Saudi Arabia

Khalid H. Zawawi
Division of Orthodontics, Faculty of Dentistry, King Abdulaziz University, P.O. Box 80209, Jeddah 21589, Saudi Arabia

Pallavi Pujar
Department of Pedodontics, Maratha Mandal's Dental College, Belgaum 590010, Karnataka, India

SuryakanthM. Pai
Department of Pedodontics, College of Dental Sciences, Davangere 577004, India

Ana Amelia Souza, Vera Cavalcanti de Araújo, Fabricio Passador Santos,
Elizabeth Ferreira Martinez, Ney Soares de Araujo and Andresa Borges Soares
Department of Oral Pathology, São Leopoldo Mandic Institute and Research Center, Rua José Rocha Junqueira 13 Ponte Preta, 13045-755 Campinas, SP, Brazil

Jose Ferreira deMenezes Filho
Instituto Tocatinense Presidente Antonio Carlos-Araguaína, Avenida Filadélfia 568, 77816-540 Araguaína, TO, Brazil

Pabbati Ravi kumar,Mandava Jyothi, Kantheti Sirisha, Khushboo Racca and Chalasani Uma
Department of Conservative Dentistry and Endodontics, GITAM Dental College and Hospital, Visakhapatnam 530045, Andhra Pradesh, India

Shipra Arora, Arundeep Kaur Lamba, Farrukh Faraz, Shruti Tandon and Abdul Ahad
Department of Periodontics and Oral Implantology, Maulana Azad Institute of Dental Sciences, New Delhi 110002, India

Ramakant Nayak, Vijayalakshmi Kotrashetti, Mayuri Kulkarni, Pradeep Somannavar and Jagadish Hosmani
Department of Oral Pathology and Microbiology, Maratha Mandal's NGH Institute of Dental Sciences and Research Centre, Belgaum, Karnataka 590010, India

Aarati Nayak
Department of Periodontology, Maratha Mandal's NGH Institute of Dental Sciences and Research Centre, Belgaum, Karnataka 590010, India

Viraj Patil
Department of Prosthodontics, Maratha Mandal's NGH Institute of Dental Sciences and Research Centre, Belgaum, Karnataka 590010, India

Meenal Nitin Gulve
Department of Conservative Dentistry and Endodontics, M.G.V.'s K.B.H. Dental College and Hospital, Mumbai Agra Road, Panchavati, Nashik 422002, India

Nitin Dilip Gulve
Department of Orthodontics, Dentofacial Orthopedics and Dental Materials, M.G.V.'s K.B.H. Dental College and Hospital, Nashik 422002, India

João Bosco Formiga Relvas and Emílio Carlos Sponchiado Jr.
Department of Endodontics, School of Dentistry, Federal University of Amazonas 69077-000 Manaus, AM, Brazil

FredsomMarcio Acris de Carvalho
Department of Endodontics, School of Dentistry, Paulista University, 69050-010 Manaus, AM, Brazil

André Augusto Franco Marques
Department of Endodontics, School of Dentistry, State University of Amazonas, 69050-030 Manaus, AM, Brazil

Lucas da Fonseca Roberti Garcia
Department of Dental Materials and Prosthodontics, Ribeirão Preto School of Dentistry, University of São Paulo, 14040-900 Ribeir˜ao Preto, SP, Brazil

Ahmad Alshadwi
Department of Oral and Maxillofacial Surgery, Boston Medical Center, Boston University, 100 East Newton Street, Boston, MA 02118, USA

Ishwar Bhatia
Department of Oral and Maxillofacial Surgery, Henry Goldman School of Dental Medicine, Boston University, 100 East Newton Street, Boston, MA 02118, USA

Sachin B. Mangalekar
Department of Periodontology, Maitri Dental College, Chattisgarh, India

Tajammul Ahmed
Department of Prosthodontics, Al Jabal Al Gharbi University, Gharyan, Libya

M. Zakirulla
Department of Pediatric Dentistry, College of Dentistry, King Khalid University, Abha, Saudi Arabia

Halawar Sangmesh Shivappa
Vasant Dada Dental College, Kavalapur, Sangli, Maharashtra, India

F. B. Bheemappa
P.M.N.M. Dental College and Hospital, Bagalkot, Karnataka, India

Chandrashekar Yavagal
Department of Pediatric Dentistry, Dr. Hedgewar Dental College, Hingoli, Maharashtra, India

Vijay Shekhar and K. Shashikala
Department of Conservative Dentistry and Endodontics, D.A.P.M.R.V. Dental College and Hospital, Bangalore, Karnataka 560078, India

Sukumaran Anil
Department of Periodontics and Community Dentistry, College of Dentistry, King Saud University, P.O. Box 60169, Riyadh 11545, Saudi Arabia

Anitha P. Krishnan
Department of Oral and Maxillofacial Pathology, College of Dentistry, Salman Bin Abdulaziz University, P.O. Box 153, Al-Kharj 11942, Saudi Arabia

R. Rajendran
College of Dentistry, King Saud bin Abdulaziz University for Health Sciences, P.O. Box 22490, Riyadh 11426, Saudi Arabia

Peeyush Shivhare, Lata Shankarnarayan, Usha, Mahesh Kumar and Malliger Basavaraju Sowbhagya
Department of Oral Medicine and Radiology, Raja Rajeswari Dental College, and Hospital, Rajiv Gandhi University, Ramohalli Cross, kumbalgodu, Bangalore, Karnataka 560074, India

A. P.Münevveroğlu
Pedodonti Ana Bilim Dalı, Di¸shekimligĭ Fakültesi, I˙stanbul Medipol Üniversitesi, 34083 Fatih, Turkey

K. C. Aydın
Diş ve Çene Radyolojisi Anabilim Dalı, Dişhekimligĭ Fakültesi Agĭz, İstanbul Medipol Üniversitesi, 34083 Fatih, Turkey

Ahmet Ercan Sekerci, Yildiray Sisman,Meryem Etoz and Duygu Goller Bulut
Department of Oral and Maxillofacial Radiology, Faculty of Dentistry, Erciyes University, 38039 Kayseri, Turkey

Syed Wali Peeran
Department of Periodontology and Oral Implantology, Faculty of Dentistry, Sebha University, Sebha, Libya

Karthikeyan Ramalingam
Department of Oral Pathology & Microbiology, Faculty of Dentistry, Sebha University, Sebha, Libya

Syed Ali Peeran
Department of Oral and Maxillofacial Prosthodontics, Faculty of Dentistry, Jazan University, Jazan 45 142, Saudi Arabia

Marei Hamed Mugrabi
Department of Periodontics, Faculty of Dentistry, Arab Medical University, Benghazi, Libya

Khaled Awidat Abdulla
Department of Oral Biology and Orthodontics, Faculty of Dentistry, Sebha University, Sebha, Libya

Shilpa Kandalgaonkar, Suyog Tupsakhare, Ashok Patil, Gaurav Agrawal
Mahesh Gabhane and Shrikant Sonune
Department Oral Pathology & Microbiology, SMBT Dental College & Hospital, Sangamner, Maharashtra 422608, India

Manas Bajpai and Deshant Agarwal
Department of Oral and Maxillofacial Pathology, NIMS Dental College, Jaipur, India

Anindya Bhalla
Department of Public Health Dentistry, NIMS Dental College, Jaipur, India
Malay Kumar
Department of Oral and Maxillofacial Pathology, Ahmedabad Dental College, Ahmedabad, India

Rakesh Garg
Department of Periodontics, NIMS Dental College, Jaipur, India

Manish Kumar
Department of Prosthodontics Crown and Bridges, NIMS Dental College, Jaipur, India

Orlando Tanaka, Wagner Oliveira, Melissa Galarza, Vanessa Aoki and Bruno Bertaiolli
Graduate Dentistry Program in Orthodontics, School of Health and Biosciences, Pontifícia Universidade Católica do Paraná, Curitiba, PR, Brazil

K. Lundin, G. Schmidt and C. Bonde
Department of Plastic Surgery, Breast Surgery and Burns Treatment, Rigshospitalet-Copenhagen University Hospital, 2100 Copenhagen OE, Denmark

Meera Sandhu, PoojaMalik and Rooposhi Saha
Pedodontics and Preventive Dentistry, ITS Center for Dental Studies and Research, C-4, ITS-CDSR, Campus, Muradnagar, Ghaziabad 201206, India

Cristian Statkievicz, Leonardo P. Faverani, Pedro Henrique Silva Gomes-Ferreira, Gabriel Ramalho-Ferreira and Idelmo Rangel Garcia-Junior
Department of Surgery and Integrated Clinic, Aracatuba Dental School, Universidade Estadual Paulista (UNESP), 16015-050 Araçatuba, SP, Brazil

Kaustubh Thakare, M. L. Bhongade, Preeti Charde, Priyanka Jaiswal and Nachiket Shah
Department of Periodontology and Implantology, Sharad Pawar Dental College and Hospital, Maharashtra, Wardha 442001, India

Aniruddha Deshpande
Department of Periodontology and Implantology, CSMSS Dental College and Hospital, Maharashtra, Aurangabad 431001, India

Sarbjeet Singh
Department of Oral Medicine & Radiology, Institute of Dental Sciences, Sehora, Jammu 181132, India

V. Sreenivasan and Kanika Garg
Department of Oral Medicine & Radiology, Subharti Dental College and Hospital,Meerut, Uttarpradesh 250002, India

Nikhel DevWazir
Department of Conservative & Endodontics, Institute of Dental Sciences, Sehora, Jammu 181132, India

Jaspal Singh Rajput
Department of Pedodontics, SGT Dental College, Hospital & Research Center, Gurgoan, Haryana 122505, India

Pawandeep Sandhu Virk
Department of Pedodontics, Desh Bhagat Dental College & Hospital, Muktsar, Punjab 152026, India

Satheesh B. Haralur and Ali Saad Al-Qahtani
Department of Prosthodontics, College of Dentistry, King Khalid University, Abha 61417, Saudi Arabia

Sérgio Kahn
Department of Periodontics, Veiga de Almeida University (UVA), Rua Ibituruna 108, Tijuca, 20271-021 Rio de Janeiro, RJ, Brazil

Walmir Júnio de Pinho Reis Rodrigues
School of Dentistry, Serra dos Órgãos University Center (UNIFESO), Avenida Alberto Torres 111, Alto, 25964-004 Teresópolis, RJ, Brazil

Marcos de Oliveira Barceleiro
Department of Dentistry, School of Dentistry, Fluminense Federal University (UFF), Rua Silvio Henrique Braune 22, Centro, 28625-650 Nova Friburgo, RJ, Brazil

Megumi Sotobori, Kohei Marukawa, Masatoshi Higuchi, Ryuichi Nakazawa, Akinori Moroi, Yuri Ishihara, Ran Iguchi, Akihiko Kosaka, Hiroumi Ikawa and Koichiro Ueki
Division of Medicine, Department of Oral and Maxillofacial Surgery, Interdisciplinary Graduate School of Medicine and Engineering, University of Yamanashi, 1110 Shimokato Chuo, Chuo-shi, Yamanashi 409-3898, Japan

Iman Parisay
Pediatric Dentistry, Dental Material Research Center, School of Dentistry, Mashhad University of Medical Sciences, Mashhad, Iran

Fatemeh Kebriaei, Bentolhoda Varkesh, Milad Soruri and Roya Ghafourifard
Department of Pediatric Dentistry, School of Dentistry, Shahid Sadoughi University of Medical Sciences, Yazd, Iran

Irla Karlinne Ferreira de Carvalho and Anibal Henrique Barbosa Luna
Paraiba Federal University (UFPB), 58091-900 João Pessoa, PB, Brazil

Carla Cristina Camilo, Manoel Brito-Júnior, Alex Carvalho Quintino and Adrianne Freire de Paula
Department of Dentistry, State University of Montes Claros, Avenue Rui Braga s/n, 39401-089 Montes Claros, MG, Brazil

André Luis Faria-e-Silva
Department of Dentistry, School of Dentistry, Federal University of Sergipe, Rua Cláudio Batista s/n, 49060-100 Aracaju, SE, Brazil

AntônioMiranda Cruz-Filho and Manoel Damião Sousa-Neto
Department of Restorative Dentistry, Faculty of Dentistry, University of São Paulo, Avenue Bandeirantes 3900, 14040-900 Ribeirão Preto, SP, Brazil

Rafaela Elvira Rozza-de-Menezes, Stefânia Jeronimo Ferreira
Diogo Lenzi Capella, Stephan Schwartz, Aline Cristina and Paulo Henrique Couto Souza
Department of Stomatology, Faculty of Dentistry, School of Health and Biosciences, Pontifical Catholic University of Paraná, Imaculada Conceição, 1155 Prado Velho, 80-215-901 Curitiba, PR, Brazil

Ana HelenaWillrich
Departament of Pathology, Erasto Gaertner Hospital, Dr. Ovande do Amaral, 201-Jardim América, 81-520-060 Curitiba, PR, Brazil

Lúcia de Noronha
Department of Pathology, School of Medicine, Pontfical Catholic University of Paraná, Imaculada Conceição, 1155 Prado Velho, 80-215-901 Curitiba, PR, Brazil

Batista Rodrigues Johann
Department ofOral Pathology, Faculty of Dentistry, School of Health and Biosciences, Pontifical Catholic University of Paraná, Curitiba, Imaculada Conceição, 1155 Prado Velho, 80-215-901 Curitiba, PR, Brazil

Rashmi Bansal, Priyanka Chowdhary, Anuraag Gurtu, Nakul Mehrotra and Abhinav Kishore
Department of Conservative Dentistry & Endodontics, Institute of Dental Sciences, Bareilly 243006, India

Pratik Dedhia and Amol Dhokar
Department of Oral Medicine and Radiology, Terna Dental College, Nerul, Navi Mumbai 400706, India

Shely Dedhia
Department of Pediatric and Preventive Dentistry, Nair Hospital Dental College, Mumbai Central, Mumbai 400008, India

Ankit Desai
Department of Periodontics, Terna Dental College, Nerul, Navi Mumbai 400706, India

Ana Amélia Souza, Eldon Guttenberg Cariri Neto, Vera Cavalcanti de Araújo, Fabricio Passador-Santos, and Andresa Borges Soares
Department of Oral Pathology, Sao Leopoldo Mandic Institute and Research Center, Rua José Rocha Junqueira13, Ponte Preta, 13045-755 Campinas, SP, Brazil

Maria Teresa de Seixas Alves
Department of Pathology, Escola Paulista de Medicina, Rua Botucatu 740, Vila Clementino, 04023-900 Sao Paulo, SP, Brazil

C. M. L. She, G. S. P. Cheung and C. F. Zhang
Comprehensive Dental Care, Endodontics, Faculty of Dentistry,The University of Hong Kong, Hong Kong

G. Siva Prasad Reddy, G. V. Reddy, I. Venkata Krishna and Shravan Kumar Regonda
Department of Oral and Maxillofacial Surgery, Panineeya Institute of Dental Sciences, Road No. 5, Kamala Nagar, Dilsukhnagar, Hyderabad, Andhra Pradesh 500060, India

Gummadapu Sarat, Nuthalapati Priyanka,Meka Purna Venkata Prabhat, Chintamaneni Raja Lakshmi, Sujana Mulk Bhavana and Dharmavaram Ayesha Thabusum
Department of Oral Medicine & Radiology, Drs. Sudha and Nageswara Siddhartha Institute of Dental Sciences, Chinoutpalli, Gannavaram Mandal, Andhra Pradesh 521286, India

Resmije Ademi-Abdyli and Feriall Perjuci
Department of Oral Surgery, Medical Faculty, University of Prishtina, Dental Branch, 10000 Prishtina, Kosovo

Teuta Bicaj
Department of Prosthetic Dentistry, Medical Faculty, University of Prishtina, Dental Branch, 10000 Prishtina, Kosovo

Yll Abdyli
Medical Faculty, University of Prishtina, Dental Branch, 10000 Prishtina, Kosovo

Thaís Borguezan Nunes, Sheyla Batista Bologna, Andréa Lusvarghi Witzel
and Silvia Vanessa Lourenço
Department of Stomatology, School of Dentistry, University of São Paulo, Avenida Professor Lineu Prestes 2227, Cidade Universitária, 05508-000 São Paulo, SP, Brazil

Marcello Menta Simonsen Nico
Department of Dermatology, Medical School, University of São Paulo, Avenida Dr. Enéas de Carvalho 255, 3o Andar, Sala 3068, 05403-000 São Paulo, SP, Brazil

Shanthan Mettu, RadhikaMuppa, Srinivas Nallanchakrava and Sri Veda Gurugubelli
Department of Pediatric Dentistry, Panineeya Institute of Dental Sciences, Kamalanagar, Dilsukhnagar, Hyderabad, Andhra Pradesh 500060, India

G. Siva Prasad Reddy
Department of Oral and Maxillofacial Surgery, Panineeya Institute of Dental Sciences, Kamalanagar, Dilsukhnagar, Hyderabad, Andhra Pradesh 500060, India

Amol Beldar and Chandrashekar Buregoni
Department of Periodontics and Implant Dentistry, Mahatma Gandhi Vidyamandir's KBH Dental College, Panchavati, Nashik 422003, Maharshtra, India

Manohar L. Bhongade
Department of Periodontics and Implant Dentistry, Sharad Pawar Dental College and Hospital Of Deemed University, Sawangi (Meghe),Wardha, Maharashtra, India

Girish Byakod
Department of Periodontics and Implant Dentistry, Rangoonwala Dental College, Pune, Maharashtra, India

G. Iannaci and R. Luise
Department of Pathology, Incurabili Hospital ASLNAPOLI1 Centro, Via Maria Longo, 50-80138 Napoli, Italy

G. Iezzi and A. Piattelli
Department of Medical, Oral and Biotechnological Sciences, University of Chieti-Pescara, Chieti, Italy

A. Salierno
Department of Oral Medicine, School of Dentistry of the Second University of the Study of Naples, Naples, Italy

Serhan Didinen, AslJ PatJrMünevveroLlu and Özlem TulunoLlu
Department of Pediatric Dentistry, Faculty of Dentistry, Istanbul Medipol University, Turkey

Didem Atabek
Department of Pediatric Dentistry, Faculty of Dentistry, Gazi University, Turkey

Gülay Kip,
Department of Anesthesia and Reanimation, Faculty of Medicine, Gazi University, Turkey
Department of Pediatric Dentistry, School of Dental Medicine, CaseWestern Reserve University, Cleveland, OH, USA

Dwarkadas Adwani and Nitin Adwani
Department of Oral & Maxillofacial Surgery, VYWS Dental College & Hospital, Amravati 444601, India

Anirudh Bhattacharya
Department of Oral & Maxillofacial Surgery, VYWS Dental College & Hospital, Amravati 444601, India
Adwani Multispeciality Dental Hospital, Ambapeth, Amravati 444601, India

Rajender Singh Arora
Department of Head & Neck Oncology, Amravati Cancer Hospital, Amravati 444601, India

Ramawatar Soni
Department of Pathology,Dr. PDMMCHospital, Amravati 444601, India

Index